Dispatches from the AIDS Pandemic

Dispatches from the AIDS Pandemic

A Public Health Story

KEVIN M. DE COCK, HAROLD W. JAFFE, AND
JAMES W. CURRAN

Edited by
ROBIN MOSELEY

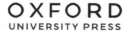

OXFORD
UNIVERSITY PRESS

OXFORD
UNIVERSITY PRESS

Oxford University Press is a department of the University of Oxford. It furthers
the University's objective of excellence in research, scholarship, and education
by publishing worldwide. Oxford is a registered trade mark of Oxford University
Press in the UK and certain other countries.

Published in the United States of America by Oxford University Press
198 Madison Avenue, New York, NY 10016, United States of America.

Library of Congress Cataloging-in-Publication Data
Names: De Cock, Kevin M., author. | Jaffe, Harold W., author. |
Curran, James W., author. | Moseley, Robin, editor.
Title: Dispatches from the AIDS pandemic : a public health story /
Kevin M. De Cock, Harold W. Jaffe, James W. Curran,
and edited by Robin Moseley.
Description: New York, NY : Oxford University Press, [2023] |
Includes bibliographical references and index.
Identifiers: LCCN 2022040714 (print) | LCCN 2022040715 (ebook) |
ISBN 9780197626528 (hardback) | ISBN 9780197626535 (epub) |
ISBN 9780197626559 (online)
Subjects: MESH: Centers for Disease Control and Prevention (U.S.) |
Acquired Immunodeficiency Syndrome—history | Pandemics—history |
United States Government Agencies—history | Communicable Disease Control—history |
Public Health Practice—history | History, 20th Century | United States
Classification: LCC RC606.6 (print) | LCC RC606.6 (ebook) | NLM WC 503 |
DDC 362.19697/92—dc23/eng/20220923
LC record available at https://lccn.loc.gov/2022040714
LC ebook record available at https://lccn.loc.gov/2022040715

DOI: 10.1093/oso/9780197626528.001.0001

Printed by Sheridan Books, Inc., United States of America

This book is dedicated to those who joined the fight against AIDS
and all who have suffered its toll.

AIDS is a war against humanity.—Nelson Mandela

So all a man could win in the conflict between plague and life was knowledge and memories.—Albert Camus

Contents

SECTION III. THE MODERN AIDS ERA

List of Figures

Contributing Authors

Mary E. Chamberland, MD, MPH, joined CDC in 1982 as an Epidemic Intelligence Service officer in New York City. She helped establish the first hospital-based AIDS surveillance system and led CDC's studies on the spectrum of HIV-related disease and HIV transmission in healthcare settings.

Bess Miller, MD, MSc, joined CDC as an Epidemic Intelligence Service officer in 1981. She participated in early AIDS investigations and directed CDC's HIV/tuberculosis activities in Africa and Asia under PEPFAR during 2003–2014.

Note to Readers

This book draws in part from oral histories and online archival materials on CDC's early AIDS response available through the GHC, an open-access platform documenting CDC's role in public health efforts against selected global infectious diseases (https://www.globalhealthchronicles.org/).

The GHC project can trace its origins to former CDC Director William Foege. He suggested collecting oral histories during the 2006 reunion of CDC professionals who worked on smallpox eradication efforts in West Africa. This successful venture led another former CDC Director, David Sencer, to spearhead the creation of a website organized as individual chronicles, each one dedicated to collecting and preserving a global public health story through oral histories and the collection of historical documents and artifacts. The GHC collection is a collaboration between the David J. Sencer CDC Museum and Emory University's Emory Center for Digital Scholarship (https://digitalscholarship.emory.edu/).

David Sencer strongly believed the story of CDC's role in the AIDS epidemic should be documented on the GHC website. As many of the CDC early AIDS public health experts and researchers were retiring, there was an urgency to capture their personal narratives and perspectives. In mid-2014, work began on the AIDS chronicle (https://www.globalhealthchronicles. org/aids). Judy Gantt, CDC Museum Director, was the project director, and Mary Hilpertshauser, the CDC Museum's Historic Collections Manager, was the project archivist. The principal investigators were Mary Chamberland and Bess Miller, retired medical epidemiologists who had worked on the CDC AIDS response (and are contributing authors to this book). Technical support was provided though informal consultation with several recognized oral historians and an advisory board. The project was supported by funding from Gilead Sciences, Inc., Abbott Laboratories, and the CDC Foundation.

The project aimed first to provide a scientific oral history, documenting the individual accounts and experiences of interviewees (narrators) from a wide range of CDC professionals and subject matter experts. The two principal investigators conducted fifty-two individual in-person interviews primarily in the CDC recording studios in Atlanta between November 2015 and

January 2019. The interviews focused on the "early years" of CDC's response to AIDS; narrators also were asked to speak on broader aspects of CDC's role and impact, on the agency's relationships with others, and on lessons for the future. The project expanded to include interviews with CDC scientists who were on the forefront of CDC's global AIDS response as leaders of its international field sites or as part of the PEPFAR program.

In addition, the project aimed to collect and catalogue archival material from the early AIDS work including photographs and other historical objects and documents. Primary source materials from the *Dr. William Darrow Collection* maintained at the David J. Sencer CDC Museum underpin many of the book's chapters.

In reflecting on his time at CDC, David Sencer recalled, "I think my favorite memory is the fact that this was an organization made up of people. It was the finest group of people you can imagine" (David Sencer interview in *CDC Connects*, August 20, 2010). We hope that this book will serve as a reminder of these people.

Frequently Used Abbreviations

AIDS	Acquired immunodeficiency syndrome
CDC	Centers for Disease Control, now Centers for Disease Control and Prevention
EIS	Epidemic Intelligence Service
Epi-Aid	Epidemiologic assistance
FDA	US Food and Drug Administration
GPA	Global Programme on AIDS, WHO
HAART, or just ART	Highly active antiretroviral therapy
HBV	Hepatitis B virus
HCW	Healthcare worker
HHS	US Department of Health and Human Services
HIV	Human immunodeficiency virus
IDU	Injection drug user
ITM	Institute of Tropical Medicine, Belgium
IV	Intravenous
KS	Kaposi's sarcoma
KS/OI	Kaposi's sarcoma and opportunistic infections
LAV	Lymphadenopathy-associated virus
MMWR	*Morbidity and Mortality Weekly Report*
MSM	Men who have sex with men
NIH	National Institutes of Health
NIR	No identified risk
OI	Opportunistic infection
PCP	*Pneumocystis carinii* pneumonia
PEPFAR	The United States President's Emergency Plan for AIDS Relief
PHA	Public health advisor
PHS	US Public Health Service
PrEP	Pre-exposure prophylaxis
STD	Sexually transmitted disease
STI	Sexually transmitted infection
TB	Tuberculosis
The Global Fund	The Global Fund to Fight AIDS, Tuberculosis and Malaria
UN	United Nations
UNAIDS	The Joint United Nations Programme on HIV/AIDS
WHO	World Health Organization

Prologue

James W. Curran

In late spring 1981, a report describing five cases of an unusual pneumonia among previously healthy homosexual men in California was submitted to the Centers for Disease Control's (CDC) *Morbidity and Mortality Weekly Report (MMWR)*. Its publication[1] on June 5th sparked calls from clinicians regarding similar cases linked to unexplained immunodeficiency and would soon be considered the first report on the HIV/AIDS pandemic. For the authors of this book and for countless others, 1981 marked personal and professional turning points. Most important are the tens of millions of individuals worldwide who prematurely lost their lives to HIV, the tens of millions more currently infected, and countless friends, relatives, and other loved ones who share the burden.

The book is told from the perspective of the authors, now retired from CDC. I (JWC) chaired the quickly assembled task force to investigate the outbreak, with Harold Jaffe as the lead for epidemiologic studies. Kevin De Cock joined a few years later, concentrating on the global impact of the virus. Although the authors have remained engaged in efforts to control HIV, the book has also been informed by firsthand accounts, told through the Global Health Chronicles (GHC),[2] of others involved in CDC's domestic and global HIV/AIDS activities. As such, the book focuses heavily on CDC, despite the innumerable individuals and organizations worldwide who have grappled with the disease from its onset.

We believe that recounting the response and perspectives of CDC staff on the front lines of the AIDS pandemic can be useful in understanding and responding to other present and future health threats. CDC's activities, though conducted during a time of government austerity, began early and focused upon data and frequent and open communications alerting the world to the problem as soon as information was known. From today's vantage point, many things would have been done and communicated differently, although "shoe-leather" epidemiology remains a crucial part of outbreak investigations.

The year 1981 was a presidential transition year in the United States; in January, Ronald Reagan succeeded Jimmy Carter as President. Reagan's successful campaign promised solutions to rising unemployment and inflation. As President, he vowed to freeze or reduce domestic government expenditures. Of course, CDC was greatly affected by the freeze in spending and hiring that ensued. Key positions could only be hired from within an already understaffed workforce, and travel and contract work were severely restricted. An outbreak of several dozen fatal infections in gay men from California and New York did not constitute a domestic priority at the highest level of the Administration.

In fact, the Administration's early indifference to the epidemic was clearly demonstrated during a White House press conference held on October 15, 1982.[3] An excerpt from the transcript of the conference includes the following exchange between Larry Speakes, the White House Deputy Press Secretary, and reporters:

Q: Larry, does the President have any reaction to the announcement—the Centers for Disease Control in Atlanta, that AIDS is now an epidemic and have [sic] over 600 cases?

MR. SPEAKES: What's AIDS?

Q: Over a third of them have died. It's known as "gay plague." (Laughter.) No, it is. I mean it's a pretty serious thing that one in every three people that get this have died. And I wondered if the President is aware of it?

MR. SPEAKES: I don't have it. Do you? (Laughter.)

Q: Does the President, does anybody in the White House know about this epidemic, Larry?

MR. SPEAKES: I don't think so. I don't think there's been any—

Q: Nobody knows?

MR. SPEAKES: There has been no personal experience here, Lester.

In fact, President Reagan did not speak of AIDS publicly until an invitation-only event at the third international conference on AIDS in Washington, DC, in 1987.

In the years immediately preceding recognition of the new disease, many of us at CDC were working closely with clinicians, investigators, and gay community leaders to understand an ongoing epidemic of hepatitis B virus (HBV) in gay men and to conduct trials of a newly developed HBV vaccine in that community. These contacts with gay men and their physicians provided great insights into the factors leading up to AIDS, as the diseases shared similar epidemiologic features. In addition, the HBV work engendered important early trust between CDC staff and many in the gay community—a consideration otherwise lacking early in the Reagan administration.

At the beginning of the outbreak, CDC had very few connections with the substance use prevention and treatment communities—both for clients and providers. The federal responsibilities were largely covered by other agencies such as the National Institute of Drug Abuse and the Substance Abuse and Mental Health Services Administration. In retrospect, this division hampered our efforts at CDC in addressing the early epidemic in minority communities of injecting drug users and their heterosexual partners and newborns.

Despite the hiring and funding restrictions, scientists and managers at CDC (and at the National Institutes of Health) responded to the growing outbreak by deploying existing staff and resources. Within days of the initial *MMWR* reports, CDC Director William (Bill) Foege, himself well-versed in the complexities of infectious diseases, formed our task force, with a charge to investigate what was then termed "Kaposi's sarcoma and opportunistic infections." A specific surveillance definition was formulated and active surveillance and case investigations began immediately, evolving as the cause of AIDS (HIV) and other factors were determined. Section I details the early years of these investigations and findings.

Within the first one to two years, it became increasingly apparent that AIDS was occurring throughout the world and that epidemiologic and clinical patterns varied. The rapid growth of the global epidemic made it imperative for CDC to conduct research and prevention work beyond the United States. Because CDC was and is a federal agency mostly funded and dedicated to protecting the health of Americans, a compelling argument was necessarily made and supported by CDC and Public Health Service (PHS) leadership to devote their science personnel and resources outside the United States. The important gaps in our scientific understanding and potential for collaborations to provide answers gave sound rationale for CDC to offer support for major scientific programs in Zaire (now Democratic Republic of Congo), Cote d'Ivoire, and Thailand. Jonathan Mann, Kevin De Cock, and Bruce Weniger, respectively, were founding directors of those projects, which, over the years, drew in hundreds of CDC staff and other colleagues from around the world. Section II describes these important projects in detail.

By the mid-1980s, we recognized that despite all the scientific and public health efforts, community activism, and individual actions, HIV was getting the upper hand and AIDS cases were rapidly increasing globally as well as domestically. Powerful tools would come, but not for nearly a decade. Although azidothymidine (AZT)[4] had been shown in 1987 to have transient efficacy for treating HIV, it was not until 1996 that highly active antiretroviral therapy (HAART, or just ART) was shown to dramatically prolong and improve the lives of those living with HIV. In the years after such treatment success, pre-exposure prophylaxis (PrEP) and voluntary male circumcision joined education, condom use and other risk-reduction methods, strategies to prevent mother-to-child transmission, and contact-tracing as effective HIV prevention tools. Finally, after two decades, the global response became robust, involving significant resource commitments including the initiative from President George W. Bush called the US President's Emergency Plan for AIDS Relief (PEPFAR).

CDC continued to play important roles throughout these eras by assigning senior scientist/physicians to the World Health Organization (Mann, Mike Merson, and De Cock) to lead their AIDS program and by participating actively in US-funded global AIDS programs through CDC's Center for Global Health. These events played out over increasing scientific understanding and advances concerning HIV and AIDS, the pandemic, and interventions to combat them. Section III of the book summarizes the current public health and clinical science of AIDS, including its origins, and describes the evolution and essentials of today's domestic and global response.

Much has been accomplished over the more than forty years of the epidemic, but much remains to be done by science and by society to control HIV. The lessons learned from the AIDS epidemic should be understood and heeded as CDC and partners address current and future global health threats.

Notes

1. CDC. *Pneumocystis* pneumonia—Los Angeles. MMWR Morb Mortal Wkly Rep 1981;30:250–252.
2. *The Global Health Chronicles*. CDC's early response to AIDS https://www.globalhealt hchronicles.org/aids.
3. Eilperin J. How attitudes toward AIDS have changed, in the White House and beyond. The Washington Post, December 4, 2013. https://www.washingtonpost.com/news/ the-fix/wp/2013/12/04/how-attitudes-toward-aids-have-changed-in-the-white-house-and-beyond/.
4. The drug first approved for HIV treatment was azidothymidine (AZT), which subsequently became known as zidovudine (ZDV).

SECTION I
FROM UNEXPLAINED ILLNESS TO EXPANDING EPIDEMIC

1

CDC and Outbreak Response

Harold W. Jaffe

The United States Centers for Disease Control and Prevention (CDC) is the nation's leading public health agency. Among its responsibilities, the agency works with public health partners to investigate unexplained illnesses and help prevent future cases. For example, CDC investigators identified the cause of a severe respiratory illness among attendees at an American Legion convention in Philadelphia in 1976 (Legionnaires' disease) and a few years later linked the newly recognized toxic-shock syndrome with the use of super-absorbent tampons by American women.[1,2] And, when reports of rare and severe diseases in previously healthy young homosexual men in the United States began appearing in the early 1980s, CDC launched investigations into what would become known as acquired immunodeficiency syndrome (AIDS).

Established in 1946 as a descendant of a World War II US Public Health Service (PHS) program called Malaria Control in War Areas, CDC is headquartered in Atlanta, Georgia, and was first called the Communicable Disease Center. Although initially focused on preventing the spread of malaria across the American South, CDC soon engaged in other infectious disease prevention efforts. Over the ensuing decades, CDC's programs gradually expanded to include environmental and occupational health, as well as chronic disease and injury prevention. Nonetheless, from the perspective of the American public, CDC has remained best known for its expertise in investigating and controlling infectious disease outbreaks.

CDC's role differs from that of the US National Institutes of Health (NIH) and the World Health Organization (WHO). Although both CDC and NIH are part of PHS and operate as divisions of the US Department of Health and Human Services (HHS), CDC, unlike NIH, does not primarily fund extramural or conduct intramural basic research in the biomedical sciences. And, although CDC and WHO, a United Nations agency, have a long history

Harold W. Jaffe, *CDC and Outbreak Response* In: *Dispatches from the AIDS Pandemic.* Kevin M. De Cock, Harold W. Jaffe, and James W. Curran and Edited by: Robin Moseley, Oxford University Press. © Oxford University Press 2023. DOI: 10.1093/oso/9780197626528.003.0001

of partnership in major international initiatives, such as disease elimination and eradication efforts, CDC's primary focus is domestic.

State and local health departments conduct most disease outbreak investigations in the United States, but they may request epidemiologic assistance ("Epi-Aid") from CDC when outbreaks are urgent, unusual, or span multiple jurisdictions. Unlike epidemiologic research, in which data collection requires approval by an institutional review board and the informed consent of participants, Epi-Aids generally are exempt from these requirements.[3]

In conducting Epi-Aids, a major CDC asset is its Epidemic Intelligence Service (EIS). Comprising CDC's "disease detectives," the EIS was created in 1951 in response to concerns about biological warfare threats arising during the Korean War. EIS officers are typically young health professionals who are accepted for training at CDC and then undertake two-year assignments in a CDC program or a CDC-sponsored position in a health department, with expectations for their participation in outbreak investigations. The EIS officer's assignment is determined through a process that seeks to match the officer's preferences as closely as possible with the needs of specific programs.

Another unique asset of CDC in responding to health threats is its cadre of public health advisors (PHAs). In the late 1940s and early 1950s, nonphysician college graduates were hired by PHS to assist states and cities with their venereal disease control activities.* PHAs were later recruited to work in tuberculosis (TB) control and immunization programs. As they gained experience, PHAs could become program managers, either in local and state programs or at CDC headquarters in Atlanta. During the global smallpox eradication program, PHAs were trained as "Operations Officers," serving two-year international tours of duty in countries where they were responsible for program logistic and management support.

When CDC participates in an outbreak investigation, its findings are first communicated directly to the health department(s) that requested assistance. To communicate to other health professionals, the public, and the media, CDC often uses its in-house publication, the *Morbidity and Mortality Weekly Report* (*MMWR*). The *MMWR* began as a summary of weekly statistics on nationally notifiable diseases produced by the National Office of Vital Statistics. But following its transfer to CDC in 1960, the *MMWR* became a

---

* The first PHAs were hired by the PHS Division of Venereal Disease, which was located in Washington, DC. The Division moved to CDC in 1957.

vehicle for rapid reporting of emerging health problems. Unlike medical journals that require outside peer review of articles before accepting them for publication, *MMWR* submissions are typically reviewed by CDC staff and editors. This practice can reduce time between submission of a report and publication to less than a week. Editorial notes that often accompany reports are used by CDC to provide commentary on the topic.

With all these assets in place, CDC (Figure 1.1) appeared to be well-positioned to respond to new threats to the nation's health. But as the narrator of Albert Camus's 1947 novel, *The Plague*, observed, "Everybody knows that pestilences have a way of recurring in the world; yet somehow we find it hard to believe in ones that crash down on our heads from a blue sky."[4] The pestilence that crashed down on CDC in June 1981 was the AIDS epidemic,

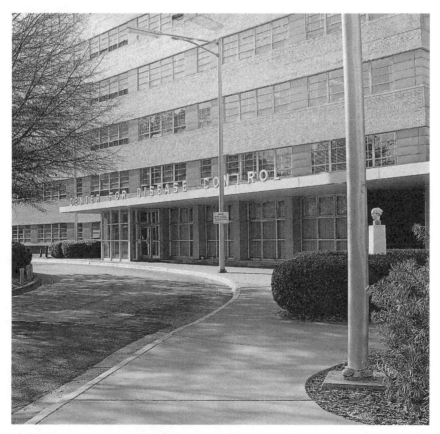

Figure 1.1. CDC headquarters, circa 1980. (CDC Public Health Image Library).

which has claimed tens of millions of lives, including hundreds of thousands of Americans, and is still with us today.

Section I of this book looks at the early days of the American AIDS epidemic through the eyes of the CDC investigators who were charged with understanding and preventing this new pestilence. It relies heavily on the first-hand accounts of these investigators, many recorded as part of CDC's AIDS oral history project, and their archived records.[5] This is the early story of a medical mystery and CDC's role in understanding it.

Notes

1. McDade JE, Shepard CC, Fraser DW, et al. Legionnaires' disease—isolation of a bacterium and demonstration of its role in other respiratory disease. N Engl J Med 1977;297:119–1203.
2. Shands KN, Schmid GP, Dan BB, et al. Toxic-shock syndrome in menstruating women—association with tampon use and *Staphylococcus aureus* and clinical features in 52 cases. N Engl J Med 1980;303:1436–1442.
3. Holt JH, Ghosh SN, Black JR. Legal considerations. In: Rasmussen SA, Goodman RA, eds., The CDC field epidemiology manual. New York: Oxford University Press; 2019:263–279.
4. Camus A. The plague. New York: Alfred A. Knopf; 1948:223.
5. *The Global Health Chronicles*. CDC's early response to AIDS. https://www.globalhealt hchronicles.org/aids.

Further Reading

Readers can find detailed histories of CDC, EIS, PHAs, and the *MMWR* in the following sources:

Etheridge EW. Sentinel for health. A history of the Center for Disease Control. Berkeley, CA: University of California Press; 1991.

Pendergrast M. Inside the outbreaks. The elite medical detectives of the Epidemic Intelligence Service. New York: Houghton Mifflin Harcourt Publishing Company; 2010.

Meyerson BE, Martich FA, Naehr GP. Ready to go: The history and contributions of U.S. public health advisors. Research Triangle Park, NC: American Social Health Association; 2008.

Shaw FE, Goodman, RA, Lindegren ML, Ward JW. A history of MMWR. MMWR Morb Mortal Wkly Rep 2011;60(Suppl):7–14.

Primary source materials on the beginnings of CDC can be found within the Malaria Chronicle on the Global Health Chronicles website (https://www.globalhealthchronic les.org/).

2

The Beginning

Harold W. Jaffe

On January 20, 1981, as cases of what would become known as AIDS were silently increasing, Ronald Reagan was sworn in as the fortieth President of the United States. In his inaugural address, Reagan described the economic challenges facing the nation and declared that "In this present crisis, government is not the solution to our problem; government is the problem." He went on to say, "It is my intention to curb the size and influence of the Federal establishment."[1]

President Reagan's statements obviously raised concerns at CDC, which was a federal agency. Would the budget be cut? Would there be hiring freezes or even layoffs? Also, would the increasingly assertive religious conservatives in the Reagan administration want to exercise more control over CDC's programs in areas such as sexual and reproductive health? As a young medical officer working in CDC's Division of Sexually Transmitted Diseases (DSTD), I[2] wasn't too worried. Given CDC's trusted reputation with the American public, I naively thought we would be spared the worst of any budget and personnel cuts or any attempts to influence our programs for political or religious purposes. And I believed that our widely admired Director, William (Bill) Foege,[3] and his senior staff members would be able to manage whatever challenges CDC might face.

Foege had been appointed CDC Director in 1977 during the administration of President Jimmy Carter. His father was a Lutheran minister, and Foege had served as a medical missionary in Nigeria before joining CDC. As an EIS officer assigned to the State of Colorado, he investigated a possible case of smallpox in a child living on the Navajo reservation in New Mexico. Although the case turned out not to be smallpox, Foege became fascinated by the disease. He later accepted a position as a CDC assignee to the WHO smallpox eradication effort and is credited for developing vaccination

Harold W. Jaffe, *The Beginning* In: *Dispatches from the AIDS Pandemic*. Kevin M. De Cock, Harold W. Jaffe, and James W. Curran and Edited by: Robin Moseley, Oxford University Press. © Oxford University Press 2023.
DOI: 10.1093/oso/9780197626528.003.0002

strategies that led to the eradication of smallpox in India.* Standing six feet seven inches tall, he was literally and figuratively a towering persona in public health.

With the widespread availability of vaccines and antimicrobial agents in the 1970s, some experts were suggesting that the era of infectious disease threats was ending, at least in high-income counties. In 1978, the eminent infectious diseases physician and educator from the University of Washington, Robert Petersdorf, wrote, "Even with my great personal loyalties to infectious disease, I cannot conceive of the need for 309 more infectious-disease experts unless they spend their time culturing each other."[4] The number 309 referred to the number of physicians who, like me, had recently taken the infectious diseases specialty board examination. But unfolding events were to prove these experts wrong.

In 1981, EIS officer Wayne Shandera[5] was working as an assignee to the Los Angeles County Health Department. Before joining EIS, Shandera had trained in internal medicine at Stanford University, where he met Michael Gottlieb. Gottlieb was completing an immunology fellowship at Stanford before moving to the UCLA Medical Center in Los Angeles. Shandera and Gottlieb remained in contact in Los Angeles, discussing possible joint research projects.

Early in 1981, Gottlieb began calling Shandera to describe some very unusual patients: young homosexual† men, who were previously healthy but had developed *Pneumocystis carinii* pneumonia (PCP). This life-threatening infection characteristically occurred in patients with an underlying immune deficiency, including persons receiving cancer chemotherapy or given drugs to prevent rejection of an organ transplant.[6] These young men were severely immunodeficient, but the cause of their immune deficiency was not apparent.

Gottlieb had seen three of these men at UCLA Hospital and was aware of another patient at Cedars-Mt. Sinai Hospital in Los Angeles. As Shandera recalled, "Mike came down to my office, and, lo and behold, there was a fifth [case report] at St. John's [Medical Center] in Santa Monica on my desk that day. I've never been able to explain if this is just some super-unnatural

* For his leadership in smallpox eradication, Foege received the 2001 Mary Woodard Lasker Public Service Award. In 2012, he was awarded the Presidential Medal of Freedom, the nation's highest civilian honor.
† The word "homosexual" reflects the standard terminology used at the time of these investigations and reports to describe men who have sex with men.

serendipity or what exactly was the case."[5] Gottlieb and Shandera agreed to submit a report of these five patients to the *MMWR*. This was a time before fax or e-mail, and Shandera stated that he and Gottlieb "had to call it in word by word to CDC."[5]

Because PCP was considered a parasitic disease,[‡] the report from Los Angeles was sent to CDC's Parasitic Diseases Branch for review. The reviewer was Dennis Juranek,[7] one of a small number of veterinarians working at CDC. Juranek supervised CDC's Parasitic Diseases Drug Service, which had been established in the late 1960s to provide American physicians access to drugs used to treat uncommon parasitic diseases. These drugs were available in other parts of the world, but demand for them was limited in the United States. As a result, pharmaceutical companies were unwilling to incur the costs associated with seeking approval for their use from the US Food and Drug Administration (FDA). In compliance with the FDA requirements for investigational new drugs, the Parasitic Diseases Drug Service had the authority to purchase these drugs overseas and provide them upon request to American physicians.

For the treatment of PCP, the Drug Service obtained the drug pentamidine isethionate from a British supplier, May & Baker. In the months preceding the report from Los Angeles, Sandra Ford, the CDC technician responsible for the day-to-day operation of the Drug Service, noticed an increasing number of requests for pentamidine to treat PCP in adult men who had no apparent cause for their immunodeficiency.[8] Juranek recalled that "Sandy Ford would bring these up, and we would discuss them. She said, 'We've got quite a few of these now,' and I said, 'Let's go ahead and make a line listing like you do as an epidemiologist. Give us the age, sex, location, and what the underlying disease was.' "[7]

With the information provided by Ford, Juranek felt the Los Angeles PCP cases were part of a larger problem and recommended publication of the report in the *MMWR*. Juranek also sent the report to DSTD, where it was reviewed by Mary Guinan,[9] a medical officer, and James (Jim) Curran,[10] head of the DSTD Research Branch. Guinan recalled Curran exclaiming "hot stuff!"[9] as he returned the report to her. They concurred with Juranek's recommendation for publication.

The report appeared in the June 5, 1981, issue of the *MMWR* (Figure 2.1).[11] Although the word "homosexual" did not appear in the title—a decision

---

[‡] The causative agent of PCP in humans was later reclassified as a fungus, *Pneumocystis jirovecii*. However, the disease is still referred to as PCP.

Dengue — Continued

Editorial Note: Dengue type 4 frequently occurs in Southeast Asia, the South Pacific, and Africa. How it was introduced onto St. Barthelemy, a small and relatively remote island in the Caribbean, remains unknown. However, French health authorities have reported to CAREC that an outbreak of dengue-like illness has been observed on St. Barthelemy, beginning in February or March, but has since declined. In the absence of reports of an ongoing outbreak of dengue in the Caribbean, the risk that travelers to this area will acquire dengue is probably small.

Dengue types 2 and 3 have been present in the Caribbean at least since the 1960ş. Dengue type 1 was first recognized in that area when an outbreak in Jamaica in 1977 was followed by numerous outbreaks on other Caribbean islands and in Central America. All these dengue types, as well as type 4, usually cause an illness that is clinically mild and typically of short duration.

Pneumocystis Pneumonia — Los Angeles

In the period October 1980-May 1981, 5 young men, all active homosexuals, were treated for biopsy-confirmed *Pneumocystis carinii* pneumonia at 3 different hospitals in Los Angeles, California. Two of the patients died. All 5 patients had laboratory-confirmed previous or current cytomegalovirus (CMV) infection and candidal mucosal infection. Case reports of these patients follow.

Patient 1: A previously healthy 33-year-old man developed *P. carinii* pneumonia and oral mucosal candidiasis in March 1981 after a 2-month history of fever associated with elevated liver enzymes, leukopenia, and CMV viruria. The serum complement-fixation CMV titer in October 1980 was 256; in May 1981 it was 32.* The patient's condition deteriorated despite courses of treatment with trimethoprim-sulfamethoxazole (TMP/SMX), pentamidine, and acyclovir. He died May 3, and postmortem examination showed residual *P. carinii* and CMV pneumonia, but no evidence of neoplasia.

Patient 2: A previously healthy 30-year-old man developed *P. carinii* pneumonia in April 1981 after a 5-month history of fever each day and of elevated liver-function tests, CMV viruria, and documented seroconversion to CMV, i.e., an acute-phase titer of 16 and a convalescent-phase titer of 28* in anticomplement immunofluorescence tests. Other features of his illness included leukopenia and mucosal candidiasis. His pneumonia responded to a course of intravenous TMP/SMX, but, as of the latest reports, he continues to have a fever each day.

Patient 3: A 30-year-old man was well until January 1981 when he developed esophageal and oral candidiasis that responded to Amphotericin B treatment. He was hospitalized in February 1981 for *P. carinii* pneumonia that responded to oral TMP/SMX. His esophageal candidiasis recurred after the pneumonia was diagnosed, and he was again given Amphotericin B. The CMV complement-fixation titer in March 1981 was 8. Material from an esophageal biopsy was positive for CMV.

Patient 4: A 29-year-old man developed *P. carinii* pneumonia in February 1981. He had had Hodgkins disease 3 years earlier, but had been successfully treated with radiation therapy alone. He did not improve after being given intravenous TMP/SMX and corticosteroids and died in March. Postmortem examination showed no evidence of Hodgkins disease, but *P. carinii* and CMV were found in lung tissue.

---

*Paired specimens not run in parallel.

Figure 2.1. First published report on what would become known as AIDS. (Harold Jaffe, personal collection).

made by the *MMWR* editor Michael Gregg—the body of the report described the five patients as "all active homosexuals." Two of the patients had died, and the three who had been tested all had laboratory evidence of severely impaired cellular immunity. The editorial note that accompanied the report stated, "The fact that these patients were all homosexuals suggests an association between some aspect of a homosexual lifestyle or disease acquired through sexual contact and *Pneumocystis* pneumonia in this population."[11]

Shortly after the June 5th publication, physicians began to contact CDC staff about other unusual illnesses appearing in homosexual men. Alvin Friedman-Kien, Professor of Dermatology at New York University (NYU) Medical Center, called to discuss cases of Kaposi's sarcoma (KS), a rare cancer predominately affecting the skin, diagnosed in thirty young homosexual men in the previous two years.[12] Some of these men also had PCP. On June 8th, Curran and I attended a national venereal disease (VD)-control seminar in San Diego, California, where we learned about similar cases in San Francisco from Robert Bolan and other physicians. I recall writing "Kaposi's sarcoma" on a slip of paper and putting it in my wallet so that I wouldn't forget the name of the disease when I returned to CDC.

On June 11th, Juranek and Curran traveled to New York City to meet with Friedman-Kien and his colleagues at NYU.[13] There, they were given a line list of KS patients, including contact information for the physicians caring for these patients. Juranek and Curran also met with Jack Weissman, a physician at Columbia Presbyterian Medical Center and Dan William, a private physician, to discuss the KS patients they had recently seen.

Curran and EIS officer Alexander Kelter made a follow-up visit to New York City on June 29th.[14] During this visit they met with additional clinicians, including the oncologists Linda Laubenstein from NYU and Bijan Safai from Memorial Sloan-Kettering Cancer Center, as well as New York City Health Department officials. While there, Curran also interviewed a patient with KS. As he described the interview,

> I can't help but remember the time I met that first patient . . . he was a handsome actor who had these blotches on his face. And he said, "Doc, from CDC, what do you think, can we get rid of these, is this going to hurt my career?" And, of course, I had never seen a case of Kaposi's sarcoma in my life, and I didn't know what to tell him. Unfortunately, he was treated with very aggressive chemotherapy, which probably hastened his disease course.

I had a chance to see him several more times before he died, and, actually, the week he died in the ICU [intensive care unit] at NYU.[10]

Kaposi's sarcoma was named for Moritz Kaposi, a Hungarian dermatologist working in Vienna, who in 1872 described five patients with "idiopathic multiple pigmented sarcomas of the skin."[15] The epidemiologic form of the disease that he described, now known as "classic" KS, was rarely seen in the United States. During the mid-1970s, only three hundred to four hundred cases were estimated to occur annually.[16] Classic KS was usually seen in elderly men, most often of southern European and Ashkenazi Jewish ancestry, and typically had an indolent clinical course. The disease was usually limited to the skin, most characteristically on the lower legs. Elderly men more often died with the disease rather than from it.

Upon microscopic examination, KS biopsy samples from young gay men and older men with classic disease appeared identical. But clinically the disease was much more aggressive in the young men, with multiple skin lesions that often increased rapidly in both size and number. There were reports of patients developing disseminated disease, with KS lesions appearing in the gastrointestinal tract (mouth, esophagus, stomach, and intestine) and in the lungs, leading to bleeding and death in some instances.

Of interest were previous reports of another form of KS seen in persons with chronic immunosuppression, most often organ transplant recipients. In one series, KS accounted for more than 3 percent of all malignancies arising in transplant recipients, with internal organ involvement in almost half of the cases.[17] Unlike classic KS, there was no male predominance in posttransplant KS cases. Reports of kidney transplant recipients in whom KS lesions regressed or disappeared following reduction or discontinuation of immunosuppressive therapy suggested a link between impaired immune function and increased KS risk.[18] But why immunosuppression predisposed a patient to the development of KS was unknown.§

The *MMWR* published descriptions of these newly reported KS cases on July 4, 1981, with the words "homosexual men" now appearing in the title.[19] The article noted that twenty-six homosexual men (twenty in New York City and six in California) had been diagnosed with KS in the previous

---

§ The etiologic agent of KS was later found to be a virus, human herpesvirus 8 (HHV-8), also known as Kaposi's sarcoma-associated herpesvirus (KSHV). Immunosuppression is thought to facilitate replication of infected cells, resulting in tumor formation. An endemic form of KS is seen in equatorial Africa, where HHV-8 infection is much more prevalent than in other parts of the world.

thirty months. The patients ranged in age from twenty-six to fifty-one years, and eight had died. Four patients developed PCP after their KS diagnosis, and several others were diagnosed with additional severe opportunistic infections (OIs, infections associated with immunosuppression), such as toxoplasmosis, a parasitic infection which can involve the brain. A review of NYU cancer registry data for KS in men under age 50 revealed three cases at NYU Medical Center from 1961 to 1971 and no cases from 1970 to 1979 at Bellevue Hospital. The report noted that

> The occurrence of this number of KS cases during a 30-month period among young, homosexual men is considered highly unusual. No previous association between KS and sexual preference has been reported. The fulminant clinical course reported in many of these patients also differs from that classically described for elderly persons.[19]

These two *MMWR* articles, published one month apart, left readers with more questions than answers. A newly reported disease, characterized by severe immune deficiency, OIs, and a rare malignancy, was killing young homosexual men in California and New York City. But was the disease really new or had it occurred earlier and not been recognized or reported? How many cases were there? Were the cases limited to California and New York City or were they appearing elsewhere? Was the disease limited to homosexual men, and, if so, why? And most importantly, what was causing the disease and how could it be prevented?

The reported disease didn't fit within the expertise of any single organizational unit at CDC, so a multidisciplinary task force was established to investigate it. Curran was selected as its leader (Figure 2.2), and the group was formally named: Centers for Disease Control Task Force on Kaposi's Sarcoma and Opportunistic Infections. As a medical student, Curran planned to become an obstetrician/gynecologist, with a specialty in family planning. However, after joining CDC and serving an assignment at the University of Tennessee to study the economic consequences of the complications of gonorrhea, he decided to change his career path and continue doing VD research at CDC.

Curran was a popular choice as the Task Force leader. As Juranek noted,

> Jim was the best-qualified person to do that because of his past history in dealing with sexually transmitted diseases. He was familiar with the

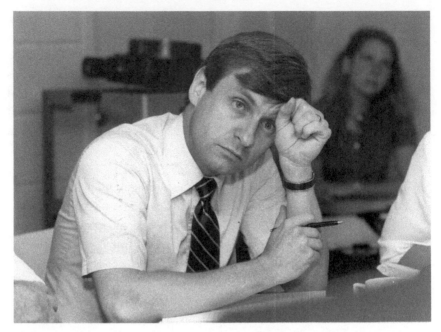

Figure 2.2. Jim Curran, 1983. (Steve Deal/*Atlanta Journal-Constitution* via AP).

systems and processes. He took it on, and it was an excellent choice. He just had the right demeanor to handle patients, the politics, and the medical community. They couldn't have picked a better person, from my perspective.[7]

The Task Force initially included about a dozen members,[20] described by Curran as

[A]n eager group of people that came from throughout the agency. People working on cancer, people working in virology, people working in STDs [sexually transmitted diseases], people working on environmental issues—and all were sort of assigned together in this ad hoc task force that we called Kaposi's sarcoma and opportunistic infections because we wanted people to think and realize that we considered this not just an epidemic of cancer, not just an epidemic of infections, but an epidemic of a conglomeration of things forming a syndrome.[10]

With one exception, the Task Force members were physicians, veterinarians, or biomedical scientists. The exception was William (Bill) Darrow,[21] a research sociologist working in DSTD. Darrow started his career as a PHA in New York City, where he worked in VD control. His job there involved interviewing patients with syphilis, eliciting the names of their sexual contacts, locating the contacts, and referring the contacts to "social hygiene" clinics for further evaluation. He was then assigned to CDC headquarters, where he received sponsorship for masters and doctoral degrees in sociology. Darrow had worked with Curran on epidemiologic studies of hepatitis B virus (HBV) infection in homosexual men, and he brought to the Task Force expertise in social and behavioral aspects of VD with a specific focus on the sexual health of homosexual men.

A critical person in facilitating the formation of the Task Force was Paul Wiesner, Director of DSTD. Wiesner was a charismatic leader who had come to CDC after training in infectious diseases at the University of Washington. As Bill Foege recounted, "One of the heroes in this story is Paul Wiesner, who immediately put people from the STD program . . . on the investigation. So, he wasted no time in responding."[3] Wiesner knew that assigning staff members to the Task Force would have a negative impact on DSTD but considered investigating this new disease to be a higher priority.

I was also personally indebted to Wiesner for helping me remain at CDC during the Reagan years. I had worked in DSTD (then known as the Venereal Disease Control Division) for three years before leaving to do an infectious diseases fellowship at the University of Chicago. Shortly after I returned to CDC, the Reagan administration announced a "reduction in force" (or "RIF") for federal employees, intended to reduce federal spending and based, in part, on seniority. For unexplained reasons, my prior federal service was not considered in assessing my seniority, and I was placed on the list of employees who could be "riffed." Although DSTD had no EIS officers, Wiesner was able to place me in EIS, which was a training program and exempt from the force reduction.

I don't specifically recall why I was asked to join the Task Force, but it may have been because of my experience working as a volunteer doctor at the Howard Brown Memorial Clinic, a facility for the medical care of gay men, while doing my fellowship in Chicago. I wasn't entirely sure that I wanted to give up my "day job" investigating antibiotic-resistant gonorrhea. But the work of the Task Force sounded interesting and important. And it seemed to me that solving this sort of problem was why CDC existed.

Notes

1. Ronald Reagan Presidential Foundation & Institute, https://www.reaganfoundation.org/media/128614/inaguration.pdf.
2. "JAFFE, HAROLD," *The Global Health Chronicles*, accessed January 8, 2023, https://www.globalhealthchronicles.org/items/show/5385.
3. "FOEGE, WILLIAM H," *The Global Health Chronicles*, accessed January 11, 2023, https://www.globalhealthchronicles.org/items/show/6480.
4. Petersdorf RG. The doctors' dilemma. N Engl J Med 1978;299:628–634.
5. "SHANDERA, WAYNE," *The Global Health Chronicles*, accessed January 29, 2023, https://www.globalhealthchronicles.org/items/show/7736.
6. Walzer PD, Perl DP, Krogstad DJ, et al. *Pneumocystis carinii* pneumonia in the United States. Epidemiologic, diagnostic, and clinical features. Ann Intern Med 1974;80:83–93.
7. "JURANEK, DENNIS," *The Global Health Chronicles*, accessed December 10, 2022, https://www.globalhealthchronicles.org/items/show/7973.
8. Schultz MG, Bloch AB. In Memoriam: Sandy Ford (1950–2015). Emerg Infect Dis 2016;22:764–765.
9. "GUINAN, MARY," *The Global Health Chronicles*, accessed January 29, 2023, https://www.globalhealthchronicles.org/items/show/5393.
10. "CURRAN, JAMES," *The Global Health Chronicles*, accessed January 24, 2023, https://www.globalhealthchronicles.org/items/show/7743.
11. CDC. *Pneumocystis* pneumonia—Los Angeles. MMWR Morb Mortal Wkly Rep 1981;30:250–252.
12. "KAPOSI'S SARCOMA," *The Global Health Chronicles*, accessed January 29, 2023, https://www.globalhealthchronicles.org/items/show/8083.
13. "KAPOSI'S SYNDROME NYC: Trip Report," *The Global Health Chronicles*, accessed January 29, 2023, https://www.globalhealthchronicles.org/items/show/8084.
14. "TRIP REPORT: Kaposi's Syndrome," *The Global Health Chronicles*, accessed January 29, 2023, https://www.globalhealthchronicles.org/items/show/8085.
15. Kaposi M. Multiple idiopathic pigmented sarcoma of the skin. CA Cancer J Clin 1982;32:342–347. Translated from the German and reprinted from Arch Dermatol Syph 1872;4:265–273.
16. Biggar RJ, Horm J, Fraumeni JF Jr, et al. Incidence of Kaposi's sarcoma and mycosis fungoides in the United States including Puerto Rico, 1973–81. J Natl Cancer Inst 1982;73:89–94.
17. Penn I. Kaposi's sarcoma in organ transplant recipients: Report of 20 cases. Transplantation 1979;27:8–11.

18. Myers BD, Kessler E, Levi J, et al. Kaposi's sarcoma in kidney transplant recipients. Arch Intern Med 1974;133:307–311.

19. CDC. Kaposi's sarcoma and *Pneumocystis* pneumonia among homosexual men— New York City and California. MMWR Morb Mortal Wkly Rep 1981;30:305–308.

20. "EMERGENCE OF KS/OI," *The Global Health Chronicles*, accessed January 29, 2023, https://www.globalhealthchronicles.org/items/show/6631.

21. "DARROW, WILLIAM," *The Global Health Chronicles*, accessed January 22, 2023, https://www.globalhealthchronicles.org/items/show/6870.

3

Surveillance

The Cornerstone of the Early Response

Mary E. Chamberland and Bess Miller

The reports of KS and PCP in homosexual men in Los Angeles, San Francisco, and New York City triggered an urgent effort to identify and characterize additional cases of this perplexing new disease. Initial priorities for the Task Force were, as Jim Curran described it, "to get a handle on what you're really investigating and to find out if it's new, who gets it, and is it going up or down . . . . These things can help lead you to finding out what the cause is, because ultimately you want to find the cause and then how to prevent the condition."[1]

Case Definition and Early Surveillance

"Getting a handle on things" through case detection and reporting activities—what in public health parlance is termed "surveillance"—was anchored in the establishment of a case definition, or a set of criteria, to standardize who would be counted as a "case." Newly minted EIS officer Harry Haverkos,[2] who joined the Task Force in July 1981, was tasked to develop the first case definition. It was a tricky assignment. For outbreaks of a new disease, it is critical that the case definition have high specificity and accuracy; in other words, that it capture only people who truly have the disease. Haverkos was a good fit for the job having recently completed an infectious disease fellowship at the University of Pittsburgh where he had done research in infections affecting immunocompromised patients. The urgency to establish a case definition compelled Haverkos to forego some of the four-week training that every incoming EIS officer was to undertake that month. Instead, he decamped to the CDC library where he scoured the published literature and framed what he termed "a three-part case definition": (1) KS

Mary E. Chamberland and Bess Miller, *Surveillance* In: *Dispatches from the AIDS Pandemic*. Kevin M. De Cock, Harold W. Jaffe, and James W. Curran and Edited by: Robin Moseley, Oxford University Press. © Oxford University Press 2023. DOI: 10.1093/oso/9780197626528.003.0003

in persons under sixty years of age; (2) the presence of at least one of five culture- or biopsy-proven infections considered to be at least moderately predictive of immune suppression (PCP, toxoplasmosis of the central nervous system, cryptococcal meningitis, disseminated or progressive herpes simplex virus infection, and invasive gastrointestinal candidiasis) in persons fifteen years of age and older; and (3) the absence of established causes of immune suppression such as malignancy, organ transplantation, or treatment with immunosuppressive drugs[2,3]. As Curran recalled:

> So, we spent quite a bit of time, meaning days to weeks, making sure that we had a handle on a very specific case definition. We were aided with this definition because the conditions were so rare and so remarkable. Men with Kaposi's sarcoma in its advanced phase or *Pneumocystis* pneumonia were often cachectic, were often like the sickest of cancer patients or disaster survivors. They were very, very, very ill. Any doctor who saw one patient would remember it. They would say, "Oh my God, this is remarkable." . . .Also, cases could be diagnosed by definitive means through open lung biopsy for *Pneumocystis* pneumonia and through a skin biopsy or tumor biopsy with Kaposi's sarcoma, or other definitive means for other fatal opportunistic infections.[1]

Passive surveillance, which relies on the willingness of healthcare providers, laboratories, and other sources to voluntarily report cases, was the mainstay of early AIDS surveillance. As described in Chapter 2, physicians who had seen similar patients began contacting the Task Force soon after the initial reports appeared in the *MMWR*. In early August 1981, CDC sent letters to state and territorial epidemiologists formally requesting that cases be reported to CDC.[4] Task Force members found themselves on the receiving end of countless calls, as recalled by Haverkos:

> I spent the whole day on the phone basically, and physicians would call. They'd tell me about their cases. I'd fill out the reports, and they'd ask me questions. . . .Patients could call, and health departments would call. I can remember we didn't have speaker phones in those days, so I would [hold the receiver]—my ears would just burn. I mean it was hot. It generates quite a bit of heat. I'd change to this ear and that ear. I was on the phone constantly. But they were looking for information, just as we were.[2]

Passive surveillance often results in delays in reporting, incomplete information, and underreporting of cases, and "getting a handle on things" required additional, resource-intensive approaches to actively search for cases.[5] By early July 1981, planning was underway to initiate multiple active surveillance activities to determine (1) the incidence of KS, PCP, and other serious OIs, both retrospectively and prospectively; (2) if groups other than homosexual men were affected; and (3) if cases were occurring in places other than New York and California.[6] Selected state tumor registries and the National Cancer Institute's Surveillance, Epidemiology, and End Results (SEER) registries in the San Francisco Bay and Atlanta areas were reviewed to determine the incidence of KS before 1980. Similarly, requests to CDC for pentamidine isethionate to treat PCP (Chapter 2) were examined from 1976 onward, with particular focus on requests for patients without an underlying medical condition.

A high priority for the Task Force was to actively survey physicians in select US cities for cases of KS and OIs. The survey was initially piloted in six cities thought to span a range of disease burden—Los Angeles, Atlanta, Miami, Rochester and Albany (New York), and Oklahoma City—and subsequently was expanded to include a total of eighteen major metropolitan areas. The Task Force relied heavily on EIS officers assigned to these cities to doggedly search for cases and to complete the two-page case report form Haverkos had developed[2,3] The officers telephoned and wrote letters to the chiefs of infectious disease, oncology, dermatology, and pathology in every hospital and contacted physicians whose practices included many homosexual men. They also reviewed medical records and searched death certificates to identify cases.[2,3,5]

The results of these early surveillance efforts were summarized in the Task Force's first peer-reviewed article, published in the *New England Journal of Medicine* in January 1982. Cases of KS and OIs were retrospectively identified as far back as 1978 and had risen steadily thereafter.[5] Nearly all of the 159 cases identified between June 1 and November 10, 1981, occurred in homosexual or bisexual men, and 77 percent were residents of New York City, Los Angeles, or San Francisco at the time of their diagnosis. Active surveillance in the fifteen other metropolitan areas failed to turn up a single case that had not been reported previously. The Task Force investigators presciently concluded that their findings suggested "the occurrence of a single epidemic of underlying immunosuppression in these men" and that the high mortality rate (38 percent overall) "indicates a serious public health problem."[5]

National Surveillance and Case Reporting

Case reports accrued relentlessly. Richard Selik[7], an epidemiologist in the Division of Sexualy Transmitted Diseases (DSTD), was (as he described) "volunteered" to join the Task Force in July 1982. His initial remit was to develop a formal, more detailed case definition suitable for national surveillance. The definition used in the eighteen major metropolitan area survey had proven useful. However, other life-threatening and often fatal infections were increasingly being diagnosed in patients with no apparent risk factors for immunodeficiency. These observations prompted serious consideration as to whether other OIs should be included in the surveillance case definition, and, if so, whether this could be done without compromising its high specificity. The outcome— the first, formal surveillance case definition for AIDS—was published in September 1982.[8] The disease list comprised KS, PCP, and an expanded list of twelve serious OIs, with a case defined as a person in whom at least one of these conditions had been diagnosed using reliable methods (e.g., histology or culture) and who had no known cause for diminished resistance to the disease.

By early 1983, a Surveillance Section had been formally established within the AIDS Activity (the programmatic name that supplanted "Task Force"). It was led by James (Jim) Allen, an epidemiologist with several years experience in CDC's Hospital Infections Program. Allen and veteran PHA Thomas (Tom) Starcher ([9]), another recent DSTD recruit to the AIDS Activity, began to assemble the essential elements of a national surveillance program for AIDS. This included the development of national guidelines for AIDS case surveillance; uniform adult and pediatric case report forms, which were typeset, printed, and distributed to state and large-city health departments; and standardized procedures for reporting cases to CDC.

One of the top priorities, as described by Starcher, was for state and large-city health departments to assume an increasingly active role in the surveillance and investigation of AIDS:

At the time I arrived in April of '83, there had been just over a thousand cases reported to CDC. . . . a lot of the reports were coming directly to CDC, and they were bypassing health departments. . . .we set up an announcement for cooperative agreements* for many major city health departments.

---

* A cooperative agreement is a legal instrument of financial assistance between a federal awarding agency and a recipient. It is distinguished from a grant in that it provides for substantial involvement

It included New York, Baltimore, Washington, DC, Chicago, Los Angeles, and San Francisco. We made awards to them for setting up surveillance. The goal was to have cases reported by doctors in clinics through those health departments on to CDC. We got back into the pattern of using the health departments out there as the true partners that they are for CDC.[9]

The Task Force had awarded the first cooperative agreement to implement active hospital-based surveillance for AIDS to the New York City Department of Health in October 1982 at an estimated first-year cost of $85,000.[10] It represented the first funding that the US Congress had appropriated for AIDS. The Task Force's decision to support enhanced surveillance in New York City reflected its importance to national surveillance. New York City accounted for nearly half of all AIDS cases in the United States at the time, and it was the only area that had reported significant numbers of cases in homosexual men as well as injection drug users (IDUs)[†] (and subsequently in their heterosexual partners).

Apart from the active review of death certificates for AIDS-related diagnoses, the New York City health department used a passive reporting system that relied on physicians and hospital infection control nurses to submit case reports in writing or by telephone (Figure 3.1). By late 1982 it was clear that "reporting fatigue" had set in; physicians and nurses were becoming overwhelmed, resulting in delays in reporting, incomplete information, and underreporting. One of the authors (MEC[11]) was an EIS officer stationed at the health department and was tapped to coordinate the implementation of a pilot program of active surveillance in fifteen New York City hospitals. Establishing surveillance in hospitals made sense, because nearly everyone with AIDS at that time required hospitalization for treatment of serious OIs.

The cooperative agreement resources also facilitated the hiring of several PHAs, who were the lynchpins to the program's success. They met weekly with each hospital's designated case reporter (typically an infection control nurse), reviewed medical records, and completed the case report forms. A subsequent study to evaluate the impact of active surveillance found that 96 percent of all patients identified with AIDS had been reported to the city's

of the Federal awarding agency in carrying out the activity contemplated by the Federal award (https://www.ecfr.gov/current/title-2/subtitle-A/chapter-II/part-200#200.1).

[†] *Injection* or *injecting drug user* and *IDUs*, along with *intravenous drug users* and *IVDUs*, were terms used at the time of these investigations and reports to describe persons who inject drugs.

PHONE REPORT FORM

Identification Number ___ ___ ___ ___ (to be assigned)

Date of Call ___ ___ ___ ___ ___ ___ ___ ___ ___ Call taken by _____
(name)

Patient

Name or initials _____

Age _____   Status: Alive _____   Dead _____

Date of Birth ___ ___ ___ ___ ___ ___   Date of Death ___ ___ ___ ___ ___ ___ ___

Sex: M___ F___   Sexual preference: M___ F___ Both ___ Unkn ___

Marital Status: Married ___   Never Married ___   Divorced ___

Widowed ___   Separated ___   Unknown ___

Race: White, not Hispanic____   Asian or Pacific Islander ____

Black, not Hispanic____   American Indian or Alaska Native ____

Haitian ____   Other country (specify) _____

Hispanic ____   Not Stated _____
Address(Street & #)_____
Residence_____
(City)   (Borough)   (State)

If hospitalized, name and location of hospital

_____   _____   _____
(Name)   (City)   (State)

Illness:	Date of Diagnosis (Month, Year)	Method of Diagnosis* (Biopsy or Culture) Yes No	Other Specimen
___ Kaposi's Sarcoma		___ ___	
___ Pneumocystis			
___ CMV Infection			
___ Progressive Herpes Simplex (duration)			
___ Toxoplasmosis (CNS)			
___ Cryptococcosis (CNS)			
___ GI candidiasis			
___ Other _____ Opportunistic Infection			
___ Other medical conditions		* Specify test	

(over)

Figure 3.1. New York City Department of Health phone report form for early cases of KS/OI, 1982. (Mary Chamberland, personal collection)

health department and the proportion of cases reported within one month of diagnosis increased from 45 percent to 69 percent.[12]

The surveillance methods piloted in New York City served as models for other US city and state health departments. The AIDS Activity transferred a cadre of some of CDC's best PHAs from across the country to Atlanta to oversee the implementation of new cooperative agreements in state, territorial, and local health departments. As part of this process, a PHA and an epidemiologist from the AIDS Activity would team up and make on-site visits to obtain first-hand accounts of progress on the ground, trouble-shoot problems, make recommendations, and gain feedback on how CDC could better support local programs. The steadfast efforts of hundreds of health department professionals combined with federal funding and technical support resulted in a national surveillance system that was remarkably robust. A 1985 evaluation in four cities that had reported 38 percent of all AIDS cases in the United States (Washington DC, New York City, Boston, and Chicago) found that the overall completeness of AIDS case reporting was 89 percent— far better than the rate for other communicable diseases.[13]

Early AIDS case surveillance played a pivotal role in flagging unusual cases. Physicians were urged to report cases that did not belong to any of the recognized risk groups. These cases triggered extensive investigations, which on occasion led to the recognition of new risk groups. An analysis of the first one thousand cases of AIDS reported in the United States between June 1981 and February 1983 found that all but sixty-one patients could be classified into established risk groups, with the authors noting that "several new groups may, however, be emerging from the study of these 61 patients."[14] Included in this group were five women with PCP who reported that they did not use intravenous (IV) drugs themselves but were the steady sexual partners of men who did. Five other patients reported receiving a transfusion of blood components in the three years prior to their illness.

Investigations of what came to be called "no identified risk" or "NIR" cases was a shared responsibility between CDC and state and local health departments. An in-person interview was an essential component of an investigation. The New York City Department of Health was renowned for its exceptional team of NIR investigators. Many had previously worked in venereal disease control programs and were instinctively adept at drawing out risk information, oftentimes eschewing the formal and lengthy NIR interview form. Kenneth (Ken) Castro[15] was the Atlanta-based CDC epidemiologist responsible for tracking NIR cases nationally in the early-mid 1980s. As he recalled,

[W]e never found alternative routes of transmission, such as through casual contact or through contact other than . . . exposure to blood and body fluids. That was in many ways reassuring . . . in spite of our dogged pursuit of these interviews. Very often, I'd say at least sixty percent of the time, when we conducted an interview, you were able to uncover risk factors, people who were heterosexual men married with children would admit under the circumstances described in the interview that, yes, they had had sex with other men and were not interested in having their family learn about that.[15]

Low-Tech Tools for Data Analysis and Dissemination

Transforming information from paper case report forms into tabulated data analyses was arduous in the pre-Internet, predesktop computing era. Health department surveillance officers mailed photocopied AIDS case report forms to CDC where each case was scrutinized to ensure it met the strict surveillance case definition criteria. As the epidemic grew, so did the crush of paper, as described by Selik:

> When I started on the Task Force [in 1981], there were only 340-some cases. When the cases came in, I was responsible for checking the case report forms to see if they met the case definition. After not very long, I was being inundated with case report forms; it was very hard to keep up with them. It felt like I was on top of a volcano that was going to explode.[7]

Selik had a keen eye for detecting incomplete data on case report forms. Health department staff, including this author (MEC), were often on the receiving end of letters with a long list of questions and requests for missing information, which Selik painstakingly wrote on lined paper in his readily identifiable block print. As he recounted,

> Communication was longhand, by pen and paper. In New York City, they were keeping track of my questions . . . in a log book that they would call the "Dear Richard book," "dear" because that was a greeting in a letter that you might get. . . . Years later, people thought that was named after Benjamin Franklin's *Poor Richard's Almanac*. They didn't know that there was a real person, me, that was the basis for that.[7]

Tabulation of national surveillance statistics relied on mainframe computing and the use of keypunched data. Curran recruited Meade Morgan, a PhD statistician from CDC's Hospital Infections Program, to lead the Analysis and Computing Section in the AIDS Activity and apply his strong logistic and informatics skills to AIDS surveillance. Morgan designed a software system to automate the process of determining which cases met the surveillance case definition and wrote early code for the national surveillance system when it became computerized.[9] He was invaluable to the program in other ways, providing statistical and modeling expertise (Chapter 11), as well as overseeing hardware and computer network installment (even removing office ceiling tiles himself to lay cabling early on).

In New York City, computerized assistance for tabulation of AIDS case data was first introduced in February 1983, coincident with the implementation of the active surveillance program. Prior to that, one of the authors (MEC) recalls that she and fellow EIS officer, Pauline (Polly) Thomas ([16]), also assigned to the city's health department, were responsible for generating "homespun" monthly surveillance reports. They used calculators to manually tabulate AIDS cases and hand-drew epidemic curves and bar graphs, carefully tracing a template designed by Thomas's architect husband (Figure 3.2).

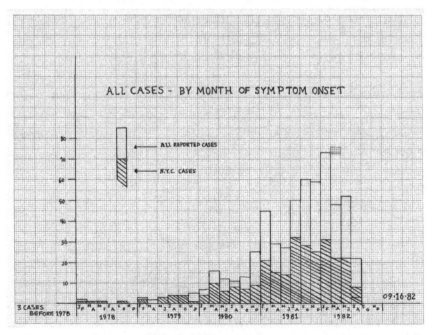

Figure 3.2. Hand-drawn epidemic curve of US and New York City KS/OI cases, September 1982. (Mary Chamberland, personal collection)

Dissemination of surveillance data at both the national and local level was an integral component of the AIDS surveillance program. Surveillance updates were published periodically in the *MMWR*, and slide sets were available without charge to anyone who asked. National AIDS surveillance data were tabulated on a weekly basis from the earliest days of the epidemic. Computerization of national surveillance data in 1983 paved the way for the *AIDS Weekly Surveillance Report* (Figure 3.3) to be printed and mailed free of charge to a distribution list that had grown to some 1,600 recipients by 1987. The *Report*, typed on an electric typewriter, included tabulations of cases by demographic characteristics, risk factors, and AIDS-related diseases. Interest in the *Report* was enormous. As Starcher recalled,

> Dr. Meade Morgan . . . was the one that fast-tracked our getting these reports together on a weekly basis. The reports generated tremendous numbers of questions. We would get calls from health departments, from the public, from newspapers, from the media, from attorneys, from everybody under the sun each week asking for those data. They followed them as religiously as we did. . . . [E]very week I was getting a call from Randy Shilts from the San Francisco Chronicle, who, of course, went on to write *And the Band Played On*, about the early days of the AIDS epidemic. He would religiously call weekly, asking for the latest numbers, asking for a breakdown for risk factors, et cetera. [9]

Persistent Generalized Lymphadenopathy in Homosexual Men

In their seminal January 1982 publication,[5] the Task Force authors suggested that the full spectrum of clinical disease likely extended beyond the severe, life-threatening opportunistic conditions included in the surveillance case definition: "If immunosuppression is the underlying cause of these conditions, then Kaposi's sarcoma and *P. carinii* pneumonia may represent the 'tip of the iceberg.' "

An increasing number of reports from clinical investigators noted conditions in homosexual men that did not meet the surveillance case definition. Examples included autoimmune blood disorders, cancers such as lymphoma, and less severe OIs such as oral thrush[14] (milder conditions were later referred to as AIDS-related complex). The case definition's specificity

ACQUIRED IMMUNODEFICIENCY SYNDROME (AIDS)
WEEKLY SURVEILLANCE REPORT - UNITED STATES

AIDS ACTIVITY
CENTER FOR INFECTIOUS DISEASES
CENTERS FOR DISEASE CONTROL
January 23, 1984

UNITED STATES CASES REPORTED TO CDC

1. PRIMARY DISEASE*	CASES	PERCENT OF TOTAL	DEATHS	PERCENT DEAD
KS without PCP	858	26.0	198	23.1
PCP without KS	1695	51.2	809	47.7
Both KS and PCP	225	6.8	145	64.4
OI without KS or PCP	530	16.0	280	52.8
Total	3308	100.0	1432	43.3

*KS = Kaposi's sarcoma
PCP = Pneumocystis carinii pneumonia
OI = other opportunistic infections

2. AGE	CASES	PERCENT OF TOTAL		3. RACE/ETHNICITY	CASES	PERCENT OF TOTAL
Under 20	17	0.5		White, not Hispanic	1910	57.7
20 - 29	733	22.2		Black, not Hispanic	847	25.6
30 - 39	1538	46.5		Hispanic	479	14.5
40 - 49	711	21.5		Other	12	0.4
Over 49	298	9.0		Unknown	60	1.8
Unknown	11	0.3				
Total	3308	100.0		Total	3308	100.0

4. Patient Characteristics**	MALES		FEMALES		TOTAL	
	CASES	PERCENT OF MALES	CASES	PERCENT OF FEMALES	CASES	PERCENT OF TOTAL
Homosexual or Bisexual	2355	76.3	0	0.0	2355	71.2
Intravenous (IV) Drug User	462	14.9	120	54.3	582	17.6
Haitian	126	4.1	21	9.5	147	4.5
Hemophiliac	21	0.7	0	0.0	21	0.6
None Apparent/Unknown	123	4.0	80	36.2	203	6.1
Total	3087	100.0	221	100.0	3308	100.0

**Patient characteristics listed are ordered hierarchically; cases with multiple
characteristics are tabulated only in the group listed first.

Figure 3.3. CDC AIDS Weekly Surveillance Report. (Mary Chamberland, personal collection)

provided a high degree of certainty that people who had one of the indicated conditions were part of the emerging epidemic; the tradeoff was that its low sensitivity excluded people who had nonspecific symptoms and diseases that were insufficiently predictive of at least moderate cellular immunodeficiency. A different approach would be needed to probe beneath the iceberg's well-defined tip.

Investigators were particularly interested in reports of young homosexual men with persistent, generalized lymphadenopathy (enlarged lymph nodes) with no identifiable cause. Could it be an early harbinger of this unexplained acquired immunodeficiency? Some of the patients had associated symptoms, such as fever, weight loss, and malaise. Reports of this syndrome from San Francisco, New York City, Los Angeles, and Atlanta increased throughout 1981.[17] CDC was interested in the epidemiology, clinical spectrum, and immunology associated with this seemingly related condition. Clinicians were beginning to develop small longitudinal studies of these cases. Donna Mildvan, Chief of Infectious Diseases at Beth Israel Hospital in New York City, requested CDC's assistance in reviewing their patients.

In February 1982, one of the authors (BM[18]) traveled to New York City with Curran to investigate the cases at Beth Israel and other hospitals in the City.[19] As a first step, a case definition was developed for this nonspecific syndrome.[‡] Patients were interviewed using an extensive questionnaire CDC had developed to investigate cases of KS and PCP (Chapter 4), and had blood drawn for immunologic testing. Among the patients were actors, musicians, dancers, businessmen, lawyers, and doctors. Their future would be heartbreaking. David Sencer, who had previously served as CDC Director[§] and was now the Commissioner of Health for New York City, offered his assistance in convening meetings with clinicians and using health department facilities for further investigations.

The findings of the investigations in New York City and of similar patients in Atlanta and San Francisco were published in the *MMWR* on May 21, 1982. The epidemiology of these patients matched that of the patients with KS and PCP. Medical histories suggesting use of nitrite inhalants and other recreational drugs were common. Immunologic studies for a small number of patients demonstrated abnormalities in cellular immune function (e.g., reduced T-lymphocyte helper-to-suppressor ratios) similar to what had been reported for patients with Kaposi's sarcoma and opportunistic infections (KS/OI) (Chapter 9).[20] The case for a relationship between this illness and

---

[‡] Persistent generalized lymphadenopathy was defined as (1) lymphadenopathy of at least three months duration, involving two or more extrainguinal sites (right and left counted separately), diagnosed by a physician; (2) absence of current illnesses or drug use known to cause lymphadenopathy; and (3) lymph node biopsy, if done, showing reactive hyperplasia (an increase in a type of white blood cells, i.e., lymphocytes, in response to an infection, autoimmune disease, or malignancy) without loss of nodal architecture.[20]

[§] David Sencer served as CDC Director from 1966 to 1977, the longest serving director in CDC history.

the KS/PCP cases was strengthening. But it wasn't known whether this syndrome was new or simply identified because our investigations were focusing on this population.

To help answer this key question, the next phase in the investigation assessed the incidence trend of persistent, generalized lymphadenopathy in homosexual men in New York City from 1977 to 1981. We determined the best method would be to review all pathology reports of isolated lymph node biopsies (i.e., one lymph node without other tissue) taken during the same period in seven large New York City hospitals. Twelve medical-record technicians were hired to help review nearly 500,000 pathology reports. It was a daunting task, but one that Curran was determined to support. One of the authors (BM) recalled Curran's motivating words to her, which were emblematic of the Task Force approach. "He said, 'Tell me what you need to do it [the study]. Do you need an airplane? Do you need a crew of a hundred people? Write down what you need, and let's get this done.'"[18] In the end, we found that the relative frequency of unexplained lymph node hyperplasia increased 75 percent during the five-year period, attributed primarily to young homosexual men.[21]

Longitudinal case studies of patients with persistent generalized lymphadenopathy would later validate the relationship between this syndrome and AIDS.[22,23] CDC epidemiologist Jonathan (Jon) Kaplan,[24] who participated in one such study in Atlanta recalled,

> We now knew what they [these patients] had, but we didn't have the HIV [human immunodeficiency virus] drugs yet. So, these men one by one coming down with these pretty awful opportunistic infections. . . . I think they were real public health heroes for helping us [understand this syndrome and disease] . . . and because of the time of history they came around [early and mid-1980s], essentially all of them have passed away.[24]

Confidentiality of AIDS Case Data

Early AIDS case reports included personally identifiable information, such as patient names, which was recorded on the case report forms that health departments mailed to CDC. Reporting by name helped to minimize duplicate reporting of the same case as it was not uncommon for patients to seek care from multiple doctors, sometimes in different states. However, community and patient advocacy groups, hospitals, and others began to raise concerns about the confidentiality of such sensitive information and the strength of legal protections to prevent its disclosure.

In response to these concerns, the New York City health department established new reporting procedures.[25] By April 1983, case report forms were being mailed to CDC with patient names blacked out and replaced with a unique New York City case number. In a separate mailing, the health department listed the case names linked to the New York City case number. In early July 1983, Sencer suspended the submission of AIDS case patient names to CDC. Instead, as described by Starcher, he lobbied for using the Soundex system[26] to encode each patient's surname as a letter followed by three numbers:

> Shortly after we got started with the active surveillance program, we met with Dr. David Sencer. . . . He suggested strongly that we look at what was called a Soundex system, an alphanumeric algorithm. . . . We switched over to the Soundex system based upon his recommendation. . . . we began converting all the previously reported cases to Soundex code, and we began the process of deleting all the personal identifiers. Tom Leonard, who was one of the Public Health Advisors working [in the AIDS Activity], was given the task of taking a razor blade and cutting out all of the personal identifiers, which he did. . . .Confidentiality was the name of the game in terms of continuing to get reports[9]

At CDC, Morgan developed a software program that automatically generated the correct Soundex code for a patient's surname. The program was copied onto compact discs and mailed to health departments to facilitate the adoption of Soundex.

Using an arcane mechanism found in the Public Health Act, CDC also sought and obtained legal protection in 1984 against disclosure of national surveillance data. This approach was the brainchild of the CDC General Counsel, Gene Matthews.[27] As he described,

> I realized that there was a chance—there was a little-known provision in the Public Health Act. It was called 308(d), that had its history in the drug abuse research that allowed people who were interviewed about their illegal drug use to be guaranteed an Assurance of Confidentiality** that the

---

** An Assurance of Confidentiality is a formal confidentiality protection authorized under Section 308(d) of the Public Health Service Act. https://www.cdc.gov/os/integrity/confidentiality/index.htm

information could never be obtained by criminal investigators and could never be used against them. It protected against subpoenas and criminal subpoenas. It was a federal law that preempted over state and local law . . . but the way the statute was written, it was for all the Public Health Service. It had only been used for the NIDA, National Institute of Drug Abuse, at the time, and then NCHS, the National Center for Health Statistics, was using it. I thought, why can't we give that a try? . . . It was one of those examples of where you glue something together in haste and hope it can get you through the next crisis cycle, and the damn thing [i.e., application of 308(d) to AIDS surveillance data] flew.[27]

A Firm Foundation for the Future

Surveillance was a fundamental component in CDC's early response to AIDS, tracking the spread of disease at the local and national level, identifying groups most at risk, and contributing to the development of prevention and control measures. CDC's surveillance work, including the formulation of case definitions, also greatly influenced AIDS surveillance practice in the rest of the world. In the decades since the first reports of AIDS, scientific and technological advances have modernized and strengthened surveillance for AIDS and HIV infection in the United States. As the epidemic continued, these advances brought a deeper understanding of HIV disease and the advent of effective therapy, necessitating further modifications to the national surveillance system as detailed in Chapter 20. Without question, however, the early experience was a cornerstone for the development of public health programs and subsequent AIDS history.

Notes

1. "CURRAN, JAMES," *The Global Health Chronicles*, accessed January 24, 2023, https://globalhealthchronicles.org/items/show/7743.
2. "HAVERKOS, HARRY," *The Global Health Chronicles*, accessed January 29, 2023, https://globalhealthchronicles.org/items/show/6897.
3. Jaffe HW. Personal records, accessed July 6, 2021.
4. "KS/OI UPDATE," *The Global Health Chronicles*, accessed December 19, 2022, https://globalhealthchronicles.org/items/show/6633.

5. Report of the Centers for Disease Control Task Force on Kaposi's Sarcoma and Opportunistic Infections. Epidemiologic aspects of the current outbreak of Kaposi's sarcoma and opportunistic infections. N Engl J Med 1982;306:248–252.

6. "KS/OI WORKGROUP BRIEFING: July 9, 1981," *The Global Health Chronicles*, accessed January 29, 2023, https://globalhealthchronicles.org/items/show/6629.

7. "SELIK, RICHARD," *The Global Health Chronicles*, accessed December 28, 2022, https://globalhealthchronicles.org/items/show/6869.

8. CDC. Update on acquired immune deficiency syndrome (AIDS)—United States. MMWR Morb Mortal Wkly Rep 1982;31:507–514.

9. "STARCHER, E. THOMAS," *The Global Health Chronicles*, accessed January 29, 2023, https://globalhealthchronicles.org/items/show/7916.

10. "COOPERATIVE AGREEMENT: New York City Health Department," *Global Health Chronicles*, accessed October 18, 2022, https://globalhealthchronicles.org/items/show/8017.

11. "CHAMBERLAND, MARY," *The Global Health Chronicles*, accessed January 29, 2023, https://globalhealthchronicles.org/items/show/7728.

12. Chamberland ME, Allen JR, Monroe JM, et al. Acquired immunodeficiency syndrome in New York City: evaluation of an active surveillance system. JAMA 1985;254:383–387.

13. Hardy AM, Starcher ET 2nd, Morgan WM, et al. Review of death certificates to assess completeness of AIDS case reporting. Public Health Rep 1987;102:386–391.

14. Jaffe HW, Bregman DJ, Selik RM. Acquired immune deficiency syndrome in the United States: the first 1,000 cases. J Infect Dis 1983;148:339–345.

15. "CASTRO, KENNETH," *The Global Health Chronicles*, accessed January 29, 2023, https://globalhealthchronicles.org/items/show/6478.

16. "THOMAS, PAULINE," *The Global Health Chronicles*, accessed January 29, 2023, https://www.globalhealthchronicles.org/items/show/7792.

17. "TASK FORCE AGENDA: January 6, 1982," *The Global Health Chronicles*, accessed January 29, 2023, https://globalhealthchronicles.org/items/show/6599.

18. "MILLER, BESS," *The Global Health Chronicles*, accessed January 29, 2023, https://www.globalhealthchronicles.org/items/show/6871 .

19. "UNEXPLAINED LYMPHADENOPATHY," *The Global Health Chronicles*, accessed January 29, 2023, https://globalhealthchronicles.org/items/show/6549.

20. CDC. Persistent, generalized lymphadenopathy among homosexual males. MMWR Morb Mortal Wkly Rep 1982; 31:249–251.

21. Miller B, Stansfield SK, Zack MM, et al. The syndrome of unexplained generalized lymphadenopathy in young men in New York City: is it related to the acquired immune deficiency syndrome? JAMA 1984;251:242–246.

22. Mathur-Wagh U, Spigland I, Sacks HS, et al. Longitudinal study of persistent generalised lymphadenopathy in homosexual men: relation to acquired immunodeficiency syndrome. Lancet 1984;323:1033–1038.

23. Abrams DI, Lewis BJ, Beckstead JH, et al. Persistent diffuse lymphadenopathy in homosexual men: endpoint or prodrome? Ann Intern Med 1984;100:801–808.

24. "KAPLAN, JONATHAN," *The Global Health Chronicles*, accessed January 29, 2023, https://globalhealthchronicles.org/items/show/8137.
25. Chamberland, Mary. Personal records, accessed September 12, 2021.
26. "CASE SURVEILLANCE CODING," *The Global Health Chronicles*, accessed January 29, 2023, https://globalhealthchronicles.org/items/show/8036.
27. "MATTHEWS, GENE," *The Global Health Chronicles*, accessed January 29, 2023, https://globalhealthchronicles.org/items/show/7965.

4

Homosexual Men

Harold W. Jaffe

As the Task Force began meeting in June 1981, one of the first questions facing us was why were all the initially reported cases of KS/OI in homosexual men. What was it about the lives of these men that was putting them at risk for this lethal disease? Two theories emerged from our discussions.

The first theory we considered was that the underlying cause of KS/OI might be a sexually transmitted infection (STI).* The decade following the 1969 Stonewall riots in New York City, a landmark event in the American gay liberation movement, saw a dramatic increase in STI rates among homosexual men. In his book, *How to Survive a Plague*, David France notes that "A tidal wave of disease followed [Stonewall]. In some quarters of the community, lengthy diagnostic profiles became bragging rights. But whether embraced or regretted, VD [venereal disease] was suddenly a fact of gay men's lives."[1] From 1969 to 1980, rates of infectious syphilis had decreased by 19 percent in American women but had increased by 50 percent in men. Further, among the men, the proportion naming male partners had increased from about a quarter to about a half. The American city with the highest syphilis rate in 1980 was San Francisco.[2]

Another infection emerging in American homosexual men was HBV. In a CDC-sponsored study of homosexual men attending VD clinics in five cities, more than 50 percent of participants had antibodies to HBV compared with 4.4 percent of volunteer blood donors.[3] The infection was associated with duration of male homosexual activity and number of nonsteady sex partners, indicating that sexual contact was the main route of transmission. Although HBV was also known to be transmitted through needle sharing among IDUs, only 8 percent of the men in the study had a history of injection drug use.

---

* Sexually transmitted infection is a term used synonymously with sexually transmitted disease and venereal disease (VD).

Harold W. Jaffe, *Homosexual Men* In: *Dispatches from the AIDS Pandemic*. Kevin M. De Cock, Harold W. Jaffe, and James W. Curran and Edited by: Robin Moseley, Oxford University Press. © Oxford University Press 2023.
DOI: 10.1093/oso/9780197626528.003.0004

If an STI were the cause, was it a new infectious agent or a new strain of an already known STI? If the latter, what STI might it be? A possible candidate STI was cytomegalovirus (CMV), a member of the herpesvirus family. The June 5, 1981 *MMWR* noted that the first five reported men with PCP had evidence of CMV disease or shedding of the virus in urine.[4] The report also noted that CMV could induce transient abnormalities in cellular immune function of healthy persons. An earlier study had reported that 94 percent of homosexual men attending a VD clinic had laboratory evidence of past CMV infection compared with 54 percent of heterosexual men attending the same clinic.[5] Further, CMV shedding in urine was only detected in homosexual patients. But why would a new strain of CMV emerge only in homosexual men? Or, more generally, if a new STI had emerged why wasn't it also affecting heterosexual men and women?

The second theory considered by the Task Force was that some sort of environmental exposure, perhaps a drug or a toxin exposure unique to homosexual men, was causing damage to the immune system. What could that be? After discussing and discarding several candidates, our interest turned to "poppers." This term referred to a class of chemicals known as alkyl nitrites, which were inhaled by some homosexual men to enhance sex by relaxing smooth muscles, including the anal sphincter, and to produce a euphoric "high." Pharmaceutical-grade amyl nitrite was used medically to treat angina—chest pain caused by insufficient blood flow to the heart—and was supplied in glass ampules. The name "poppers" derived from the sound made when an ampule was snapped open. But we would need to learn more about poppers, including whether they were used recreationally by heterosexuals, before deciding whether this lead was worth pursuing.

Another explanation for KS/OI, not thought likely by the Task Force but discussed by other researchers, was the theory of "immune overload." These researchers suggested that there was no single etiology of this illness; rather, immunodeficiency resulted from the cumulative effects of multiple infectious agents, environmental toxins, and perhaps other factors, such as semen exposure. A leading proponent of this theory, Joseph Sonnabend, later wrote, "Promiscuity, the resulting exposure, and immune responses to infectious agents and sperm are proposed to be the initiating and sustaining factors [of the disease]."[6]

A classic epidemiologic approach to finding the possible cause of a disease is to conduct a case-control study. In this type of study, the exposure histories of persons with the condition of interest (cases, or case patients) are compared with exposure histories of persons without the condition (controls, or control patients). One or more controls are selected for each case and may be matched with the case by demographic variables such as age, sex, and race/ethnicity. The Task Force agreed on the need for a case-control study of KS/OI but felt that more information about the cases was needed before designing such a study.

To collect this exploratory information, Bill Darrow and I drafted an extensive questionnaire to examine possible risk factors for KS/OI, including medical, occupational, and travel histories; chemical exposures (including nitrite inhalants); illicit drug use; and sexual behaviors. In mid-summer 1981, we worked with local health departments and clinicians to arrange for Task Force physicians to conduct these exploratory interviews with KS/OI patients.

Mary Guinan (Chapter 2), now assigned to the Task Force by the the Division of Sexually transmitted Diseases (DSTD), and Polly Thomas (Chapter 3) were asked to interview patients in New York City. As Guinan recalled, "We had this huge interview form that we had devised because we really didn't know what it [the condition] was. So, it was about 35 pages, I think, of questions, of every kind of question, because we had no idea [of what we were looking for]."[7] Thomas provided more details on the interviews:

Mary Guinan came to New York to do interviews. . . I was able to join her, and they [Darrow and Jaffe] had developed a sort of a "fishing" interview. . . We went and started interviewing the patients in the hospitals mainly. I did my first couple with Mary. Because she had worked in STDs, she was comfortable with some of the questions, which were pretty graphic sexual practice questions. . . I did interview one gentleman—a gentleman in a shop in Greenwich Village. He said to me, "Is this the first time you're asking these questions?" He turned out to be someone who was producing poppers [amyl nitrite] in his bathtub in his home. He was manufacturing.[8]

I traveled to San Francisco, where I met Paul Volberding, a young oncologist at San Francisco General Hospital, and Marcus Conant, a dermatologist in private practice, both of whom had cared for patients with KS. Volberding kindly gave me permission to talk to several of his hospitalized patients. Seeing the illness for the first time, I was shocked by its severity. Young, previously healthy men were so wasted that they looked like concentration camp survivors. I recall one patient whose face was almost entirely covered with the purple blotches of KS. But despite the severity of their illnesses, these men were extremely cooperative and did their best to answer my questions.

One of the things we learned from these early interviews was that these men were buying nitrite inhalants from gay bathhouses, bookstores, and bars. What they bought was not pharmaceutical-grade amyl nitrite in glass ampules; rather, they purchased small screw-top glass bottles, some labeled with names like "Rush" or "Locker Room," and others with no labels. When one of the men I interviewed told me the name of the bar where he obtained his bottles, I asked Carlos Rendon, a San Francisco Health Department disease investigator, to drive me there so that I could buy some bottles for analysis at CDC. But when we pulled up to the bar, I lost my nerve and told Carlos that I didn't want to go inside. Without hesitation, Carlos entered the bar and emerged a few minutes later with several bottles.

The bottles that I brought back from San Francisco, as well as those purchased in New York City and Atlanta, were sent to CDC laboratories for analysis. The microbiology laboratory reported no contamination of the inhalants by either bacteria or fungi.[9] The toxicology laboratory performed qualitative analyses on twenty-one samples and found that the primary ingredients were either amyl nitrite or butyl nitrite,[10] compounds with similar biological effects. The immunology laboratory also drafted a protocol for assessing the immunotoxicity of nitrite inhalants in mice.[11]

At CDC, we analyzed our exploratory interview data from thirty-five KS/OI patients living in New York, San Francisco, and Atlanta. Curiously, a document summarizing the findings mentions that one of the patients was female but provides no further details.[12] The median age of the patients was thirty-five years, and thirty of the thirty-five patients were white. Use of marijuana, cocaine, and amphetamines was common, and 85 percent of patients reported using nitrite inhalants at least monthly. About two-thirds of the patients had a history of syphilis. These patients were highly sexually active, with a median of eighty-seven different male partners during the year before symptom onset, and much of their sexual contact took place in gay bathhouses and bars.

In anticipation of the formal case-control study, Darrow also coordinated a survey of the behaviors of homosexual and heterosexual men without KS/OI attending VD clinics in New York City, San Francisco, and Atlanta.[13] The homosexual patients at the clinic had many more sex partners per year than the heterosexual patients and were much more likely to report using nitrite inhalants. Comparing thirty of the previously interviewed KS/OI patients with thirty homosexual VD clinic patients, Darrow found that the KS/OI patients were much more sexually active than the clinic patients, averaging twice as many sex partners per year, and they were more likely to have "one-time" partners from bathhouses. The KS/OI patients were also more likely to have used nitrite inhalants and to have used them for a longer time. Presciently, Darrow wrote that similar results should be expected from the planned case-control study.[13]

As these preliminary data were being analyzed, Jim Curran asked me to develop a protocol for a national case-control study to begin no later than October 1, 1981. Having never worked on a case-control study, I was a bit nervous about taking this on. But with help from Task Force colleagues, especially Darrow, I wrote a draft protocol.[14] Some aspects of the protocol were straightforward. We would conduct in-person interviews with cases, defined as patients with KS and/or PCP, in New York City, San Francisco, Los Angeles, and Atlanta using a shorter version of the questionnaire developed in the pilot survey of thirty-five KS/OI patients.[15] But selection of control patients was much more problematic. We agreed that controls should primarily be homosexual men without KS/OI,[†] matched with cases by race/ethnicity and city of residence and within an age range. But how would these men be selected?

Ideally, the control patients should have come from a random sample of homosexual men living in the four cities. Creating a random sample did not seem feasible, so we had to come up with other options. Given that no single group of control patients was optimal, we decided to try recruiting multiple control groups. One group would come from practices of internists or family physicians serving mainly gay men, while another would be recruited from VD clinics. We knew the latter group would be biased toward men who were highly sexually active and would possibly obscure sexual activity as a risk factor for KS/OI. A third control group would consist of male homosexual friends of the case patients who were not their sexual partners.

The laboratory members of the Task Force also requested that we obtain specimens from the participants for further study. Blood would be needed for immunologic studies and for tests for antibodies to syphilis and to a variety of viruses and parasites. Urine, as well as mouth and rectal swab specimens,

---

[†] The original protocol proposed recruiting some heterosexual male control patients, but we later decided against including them.

would be collected to test for CMV, herpes simplex virus, and adenovirus infections.

Logistical aspects of the study, including identifying potential cases and controls, finding appropriate interview locations, and arranging for specimen shipments to Atlanta, also had to be addressed. Fortunately, Wilmon Rushing, a soft-spoken Mississippian who was working as a PHA in CDC's TB control division, had been recruited to serve as a management officer for the Task Force. Rushing identified PHAs who were assigned to the relevant health departments to work out these important details.

The interviews would be conducted by physicians from the Task Force and EIS officers assigned to the relevant health department. Because none of us had been trained to do this sort of interviewing, Darrow arranged a training session. As he recalled,

> When it came time to do the study, we called [a meeting]. . . as I remember everybody came in, and we only had a few days to train them. . . I can remember interviewing a confederate [another PHA], and I said, "You give me as hard a time as possible. . . We're going to role-play this in front of the people, so they can see the whole thing happening and then can ask questions: why did you do this, why did you do that. It worked very well.[16]

In early September, as the details of the case-control study were being finalized, I asked Darrow if there might be a way to arrange a "field trip" to a bathhouse. Having sex partners in bathhouses was emerging as a possible risk factor for KS/OI, and I thought it would be helpful to learn more about these venues. A few days later Darrow had gotten permission from the manager of the Club Baths in Atlanta for us to visit and interview some of its patrons. Attired in blazers and ties, Bill and I were rather obvious amid men wearing nothing or, at most, bath towels. I felt extremely awkward sitting at a card table, asking the men who walked by if they would mind talking to us for a few minutes. Much to my relief, however, once we explained what we were doing, many of the men were willing to be interviewed. For example, one told us that he was a microbiologist employed by Emory University Hospital, right down the street from CDC, and was very curious about what we were discovering. These men had heard about this new disease and wanted to help us.

Although the Club Baths had some bathing facilities, the men we spoke to were not there to bathe. They were there to have sex with men they had never met and might never meet again. Some patronized the bathhouse several times a week and had multiple partners at each visit. Nitrite inhalants, an integral part of sex for many of the men, were sold in the bathhouse. Coincidentally, we happened to be there on "Popper Night," when all inhalants were on sale.

In mid-September, I was feeling optimistic about our preparations for the case-control study and decided that I could take time to attend a meeting on KS at NIH's National Cancer Institute (NCI). I was disappointed that the meeting was largely focused on previous NCI studies of KS in Africa. But at a meeting break, I asked an NCI epidemiologist how he would do the study that we were planning. He told me it would take three years—a year to design the study, a year to conduct it, and a year to analyze the data. When I said that we were going to do the whole thing in a few months, he replied that wasn't possible. My optimism about our study faded.

Despite my concerns, the study went well. We split the interviewers into teams: the team for New York City was headed by Curran, and I led the California team. We did the New York and San Francisco interviews and specimen collections in hotel rooms. One investigator would interview a case patient and that patient's matched controls. We expected that the case and control patients, all homosexual men, would have reservations in sharing the intimate details of their lives with researchers from the federal government. But once a level of trust was established, we found these men to be remarkably candid and cooperative. They were scared—case patients knew that they were seriously ill and control patients often knew others with the disease—and wanted to do everything they could to help us find the cause.

Martha Rogers,[17] a pediatrician and an Atlanta-based EIS officer assigned to the Task Force from the Division of Viral Diseases was part of the study's New York City interview team. As she remembered,

We were staying in the Barbizon Hotel, it used to be the Barbizon Hotel for Women, but I don't think it was just for women at that point. We were staying in that hotel and had rented another room where we did the interviews and also collected all the biologic specimens. So, we often had men who would come to the hotel and call up for us at the front desk. They [hotel staff] would be seeing these young women coming down the elevator and getting these very handsome young men and taking them back up to this room where we did all the interviewing. That hotel had a person standing, we called him the elevator guy, and he would look at us askance as we began bringing up all these young men.[17]

Mary Guinan and I did the interviews in San Francisco. All was going well until, as Guinan recalled,

> Then I had a problem with—there was a young man with AIDS who was very tall and built like a football player. He agreed to give blood, and so he sat on the stool and put his arm on the kitchen counter there, the kitchen-ette counter. I drew the blood from him, and as I was drawing the blood he fainted, and he fell on top of me. I couldn't get the tourniquet off. Then when he fell on top of me, I pulled the needle out and stuck it in my hand. But all I could think of was here was this person unconscious on the floor. I pulled the tourniquet off, and I washed the blood out of my hand. But here was this unconscious person on the floor, and I was wondering, "How am I going to explain this?" Subsequent to that, two years later I had had a child, and I found on my arm a lesion that looked like Kaposi's sarcoma. So, I remembered the needle stick, and it was the hand that I had gotten the needle stick in. My heart stopped.[7]

Fortunately, the skin lesion was not KS and disappeared without treatment.

We finished our interviews in December 1981 and returned to CDC with data on fifty case patients (out of the seventy nationally reported patients with KS and/or PCP) and 120 control patients (seventy-eight recruited in VD clinics and forty-two from private medical practices). Because not even half the cases could name friends who met our definition for control patients, this control group was excluded from the analysis. The Task Force did not have a statistician, so we were asked to work with Keewhan Choi, a statistician in CDC's Epidemiology Program Office. The arrangement was a bit awkward given that Choi did not report directly to Curran and had other responsibilities. We therefore relied on Darrow to perform interim analyses, and his office rapidly filled with large paper printouts from CDC's mainframe computer.

In the final analysis, done by Choi, case patients were found to be highly sexually active with a median of sixty-one male partners per year, more than twice as many as either group of control patients. An average of half of the cases' partners were from bathhouses. Although case patients reported using more kinds of illicit drugs (such as cocaine and amphetamines) compared to control patients, almost all cases and control patients reported using nitrite inhalant. In an analysis that looked at the effects of multiple variables, those associated with having many sexual partners were most strongly correlated with having KS and/or PCP. Nitrite inhalant use emerged as a relatively unimportant risk factor. We were cautious in drawing conclusions from the study, however, and wrote, "Although the number of sexual partners seems to be the most important risk factor, we cannot exclude the possibility that other highly correlated variables, such as illicit drug use, play some part in the development of these diseases."[18]

Rogers coordinated the laboratory component of the study.[19] As expected, the case patients had evidence of severe cellular immune deficiency. Interestingly, some of the control patients also had abnormal immunologic findings, perhaps suggesting they were also at risk for developing KS or PCP. Case patients also had higher levels of antibodies to two herpesviruses, CMV and Epstein-Barr virus (EBV), and a higher frequency of detection of CMV in urine and throat swab specimens. Herpesviruses were known, however, to cause latent infections that could reactivate when persons received drugs that suppressed the immune system. Therefore, as noted by the study authors, they could not determine whether the CMV and EBV findings were the cause or consequence of immunosuppression. Further studies of the CMV isolates from case and control patients showed a variety of viral strains, with no strain unique to the cases. Case patients also were more likely to have laboratory evidence of past syphilis and hepatitis A virus infection, consistent with their higher level of sexual activity and more frequent sexual exposure to feces[‡] compared to the control patients.

As the CDC study was being analyzed, researchers at New York University (NYU) Medical Center were conducting another case-control study.[20] This study was limited to twenty KS patients in New York City and forty male homosexual control patients from a single medical practice. The results of this study were generally similar to those of the CDC study, although the NYU researchers found that the number of lifetime uses of amyl nitrite was more strongly associated with KS than was number of sex partners per month.

What was the behavior leading to KS/OI? Was sexual activity spreading a new infection, or was it the use of illicit drugs, possibly inhalants? While the CDC study favored the former hypothesis and the NYU study supported the

---

‡ Hepatitis A virus is primarily transmitted by the fecal-oral route.

latter, neither of the studies could reach a definitive conclusion because these behaviors were so highly correlated with each other. We needed a new lead.

In early 1982, that lead came from David Auerbach,[21] the EIS officer who had taken Wayne Shandera's (Chapter 2) place at the Los Angeles County Health Department. Auerbach had some familiarity with KS/OI before joining EIS and recalled, "I think the betting might have been on a toxic exposure. After all, I think a completely new disease entity, infectious entity, in North America would be virtually unprecedented in modern medicine."[21] He had done interviews in Los Angeles for the CDC case-control study and had made contacts with the local gay community. Then one day he got a call from a person who, as he recalled, "must have been someone in the gay community or perhaps in the health department or a gay community center, I'm not sure, mentioning somewhat anecdotally that there were a number of the patients who had had [sexual] contact either with each other or with another individual."[21]

Auerbach called CDC to discuss how to pursue this lead. It was decided that Darrow would go to Los Angeles and work with Auerbach. Darrow and Auerbach proved to be an excellent team. As Auerbach said,

> Bill was terrific in every way. Bill is not a clinician. His graduate degree is in—he has a PhD in sociology, but really to the point, Bill was probably the most naturally gifted interviewer I've ever worked with. We started to find that, in fact, there were linkages between these, at least some of the patients. Also, notably many of them had contact with a single individual not from Los Angeles, who became known as the Patient Zero. I think there were nineteen known patients in the Los Angeles area. We could interview thirteen of the nineteen. The others, I think, were no longer alive. Of those thirteen, there were connections among nine.[21]

Darrow added the following:

> I think this was in April of 1982 that I flew out to Los Angeles to spend a week with David Auerbach. I think we were able to talk to thirteen or fourteen of the cases or somebody who knew them and ask them about their partners. There was this one particular day, I think it was the second or third day I was there, we had three different interviews scheduled—one in the morning, one in the afternoon, and one in the evening—all with people who were involved and either had what we now know is AIDS or

they had a very close lover or friend who had AIDS. The first two of these men mentioned the same sex partner, "There was this very handsome, debonair flight attendant for Air Canada that I met, and oh God, he was such a nice guy." When the third patient named the same sex partner, I dropped my pencil, and Dave [Auerbach] almost fell off his chair. We looked at each other with our mouths open and said, "How could this be?" The same person is named three times. I ended up calling this person the "Out-of-California" case because everybody else either resided in California, in Los Angeles, or somewhere in California. I labeled him "O" for being outside of California—the flight attendant from Air Canada.[16]

According to Darrow, when he returned to Atlanta, he said to Guinan, "You know, I think this guy is responsible for cases in San Francisco and New York and elsewhere. I think we need to pursue this. He might give me a list of more names if I can talk to him. What do you know about him?"[16] Guinan had conducted an exploratory interview with this individual during the summer of 1981, and Darrow recalled that she replied, "Oh, he's a patient of Dr. Friedman-Kien. Let's call Dr. Friedman-Kien and see if they'll set up something for you to go up there and talk to him."[16]

Darrow interviewed the patient in Friedman-Kien's office in New York. The patient, who was being treated for KS, was very cooperative, but said that he would need to consult his "black book" before he could name his sex partners. Darrow said he called the patient later that day and the patient "started reading all the names, and he read, as I remember, seventy-two. . . a small fraction of the numbers of sex partners that he had. It turned out that eight of them had been reported to us as having Kaposi's sarcoma or an opportunistic infection."[16]

The cluster of patients from southern California was reported in the June 18, 1982, issue of the *MMWR*.[22] The report noted that data on sex partners was obtained from thirteen patients with KS or PCP, of whom nine had sexual contact with another KS/PCP patient within the previous five years. Several of the patients reported having sex with the patient who was not a resident of California. A subsequent report of the extension of the cluster investigation outside of California described forty patients in ten North American cities who were linked by sexual contact[23] (Figure 4.1). Eight patients, four from southern California and four from New York City, were sexual contacts of the Air Canada flight attendant. The forty cluster patients represented 16 percent of all homosexual male cases reported to CDC at the time of the

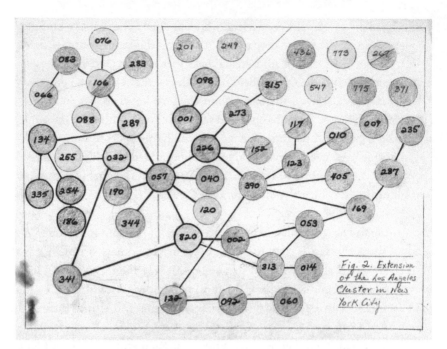

Figure 4.1. Draft diagram of sexually linked KS/OI patients drawn by Bill Darrow. Patients are identified by CDC case numbers. Patient #057 is the out-of-California KS patient who became known as Patient Zero. (Dr. William Darrow Collection, David J. Sencer CDC Museum)

investigation. The report noted that the cluster findings were consistent with the infectious-agent hypothesis for the disease and that, if true, the flight attendant "may be an example of a 'carrier' of such an agent."[23]

Darrow recalled, "My fondest memory after I described the study to an in-house audience [at CDC] [Figure 4.2] came from Task Force member Bruce Evatt [[24]] [Chapter 8], who said, 'I'm willing to bet a six-pack of beer with anyone here that we are dealing with a sexually transmitted agent.' All I could think of was, 'It's Miller time.'"[25]

In Darrow's initial presentations of the cluster investigation, he was careful to refer to the flight attendant as Patient O (the letter), the outside-of-California case. But the letter O soon morphed into the number 0, and the flight attendant became known at Patient Zero. Indeed, a careful look at the report of the forty-patient cluster shows the use of the number zero.

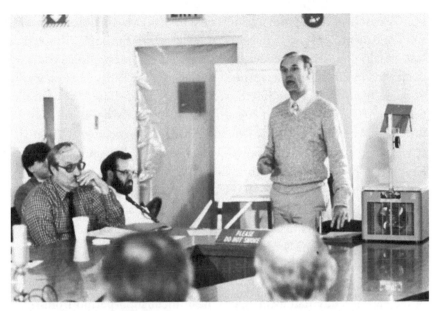

Figure 4.2. Bill Darrow presenting at a Task Force meeting. Visible seated participants: PHA Larry Zyla at left and epidemiologist Peter Drotman. (Courtesy of Bill Darrow)

The story of Patient Zero was carefully researched by the medical historian Richard McKay.[26] McKay recounts a visit made to CDC by the journalist Randy Shilts, who was conducting research for his popular book about the early AIDS epidemic, *And the Band Played On.*[27] During that visit, Shilts recalled "[T]hey [CDC investigators] started talking about Patient Zero. I thought, *'Ooh, that's catchy'.*"[27] Although CDC never revealed Patient Zero's name, McKay concluded that Shilts learned from his contacts in the gay community that Patient Zero was a French Canadian named Gaetan Dugas and used the name in his book.

As Darrow recalled,

When Randy interviewed me at CDC, he said, "You don't have to tell me anything about the cluster study. I know all about it." Later, I discovered Randy was using names. I told him he could use my name and the names of other "public figures," but he should not name AIDS patients without their consent. It could cause problems. He refused to take my advice.[28]

McKay describes a proposal by Shilts's editor at St. Martin's Press to use the story of Patient Zero as a "promotional hook" to sell the book. Although he was initially opposed to the idea, Shilts relented. The promotional effort was successful, leading to extensive media coverage of the Patient Zero story. For example, the *New York Post* ran the story under the headline "The Man Who Gave Us AIDS."[29] CDC never suggested that Patient Zero was the source of the North American epidemic. In fact, subsequent genetic analysis of HIV strains from archived serum samples collected from Patient Zero and very early AIDS patients in New York City and San Francisco established that he was not the "primary case" in the United States.[30] However, it would not require many men like him—very sexually active and highly mobile—to spread a sexually transmissible agent to large numbers of men who have sex with men (MSM) in the United States.

Did the cluster investigation prove that an STI was the cause of the KS/OI epidemic in homosexual men? Based on six pairs of patients, the authors of the cluster study had estimated a mean incubation period from sexual contact to symptom onset of 10.5 months. But studies done following the discovery of HIV have shown the time between infection and disease to be much longer, an average of about ten years for young adults.[31] One might argue therefore that many of the cluster patients acquired their infection years before their sexual partnerships with other members of the cluster. On the other hand, these patients were among the earliest KS/OI patients to occur after the introduction of HIV into the United States.[§] By definition, they would have relatively short incubation periods. Whether the cluster represented an infection transmission network or simply a sexual network cannot be determined.

Although neither the CDC case-control study nor the cluster study was considered definitive proof by itself, taken together they strongly indicated that sexual activity, rather than nitrite use, was the primary risk factor for KS/OI in American homosexual men. The epidemiologic evidence was supported by CDC laboratory studies that found no evidence of immuno-deficiency in mice exposed to isobutyl nitrite vapors.[32] Although subsequent epidemiologic studies suggested that nitrite use might be a cofactor for the development of KS in immunosuppressed men,[33] nitrites were not the cause

---

[§] Based on molecular analysis of early HIV infections, the virus is thought to have entered the United States from the Caribbean in the early 1970s.[29]

of KS/OI. Sexual activity was spreading an unidentified infection causing immunodeficiency.

The first PHS recommendations for prevention of what had become known as AIDS were published on March 4, 1983, and stated, "Sexual contact should be avoided with persons known or suspected to have AIDS. Members of high-risk groups should be aware that multiple sexual partners increase the probability of developing AIDS."[34]

And if sexual activity was a risk factor for AIDS in homosexual men, were heterosexual men and women also at risk?

Notes

1. France D. How to Survive a Plague. The Story of How Activists and Scientists Tamed AIDS. New York: Random House; 2017.

2. CDC. Syphilis trends in the United States. MMWR Morb Mortal Wkly Rep 1981;30:441–444.

3. Schreeder MT, Thompson SE, Hadler SC, et al. Hepatitis B in homosexual men: prevalence of infection and factors related to transmission. J Infect Dis 1982;146:7–15.

4. CDC. *Pneumocystis* pneumonia—Los Angeles. MMWR Morb Mortal Wkly Rep 1981;30:250–252.

5. Drew WL, Mintz L, Miner RC, Sands M, Ketterer B. Prevalence of cytomegalovirus infection in homosexual men. J Infect Dis 1981;143:488–492.

6. Sonnabend J. Witkin SS, Purtilo DT. Acquired immunodeficiency syndrome, opportunistic infections, and malignancies in male homosexuals. A hypothesis of etiologic factors in pathogenesis. JAMA 1983;249:2370–2374.

7. "GUINAN, MARY," The Global Health Chronicles, accessed January 29, 2023, https://www.globalhealthchronicles.org/items/show/5393.

8. "THOMAS, PAULINE," The Global Health Chronicles, accessed January 29, 2023, https://www.globalhealthchronicles.org/items/show/7792.

9. "CULTURE RESULTS: Nitrite Samples," The Global Health Chronicles, accessed January 29, 2023, https://www.globalhealthchronicles.org/items/show/8096.

10. "UNKNOWN ORGANONITRITE: Qualitative Analysis," The Global Health Chronicles, accessed January 29, 2023, https://www.globalhealthchronicles.org/items/show/8093.

11. "INHALATION STUDY: Protocol," The Global Health Chronicles, accessed January 29, 2023, https://www.globalhealthchronicles.org/items/show/8094.

12. "DATA SUMMARY: 35 Interviews," The Global Health Chronicles, accessed January 29, 2023, https://www.globalhealthchronicles.org/items/show/6606.

13. "INHALANT USE," The Global Health Chronicles, accessed January 29, 2023, https://www.globalhealthchronicles.org/items/show/6639.

14. "CASE-CONTROL STUDY—DRAFT PROTOCOL," *The Global Health Chronicles*, accessed January 29, 2023, https://www.globalhealthchronicles.org/items/show/6528.

15. "CASE-CONTROL STUDY: INTERVIEW FORM," *The Global Health Chronicles*, accessed January 29, 2023, https://www.globalhealthchronicles.org/items/show/6558.

16. "DARROW, WILLIAM," *The Global Health Chronicles*, accessed January 29, 2023, https://globalhealthchronicles.org/items/show/6870.

17. "ROGERS, MARTHA," *The Global Health Chronicles*, accessed January 29, 2023, https://www.globalhealthchronicles.org/items/show/5395.

18. Jaffe HW, Choi K, Thomas PA, et al. National case-control study of Kaposi's sarcoma and *Pneumocystis carinii* pneumonia in homosexual men: Part 1. Epidemiologic results. Ann Intern Med 1983;99:145–151.

19. Rogers MF, Morens DM, Stewart JA, et al. National case-control study of Kaposi's sarcoma and *Pneumocystis carinii* pneumonia in homosexual men: Part 2. Laboratory results. Ann Intern Med 1983;99:151–158.

20. Marmor M, Friedman-Kien AE, Laubenstein L. Risk factors for Kaposi's sarcoma in homosexual men. Lancet 1982;1:1083–1087.

21. "AUERBACH, DAVID," *The Global Health Chronicles*, accessed January 29, 2023, https://www.globalhealthchronicles.org/items/show/8135.

22. CDC. A cluster of Kaposi's sarcoma and *Pneumocystis carinii* pneumonia among homosexual male residents of Los Angeles and Orange Counties, California. MMWR Morb Mortal Wkly Rep 1982;31:306–307.

23. Auerbach DM, Darrow WW, Jaffe HW, Curran JW. Clusters of cases of the acquired immune deficiency syndrome. Patients linked by sexual contact. Am J Med 1984;76:487–492.

24. "EVATT, BRUCE," *The Global Health Chronicles*, accessed January 29, 2023, https://www.globalhealthchronicles.org/items/show/6479.

25. Darrow WW. Personal communication, July 20, 2020.

26. McKay RA. Patient Zero and the Making of the AIDS Epidemic. Chicago: The University of Chicago Press; 2017.

27. Shilts R. And the Band Played On. Politics, People, and the AIDS Epidemic. New York: St. Martin's Press; 1987.

28. Darrow WW. Personal communication, April 14, 2022.

29. The Man Who Gave Us AIDS. New York Post, October 6, 1987.

30. Worobey M, Watts TD, McKay RA, et al. 1970s and "Patient 0" HIV-1 genomes illuminate early HIV/AIDS history in North America. Nature 2016;539:98–101.

31. Collaborative Group on AIDS Incubation and HIV Survival including CASCADE EU Concerted Action. Time from HIV-1 seroconversion and death before widespread use of highly-active antiretroviral therapy: a collaborative re-analysis. Lancet 2000;355:1131–1137.

32. CDC. An evaluation of the immunotoxic potential of isobutyl nitrite. MMWR Morbid Mortal Wkly Rep 1983;457–458.

33. Haverkos H, Pinsky P, Drotman DP, Bregman DJ. Disease manifestations among homosexual men with acquired immunodeficiency syndrome: a possible role of nitrites in Kaposi's sarcoma. Sex Transm Dis 1985;12:203–208.
34. CDC. Prevention of acquired immune deficiency syndrome (AIDS): report of interagency recommendations. MMWR Morb Mortal Wkly Rep 1983;32:101–104.

5

Heterosexual Men and Women and Injection Drug Users

Harold W. Jaffe

Given the evidence that KS/OI was likely caused by an infectious agent that was sexually transmitted between homosexual men, was there a known STI that might serve as a model for the spread of this agent? The most likely model appeared to be HBV, which can be transmitted sexually and through parenteral (nonoral) blood exposure and was endemic in homosexual men in the 1970s and 1980s.[1,2] If HBV were the correct model, KS/OI would likely appear in the female sex partners of bisexual men and in IDUs exposed to blood through sharing of needles and other drug-related paraphernalia. Infected IDUs, both men and women, could transmit the agent to their sex partners. By establishing a national KS/OI surveillance program (Chapter 3), CDC hoped to identify any new groups at risk for the disease and determine routes of transmission of the causative agent.

Indeed, as national surveillance for KS/OI expanded during the summer of 1981, the first cases of KS/OI in persons who were not homosexual or bisexual men were identified. The August 28, 1981, issue of the *MMWR* reported a cumulative total of 108 KS/OI patients, of whom six were described as heterosexual men and one as a woman.[3] The report provided no additional information about these patients.

In reviewing the interviews and documents available through the Global Health Chronicles,[4] I found no other mention of these first heterosexual male patients but did note a description by Mary Guinan of an early female patient. Whether this was the same woman reported in the *MMWR* is not clear. As Guinan remembered,

There was this rumor that women couldn't get it. Of course, we in STD said, "Whoever heard of a sexually transmitted disease that could only be transmitted by one sex, you know?" But there was this feeling that

Harold W. Jaffe, *Heterosexual Men and Women and Injection Drug Users* In: *Dispatches from the AIDS Pandemic*. Kevin M. De Cock, Harold W. Jaffe, and James W. Curran and Edited by: Robin Moseley, Oxford University Press.
© Oxford University Press 2023. DOI: 10.1093/oso/9780197626528.003.0005

women couldn't get it. There was this one woman that was reported with *Pneumocystis* pneumonia. I got a call from her doctor in Philadelphia, and she had no risk factors that anyone could think of for her . . . I had interviewed the patient. About a month later, the woman's physician called me and told me that she had lymphoma, so she wasn't a case.* [5]

The first insight into a new risk factor for KS/OI came in a study of eleven men with PCP authored by Henry Masur and colleagues from hospitals in New York City and published in December 1981.[6] Although it was primarily an immunologic study, the authors noted that five of the eleven men were heterosexual. Further, four patients—two homosexuals and two heterosexuals, had histories of IV heroin use. The authors noted, "Narcotic abuse has been reported to cause *in vitro* immune defects similar to those described here, yet it has not previously been associated with pneumocystosis [PCP]."[6] The authors did not speculate on other reasons that IDUs might be at risk for PCP.

The next update from CDC, reporting KS/OI surveillance data through November 10, 1981, was published in January 1982.[7] Only one of the 159 KS/OI patients was a woman, while twelve men were reported to be heterosexual. Again, no details of these cases were provided. However, Guinan subsequently updated the surveillance analysis through December 28, 1981, and provided additional data on the then twenty-six patients (twenty men and six women) reported to be heterosexual.[8] Thirteen of the men and four of the women were reported to be IDUs. The majority of these IDU patients were Black or Hispanic and resided in New York City. No risk factors were described for the other nine heterosexual patients. Because many of these twenty-six patients had died before they could be interviewed, it was not always possible to verify their sexual and drug-use histories.

Along with Guinan, Harry Haverkos was looking at patients reported to be heterosexual. On March 12, 1982, Haverkos received a call from John Hanrahan, an EIS officer assigned to the New York State Health Department, and Gary Wormser, Chief of Infectious Diseases at Westchester County Medical Center in Valhalla, New York, informing CDC of three prisoners at the nearby Taconic Correction Facility who had been diagnosed with PCP and were now hospitalized at the Medical Center.[9]

---

* The KS/OI case definition specified that an underlying malignancy would exclude a patient from being considered a case.

Haverkos and Guinan traveled to Valhalla, where they met with Hanrahan and interviewed the three Taconic inmates. The three patients were white men; two denied homosexual activity, while the third said he had one homosexual contact in 1974. All had used IV drugs before incarceration, and one reported "renting needles" from other inmates while previously incarcerated at the Sing Sing Correctional Facility in Ossining, New York. Hanrahan also described four KS/OI patients in other New York State correctional facilities and one in Riker's Island (a New York City facility). From Isabel Guerrero, a former EIS officer now working for the New Jersey State Health Department, Hanrahan had learned of two additional cases in New Jersey correctional facilities. These seven inmates were all men, all but one was Black or Hispanic, and all had used IV drugs.

On June 11, 1982, CDC published a one-year update on KS/OI in the *MMWR*.[10] Of the 355 cases reported since the previous June, forty-one of them (12 percent) were in heterosexual men and thirteen (4 percent) were in heterosexual women. PCP accounted for a higher proportion of the diagnoses in both heterosexual men and women than in homosexual men, in whom KS was proportionately more frequent. Both male and female heterosexual PCP patients were more likely than homosexual patients to be Black or Hispanic, and more than half had used IV drugs. The accompanying editorial note urged caution in interpreting the sexual orientation data for men because this information was largely obtained from reporting physicians and had not been confirmed. No comment was made about how IV drug use might be a risk factor for KS/OI. Nonetheless, the note stated, "Similarities between homosexual and heterosexual cases in diagnoses and geographic and temporal distribution suggest that all are part of the epidemic."[10] The note further concluded that "differences in race, proportion of PCP cases, and IV drug use suggest that risk factors may be different for these groups."[10]

About six weeks after the publication of the *MMWR* update, I received a call from Gerald (Jerry) Friedland and Robert Klein, infectious diseases physicians at Montefiore Medical Center in the Bronx, New York. They were calling to let CDC know that they were caring for two male KS/OI patients whose female sexual partners had unexplained immunodeficiency (couples 1 and 2). Both men were thought to be heterosexual, and one had a history of IV drug use. Both women denied IV drug use; one had generalized lymph node enlargement and laboratory evidence of cellular immunodeficiency, and the other was being treated for probable PCP. Friedland and Klein asked for assistance to confirm the drug use and sexual histories of these women.

I replied that I would see if Bill Darrow might be available to assist and asked them to keep CDC informed as they learned more about these couples.

In a subsequent call, Carol Harris, an infectious disease fellow working with Friedland and Klein, told me that the couples' investigation had been expanded beyond Montefiore to include several other hospitals affiliated with The Albert Einstein College of Medicine. The expanded investigation had identified additional female sex partners of men with KS/OI. Darrow agreed to travel to the Bronx to assist in interviewing the members of these couples.

Of the eight couples under investigation, Darrow was able to interview four men with KS/OI and six of the female partners. He established that two of the men with KS/OI were bisexual, including one of the men initially described as heterosexual in the call from Friedland and Klein, while the other two interviewed men were IDUs.[11] The six interviewed female partners all denied IV drug use. The diagnosis had been confirmed in the female partner initially described as having probable PCP. Two of the other female partners had lymph node enlargement, and one had abnormally low white blood cell counts.

The Montefiore team reported the results of the investigation of couples 1 and 2 in the January 3, 1983, issue of the *MMWR*[12] and followed up with a more detailed report of seven female partners of men with KS/OI.[†] [13] Of the seven women, only one was immunologically normal. Citing the earlier cluster study of homosexual men by David Auerbach and Darrow,[14] the Montefiore authors restated the hypothesis that "an agent transmissible to sexual contacts may be responsible for the abnormalities in cellular immunity present in this syndrome" and concluded that "This study suggests AIDS[‡] may be sexually transmitted between heterosexual men and women."[13]

The Montefiore investigators and Darrow went on to characterize a study population of IDUs with AIDS and related immunodeficiency as well as "healthy" drug users in the Bronx.[15] The great majority of study subjects were young, nonwhite, and of lower socioeconomic

[†] At the time of these studies, the *New England Journal of Medicine* (*NEJM*) was following the "Ingelfinger Rule" (named for the former Editor-in-Chief, Franz Ingelfinger), which advised authors that the journal would not accept articles if the substance of their findings had been published elsewhere. Jim Curran called Arnold Relman, the *NEJM* Editor-in-Chief at the time the *MMWR* report appeared, to ask for an exception to the rule to allow the Montefiore group to submit their complete findings to the journal. Relman agreed.

[‡] The name "KS/OI" was replaced with acquired immunodeficiency syndrome (AIDS) in July 1982 (Chapter 8).

status; about 20 percent were homosexual or bisexual men. In contrast to middle-class white homosexual men with KS/OI who were often highly mobile, these IDUs rarely traveled to other cities.[§] All study subjects used IV heroin and cocaine, either alone or in combination. Needle sharing was almost universal and often took place in "shooting galleries," settings such as abandoned buildings, where needles were shared with multiple anonymous partners. Sharing of needles among heterosexual and homosexual IDUs was commonly reported. The authors noted that "Needle sharing is also the likely epidemiologic connection between the homosexual and heterosexual AIDS populations, since homosexual IV drug abusers admit to using 'shooting galleries' and sharing needles at the same high rate as heterosexual IV drug abusers."[15] Although not stated by the authors, "shooting galleries" and bathhouses could be seen as having analogous roles in the spread of the putative "AIDS agent" through blood and sexual contact, respectively.

In another follow-up study led by Guinan,[16] AIDS patients reported to CDC as heterosexual were interviewed using a questionnaire modeled after the one used in the CDC case-control study of homosexual men described in Chapter 4. Of the thirty-one interviewed patients (twenty-four men and seven women), twenty-two were IDUs, four were Haitians (a population that had been classified as a risk group [Chapter 6]), and the remaining five did not belong to an identified risk group. Compared with the fifty homosexual men interviewed in the case-control study, the heterosexual patients were more likely to be nonwhite and of lower socioeconomic status and were less likely to have KS. Heterosexuals were also less likely to have had other STIs and were much less sexually active than homosexuals. Testing of serum samples found that the heterosexual patients were less likely to have evidence of past syphilis infection than the homosexual patients, while laboratory markers for HBV infection were found frequently in both homosexuals (96 percent) and heterosexuals (84 percent).

As heterosexual AIDS patients were being investigated in the United States, the first African AIDS patients were being reported from Belgium and France.[17,18,19,20] These patients, who were seeking medical care, came from Central Africa (Zaire[**] and Chad) and West Africa (Mali) and reported neither drug use nor homosexual activity.

[§] An exception were Puerto Rican IDUs living in New York and New Jersey who traveled to Puerto Rico.

[**] Now, the Democratic Republic of Congo (DRC). Both names are used in this book.

The AIDS epidemic was rapidly worsening. An *MMWR* update published in September 1982 noted that reported cases were doubling approximately every six months.[21] The overall case-fatality ratio (the proportion of cases known to have died) was 41 percent and exceeded 60 percent for persons followed for at least a year after diagnosis. Although the causative agent of AIDS remained unknown, the available information was consistent with its transmission through sexual contact and blood exposure. The risk of AIDS could also potentially extend to recipients of blood and blood products, as well as to health-care workers with occupational blood exposures and infants born to infected mothers.

Was there a single moment of clarity at which all these risks came into sharp focus for the Task Force? If there was such a moment, I can neither remember it nor find documentation that it occurred. Instead, I think that as more epidemiologic information became available, the more confident we became that HBV was the correct model for AIDS. There would be nothing to stop the epidemic from expanding through both sexual and blood exposures and taking the lives of millions of people around the world. Perhaps this vision was too frightening to comprehend at the time, but it tragically proved to be correct.

Notes

1. Schreeder MT, Thompson SE, Hadler SC, et al. Hepatitis B in homosexual men: prevalence of infection and factors related to transmission. J Infect Dis 1982;146:7–15.
2. Seef LB. Hepatitis in the drug abuser. Med Clin N Am 1975;59:843–848.
3. CDC. Follow-up on Kaposi's sarcoma and *Pneumocystis* pneumonia. MMWR Morb Mortal Wkly Rep 1981;30:409–410.
4. *The Global Health Chronicles.* https://globalhealthchronicles.org/aids.
5. "GUINAN, MARY," *The Global Health Chronicles*, accessed January 29, 2023, https://www.globalhealthchronicles.org/items/show/5393.
6. Masur H, Michelis MA, Greene JB, et al. An outbreak of community-acquired *Pneumocystis carinii* pneumonia: initial manifestations of cellular immune dysfunction. N Engl J Med 1981;305:1431–1438.
7. Centers for Disease Control Task Force on Kaposi's Sarcoma and Opportunistic Infections. Special Report. Epidemiologic aspects of the current outbreak of Kaposi's Sarcoma and opportunistic infections. N Engl J Med 1982;306:248–252.
8. "HETEROSEXUAL CASES," *The Global Health Chronicles*, accessed January 29, 2023, https://www.globalhealthchronicles.org/items/show/8011.

9. "PNEUMOCYSTIS CARINII PNEUMONIA: Prison Cases," *The Global Health Chronicles*, accessed January 29, 2023, https://www.globalhealthchronicles.org/items/show/6543.

10. CDC. Update on Kaposi's sarcoma and opportunistic infections in previously healthy persons—United States. MMWR Morbid Mortal Wkly Rep 1982:31:294–301.

11. "MONTEFIORE MEDICAL CENTER: Heterosexual Cases," *The Global Health Chronicles*, accessed December 15, 2022, https://www.globalhealthchronicles.org/items/show/8073.

12. CDC. Immunodeficiency among female sexual partners of men with acquired immune deficiency syndrome (AIDS)—New York. MMWR Morbid Mortal Wkly Rep 1983;31:697–698.

13. Harris C, Butkus Small C, Klein RS, et al. Immunodeficiency in female sex partners of men with the acquired immunodeficiency syndrome. N Engl J Med 1983;308:1181–1184.

14. Auerbach DM, Darrow WW, Jaffe HW, Curran JW. Clusters of cases of the acquired immune deficiency syndrome. Patients linked by sexual contact. Am J Med 1984;76:487–492.

15. Friedland GH, Harris C, Butkus-Small C, et al. Intravenous drug abusers and the acquired immunodeficiency syndrome (AIDS). Demographic, drug use, and needle-sharing patterns. Arch Intern Med 1985;145:1413–1417.

16. Guinan M, Thomas PA, Pinksy PF, et al. Heterosexual and homosexual patients with the acquired immunodeficiency syndrome: a comparison of surveillance, interview, and laboratory data. Ann Intern Med 1984;100:213–218.

17. Clumeck N, Mascart-Lemone F, de Maubeuge J, Brenez D, Marcelis L. Acquired immunodeficiency syndrome in black Africans. Lancet 1983;1:642.

18. Brunet JB, Bouvet E, Leibowitch J, et al. Acquired immunodeficiency syndrome in France. Lancet 1983;1:700–701.

19. Vittecoq D, Modai J. AIDS in a black Malian. Lancet 1983;2:1023.

20. Offenstadt G, Pinta P, Hericord P, et al. Multiple opportunistic infections due to AIDS in a previously healthy black women from Zaire. N Engl J Med 1983;308:775.

21. CDC. Update on acquired immune deficiency syndrome (AIDS)—United States. MMWR Morb Mortal Wkly Rep 1982;31:507–514.

6

Haitian Americans and Haiti

Harold W. Jaffe

While the CDC Task Force worked to understand the spread of KS/OI in the United States, we had no idea that the disease was also occurring in Haiti— less than eight hundred miles from US shores. The 1970 US census estimated that about 28,000 Haitian-born persons resided in the United States,[1] many in Haitian American communities that had been established in New York City and south Florida. Haitians had left their country to escape poverty (Haiti was and still is the poorest country in the Western Hemisphere) and the repressive rule of François "Papa Doc" Duvalier and his son, Jean-Claude "Baby Doc." Migration surged during the years 1978 to 1981, when tens of thousands of Haitians arrived in the United States, often traveling by boat ("boat people") and frequently settling in Miami.[2])

The University of Miami/Jackson Memorial Medical Center (JMMC) was the only public hospital serving indigent patients in Miami and where many Haitian immigrants sought care. In May 1981, George Hensley, a pathologist at JMMC, diagnosed toxoplasmosis in an autopsy sample of brain tissue taken from a Haitian resident of Miami.[3] Toxoplasmosis is caused by the parasite *Toxoplasma gondii*, which infects millions of people throughout the world. Most infections cause mild or no symptoms, although infants born to mothers infected during pregnancy may suffer serious damage. But like other OIs, toxoplasmosis may reactivate in immunosuppressed patients causing severe disease including brain infection (encephalitis). Hensley reported, however, that "no evidence of any unusual predisposing condition or therapy was found in this patient."[3]

Harry Haverkos recalled that Hensley was performing autopsies on additional Haitian American patients dying of encephalitis and sending brain specimens to the laboratory of Jack Remington at Stanford University.[4] Remington, a leading authority on toxoplasmosis, reported finding evidence of *Toxoplasma* encephalitis (TE) in these specimens. Remington knew Dennis Juranek (Chapter 2) from CDC's Division of Parasitic Disease and

Harold W. Jaffe, *Haitian Americans and Haiti* In: *Dispatches from the AIDS Pandemic*. Kevin M. De Cock, Harold W. Jaffe, and James W. Curran and Edited by: Robin Moseley, Oxford University Press. © Oxford University Press 2023. DOI: 10.1093/oso/9780197626528.003.0006

contacted him (Juranek) to discuss the Miami cases. According to Haverkos, Remington told Juranek that he not only had the Miami cases but that he had two other TE biopsies from Haitian men, one from Montreal and one from New York City, and asked him if he didn't think it was a little strange: "Nine cases, I mean, this is a fairly rare disease in the US."[4] Assuming these patients had not received immunosuppressive therapy, they would have met CDC's case definition for KS/OI.

Haverkos continued to monitor possible KS/OI cases in Haitian Americans, and in November 1981, five months after the first *MMWR* report on *Pneumocystis* pneumonia in homosexual men, he sent a memo to the Task Force titled "The Haitian Connection."[5] In it, he wrote:

> We have heard of ten cases of opportunistic infections or Kaposi's sarcoma in Haitian persons at Jackson Memorial Hospital in Miami, and one case of *Pneumocystis carinii* pneumonia in a Haitian now living in Los Angeles. Four of these cases have evidence of steroid therapy prior to diagnosis [which would potentially exclude them as patients meeting the KS/OI case definition] . . . Five have evidence of tuberculosis—four disseminated. Eight cases were diagnosed at autopsy.[5]

He noted Hensley's plan to review all autopsies done on Haitians dying at JMMC and went on to write, "Why are these infections occurring in Haitians now? We are looking into rates of these infections on the Island of Haiti through Dr. Alain Roisin."[5]

Roisin, a Belgian national, had worked for WHO as an epidemiologist in Haiti before joining CDC as an EIS officer assigned to the health department in Rochester, New York. In December 1981, Roisin was visiting friends in Haiti and called Task Force member Richard Sattin to report that a dermatologist in Haiti had seen patients with KS. The dermatologist was Bernard Liautaud, who subsequently reported the patients at a congress of French-speaking physicians held in Port-au-Prince.[6] In his report, Liautaud noted that while he and his colleagues were aware of only one Haitian patient with KS during the prior decade, they had recognized eleven cases between June 1979 and November 1981. Of the eleven patients, nine had disseminated disease and a rapidly fatal outcome. Only one patient was a homosexual man, and none had a history of drug abuse. He concluded his report by writing, "The appearance of an 'outbreak' [of KS] has been demonstrated among American homosexuals; it must be seriously considered in Haiti. Although our Haitian cases are contemporaneous with the small 'epidemic' among American homosexuals, there is no obvious correlation between the two foci."[6]

These reports strongly suggested that KS/OI was occurring in Haiti and in Haitians living in the United States but left many questions unanswered. Why were some Haitians at risk for KS/OI? If the disease was caused by an infectious agent, how was it being transmitted in Haiti? Had the infection spread from one country to the other? If so, what was the direction of the spread? To help answer these questions, we needed more firsthand information.

Peter Drotman,[7] a recent EIS graduate, had been working in CDC's Division of Sexually Transmitted Diseases when he was assigned to the Task Force. He and Haverkos informally agreed to split the investigations of Haitian patients: Haverkos would be responsible for the domestic work, while Drotman would go to Haiti. Although Drotman had seen extreme poverty while working with the WHO smallpox eradication program in Bangladesh, he was taken aback by what he saw on his arrival in Port-au-Prince. He recalled, "[T]he first thing you see in the town is the presidential palace, which is enormous and looks very much like the White House does in Washington, DC, except it's surrounded by disheveled buildings that are crumbling."[7] As a representative of CDC, he first met with the Haitian Minister of Health. According to Drotman, the Minister was very welcoming and told him that "[A]ll the facilities of the Ministry of Health are at your disposal."[7] Drotman then entered the Ministry of Health building, where he observed, "there was literally nothing there."[7] The only person he found in the building was Alain Roisin.

Drotman and Roisin were joined by the JMMC pathologist George Hensley and formed a team to visit physicians and hospitals that had reported seeing KS/OI patients. While Drotman and Roisin spoke with patients and reviewed medical records, Hensley examined biopsy materials obtained from the patients. Drotman also collected patient blood samples and shipped them to the CDC immunology laboratory. The immunologic profile of the Haitian patients was like that seen in American KS/OI patients. Regarding possible risk behaviors, Drotman concluded:

There may have been a heterosexual transmission component there. There probably was a homosexual transmission component, but it was much more difficult to get the kind of history questionnaire response from the

Haitian patients in Haiti than I had become used to in traveling around the United States.[7]

Taking the lead on domestic investigations, Haverkos traveled to Miami in April 1982 to learn more about the Haitian Americans there who had been diagnosed with KS/OI. He saw several patients with PCP as well as a patient with KS. But like Drotman, he had little success in eliciting information on possible risk behaviors. On a return visit to Miami, Haverkos reviewed reports of nineteen Haitian American patients seen at JMMC. These patients had been diagnosed with a variety of OIs and had no apparent cause for their underlying immunosuppression.[8] Haverkos noted extreme weight loss in many of these patients and commented on their high rate of TB.

On July 9, 1982, CDC published an *MMWR* summary of what the Task Force had learned about KS/OI in Haitians residing in the United States.[9] The report included the nineteen patients with OIs that Haverkos had reviewed in Miami, a Miami KS patient, ten other patients residing in Brooklyn, New York, and four patients living elsewhere. All but four of the thirty-four patients were male; of the twenty-three men interviewed, none reported homosexual activity. Of the twenty-six patients for whom drug-use information was given, only one reported a history of IV drug use. Patients ranged in age from twenty to forty-five years, with the majority having lived in the United States for less than two years. At least one patient had an onset of illness before leaving Haiti. Nearly half the patients had died. The editorial note stated, "It is not clear whether this outbreak is related to similar outbreaks [in the United States] among homosexual males, IV drug abusers, and others, but the clinical and immunologic pictures appear quite similar."[9]

Following the *MMWR* report, investigators from Miami (JMMC) and Brooklyn (State University of New York Downstate Medical Center) published more details about their KS/OI patients. Thomas (Tom) Spira,[10] a CDC immunologist and Task Force member (Chapter 7), performed the immunologic assays for both groups. The Miami investigators noted that seven of their twenty patients had developed disseminated TB preceding other infections by two to fifteen months, and the Brooklyn investigators reported extrapulmonary (outside of the lung) TB in five of their ten patients ([11,12]). Like many low-income countries, Haiti had high rates of TB infection. In healthy persons the immune system usually controls the infection, but in KS/

OI patients that control was lost. Later we would learn that TB was the most common OI seen in the global AIDS epidemic.

Although CDC reports had described KS/OI in the United States and Haiti as separate outbreaks, Haitian authorities were clearly concerned that Haiti might be portrayed as the source of the disease. In a memorandum to the Task Force, dated September 8, 1982, Alain Roisin summarized a phone call he had with Volvick Remy Joseph, the Haitian Minister of Health:

1. He (Joseph) is concerned about the use of information from Haiti. He agrees that cases occurred in the country, but that so far, it is impossible to determine where the problem began. The investigation is still in progress.
2. All future investigations will be supervised by the Ministry of Health.
3. All publications from Haiti will need to go through his office.[13]

Roisin also added his own observation:

If we would like to continue to collaborate and work with the Ministry of Health, we need to be really careful about our comments regarding the situation in Haiti. Two possible points are:

1. Possible misassoc[i]ation between groups (Haitian–Drug addict–Homosexual)
2. The hypothesis that the problem originated in Haiti.[13]

Tensions between the United States and Haiti further escalated with the March 4, 1983, *MMWR* publication of the first guidelines for prevention of what now was called AIDS.[14] Although the report acknowledged that "Very little is known about risk factors for Haitians with AIDS," it listed Haitian entrants to the United States as being at increased risk for AIDS along with homosexual or bisexual men with multiple sex partners and IV drug abusers.[14] Further, as will be discussed in more detail in Chapter 8, the PHS guidelines recommended that "As a temporary measure, members of groups at increased risk for AIDS [which would include Haitian entrants] should refrain from donating plasma and/or blood."[14] Although the "risk group" designation was applied to homosexual men and IV drug abusers because of their specific risk behaviors, no such behaviors had been identified for Haitian entrants.

Listing Haitians as a risk group resulted in multiple unintended consequences. In a *New York Times* article published on July 31, 1983, the medical reporter Lawrence Altman (a former EIS officer) wrote, "An international controversy has arisen over whether American health officials have unfairly categorized residents of Haiti and Haitians in the United States as having an increased risk of contracting acquired immune deficiency syndrome, or AIDS."[15] He cited the assertion of Saidel Laine, president of the Haitian Medical Association, that "American health officials had used unscientific methods in their investigations."[15] Laine called the studies "racist," and said the findings "had left a whole nation of people unduly alarmed and unfairly stigmatized."[15] Altman also quoted a report from a New York AIDS task force to Governor Mario Cuomo that "expressed concern about Haitian-American civil rights, saying, in part, 'Haitians are being fired from their jobs for no reason other than their national origin.'"[15] Altman noted that tourism to Haiti had dropped by 20 percent.

Given these unintended consequences, were the PHS guidelines right in listing Haitians as an AIDS risk group? The answer probably depends on who is asked the question. But from the perspective of US public health officials, whose priority was to assure the safety of donated blood in the absence of a test for the putative AIDS agent, the PHS recommendations were justified.

Fortunately, studies by Haitian investigators were underway to better understand AIDS and its risk factors. Leading these studies was the highly respected Haitian physician/scientist Jean "Bill" Pape. Born in Haiti, Pape studied medicine at Cornell Medical College in New York before returning home. In Haiti, Pape put together a team of clinicians, The Haitian Study Group, which included Bernard Liautaud, to review the AIDS patients they had seen in Port-au-Prince.[16] The team identified sixty-one patients seen between June 1979 and October 1982, forty-five of whom had OIs, fifteen had KS, and one had both KS and an OI. Most patients had died within six months following their diagnosis. The patients came from throughout Haiti, and 85 percent were men. Examination of the medical records of thirty-one of the men found that only two had a history of bisexuality; however, five of the twenty-one men interviewed by a Study Group member said they were bisexual. None of the nine female patients reported working as prostitutes, and all patients denied illicit drug use. Pape wrote that "The identification of bisexual Haitian patients who had sexual relations with American homosexuals in New York and Miami also provides a link between the two populations."[16] He also noted a relatively high prevalence of AIDS in Carrefour, a suburb of Port-au-Prince, describing it as being "recognized as the principal center of male and female prostitution in Haiti."[16]

Pape and his colleagues went on to conduct a case-control study to better understand the risk factors for AIDS in Haiti.[17] They administered a questionnaire to 128 AIDS patients (cases) and to 112 same-sex siblings and friends of the patients in comparable age groups (controls). Of the ninety-three male AIDS patients, 36 percent were bisexual and one had a history of IV drug use, while 40 percent of the thirty-five female patients had received transfusions within four years of their onset of illness. Comparisons of cases (with or without these other risk factors) to controls revealed two significant differences. First, both male and female case patients had a greater number of heterosexual sex partners than control patients. Second, the case patients were more likely to have received intramuscular injections of medications in the five years before their onset of symptoms, to have received a greater number of injections, and to have received them from nonmedical sources. Pape noted that intramuscular injections of medications were commonly given in Haiti to persons "not feeling well" and that needles and syringes may be reused without sterilization.[17] He wrote, "These findings are consistent with the hypothesis that transmission of the syndrome is similar to that of hepatitis B."[17] He also concluded that "heterosexual transmission of AIDS is important in Haiti."[17]

CDC also planned a case-control study of AIDS in Haitian Americans,[18] led by Joyce Johnson, who had previously served as an EIS officer in CDC's viral hepatitis program. The study promised to be difficult. As described previously, Haitian Americans were feeling the stigma of AIDS. Enrolling them in a study sponsored by the US government was likely to be a challenge. Further, the academic centers caring for most of the Haitian Americans with AIDS were rivals, not anxious to share their data.

To address the issues of cultural sensitivity of the study, Johnson turned to the Association of Haitian Physicians Abroad for advice. In turn, the Association provided three physicians as consultants to the study. Although these physicians all spoke Haitian Creole, they advised Johnson to contract with a Haitian linguist to be sure the translation of the study questionnaire was accurate, particularly for topics such as homosexuality. I remember asking the linguist how he would approach the sensitive issue of sexual orientation. After explaining the Haitian Creole words he would use, he added that it was not just the questions that are important, it's the patient's expression when asked the questions that really count. Wow, I thought, this is really going to be hard.

After prolonged negotiations, Johnson secured agreements with both the Miami and Brooklyn groups to enroll their Haitian American AIDS patients in the study and to provide Haitian American control patients from their hospital wards, outpatient clinics, and private physicians' offices. Unfortunately, Johnson's one-year attachment to the Task Force ended before the study was finished, and she returned to clinical training.[*] Her replacement on the study was Ken Castro (Chapter 3). Castro was born in Puerto Rico and had trained in medicine at Montefiore Medical Center in New York City. He saw the study through to its conclusion and publication.[19]

A total of fifty-five case patients (forty-five men and ten women) and 242 control patients (164 men and 78 women) were enrolled. Of the case patients, one man was homosexual, and no one reported IV drug use. Compared with the male controls, male cases had entered the United States more recently, were more likely to have a history of gonorrhea and a positive blood test for syphilis, and more often reported sex with female prostitutes. Compared with female controls, female cases were more likely to have been offered money for sex and were more likely to have voodoo-priest friends. There was no significant difference between cases and controls in their histories of receiving intramuscular injections in Haiti.

Although the significance of the voodoo priests was unclear, the rest of the study findings pointed to heterosexual transmission of HIV as the main risk factor for AIDS in these Haitian Americans. Castro recalled that because of the study, "[W]e ended up with enough evidence to inform a policy decision by CDC to drop the Haitian category as a separate risk group, . . . acknowledging that it was mostly sexually acquired."[†] [20]

In retrospect, some aspects of the early AIDS epidemics in Haitian Americans and in Haiti can now be seen more clearly. First, virtually all cases of AIDS in Haitian Americans were in persons who had recently arrived in the United States. Given that the average incubation period between HIV infection and AIDS is about ten years in adults,[21] these persons almost certainly had become infected in Haiti. Second, the early AIDS epidemics in

---

[*] In 1997, Johnson became "Surgeon General" [Director of Health and Safety] of the US Coast Guard.

[†] The exclusion of Haitian Americans as blood donors remained in place until 1990, several years after the implementation of blood bank screening for HIV (Chapter 8).

Haiti and the United States may have been linked through sexual contacts between bisexual Haitian men and homosexual American men. Although recent phylogenetic analysis of Haitian and US HIV strains indicated the virus was present in Haiti before it appeared in the United States,[22] the role of these bisexual Haitians in the start of the American epidemic remains unknown. Third, as time passed and heterosexual transmission became the major route of HIV spread in Haiti, the Haitian epidemic came to resemble more closely the epidemic in sub-Saharan Africa than the American epidemic. But fortunately, Haiti never experienced the severe "generalized" heterosexual epidemic seen in sub-Saharan Africa.

Notes

1. Gibson C, Jung K. Historical census statistics of the foreign-born population of the United States: 1850-2000. US Census Bureau, Population Division, Working Paper No 81. February 2006. https://www.ccnsus.gov/content/dam/Census/library/working-papers/2006/demo/POP-twps0081.pdf.
2. Gutekunst CP. Interdiction of Haitian migrants on the high seas: a legal and policy analysis. Yale J Intl Law 1984;10:151–184.
3. Moskowitz LB, Kory P, Chan JC, Haverkos HW, Conley FK, Hensley GT. Unusual causes of death in Haitians residing in Miami. High prevalence of opportunistic infections. JAMA 1983;250:1187–1191.
4. "HAVERKOS, HARRY," The Global Health Chronicles, accessed January 29, 2023, https://www.globalhealthchronicles.org/items/show/6897.
5. "KAPOSI'S SARCOMA IN HAITI," The Global Health Chronicles, accessed January 29, 2023, https://www.globalhealthchronicles.org/items/show/8058.
6. Liautaud B, Laroche CL, Duvivier J, Pean-Guichard CL. Kaposi sarcoma: incidence in Haiti. Presented at the 18th Congress of French-speaking Physicians of the Western Hemisphere, Port-au-Prince, April 12–16, 1982 (translated from the French).
7. "DROTMAN, PETER," The Global Health Chronicles, accessed January 29, 2023, https://www.globalhealthchronicles.org/items/show/7958.
8. "OPPORTUNISTIC INFECTIONS: Haitian Refugees," The Global Health Chronicles, accessed January 29, 2023, https://www.globalhealthchronicles.org/items/show/8066.
9. CDC. Opportunistic infections and Kaposi's sarcoma among Haitians in the United States. MMWR Morb Mortal Wkly Rep 1982;31:353–354, 360–361.
10. "SPIRA, THOMAS," The Global Health Chronicles, accessed January 29, 2023, https://www.globalhealthchronicles.org/items/show/5396.
11. Pitchenik AE, Fischl MA, Dickinson GM, et al. Opportunistic infections and Kaposi's sarcoma among Haitians: evidence of a new acquired immunodeficiency state. Ann Intern Med 1983;98:277–284.

12. Veira J, Frank E, Spira TJ, Landesman SH. Acquired immune deficiency in Haitians. Opportunistic infections in previously healthy Haitian immigrants. N Engl J Med 1983;308:125–129.
13. Memorandum to AIDS Task Force Coordinator from Alain Roisin, M.D., September 8, 1982 (Author's archives).
14. CDC. Prevention of acquired immune deficiency syndrome (AIDS): Report of inter-agency recommendations. MMWR Morb Mortal Wkly Rep 1983;32:101–104.
15. Altman, LK. Debate grows on U.S. listing of Haitians in AIDS category. New York Times, July 31, 1983. https://www.nytimes.com/1983/07/31/us/debate-grows-on-us-listing-of-haitians-in-aids-category.html (Accessed September 4, 2021).
16. Pape JW, Liautaud B, Thomas F, et al. Characteristics of the acquired immunodefi-ciency syndrome (AIDS) in Haiti. N Engl J Med 1983;309:945–950.
17. Pape JW, Liautaud B, Thomas F, et al. The acquired immunodeficiency syndrome in Haiti. Ann Intern Med 1985;103:674–678.
18. "HAITIAN AIDS STUDY: Protocol Draft," *The Global Health Chronicles*, accessed January 29, 2023, https://www.globalhealthchronicles.org/items/show/8064.
19. The Consortium Study Group of AIDS in Haitian-Americans. Risk factors for AIDS among Haitians residing in the United States. Evidence of heterosexual transmission. JAMA 1987;257:625–629.
20. "CASTRO, KENNETH," *The Global Health Chronicles*, accessed January 29, 2023, https://www.globalhealthchronicles.org/items/show/6478.
21. Collaborative Group on AIDS Incubation and HIV Survival including CASCADE EU Concerted Action. Time from HIV-1 seroconversion and death before wide-spread use of highly-active antiretroviral therapy: A collaborative re-analysis. Lancet 2000;355:1131–1137.
22. Worobey M, Watts TD, McKay RA, et al. 1970s and "Patient 0" HIV-1 genomes illu-minate early HIV/AIDS history in North America. Nature 2016;539:98–101.

7

Mothers and Infants

Harold W. Jaffe

In mid-1982, the CDC Task Force began receiving reports of unexplained immunodeficiency in infants. Congenital immunodeficiencies (i.e., impaired immune function present at birth) were well known at the time, causing syndromes characterized by specific defects in the immune system. Often these syndromes were inherited, and some were associated with birth defects. But the reports reaching us were different. Most of the mothers of these immunodeficient infants either had AIDS or were known to be in groups at risk for the disease. Others were found to be the sex partners of at-risk men.

On July 28, 1982, I wrote in my CDC notebook, "20-month-old male has mucocutaneous candidiasis and now has disseminated *M. avium*. Previous immunologic studies showed no specific defect. Mother is [patient name] (case #198) IV drug addict with PCP. Hospitalized at N.Y. hospital. (Dr. O'Reilly). Spira will call."[1] This note requires some decoding. Mucocutaneous candidiasis is a fungal infection involving the mucous membranes (e.g., the linings of the mouth and throat) and skin. Although not unusual in infants, oral candida infections were also frequently seen in adults with AIDS. Disseminated infection with *Mycobacterium avium*, a relative of the bacterium that causes TB, was a much rarer condition that had also been reported in adult AIDS patients. The case number indicated that the mother had been reported to CDC as having AIDS. Richard O'Reilly was a physician and researcher at Memorial Sloan-Kettering Cancer Center (MSKCC) in New York City, who was known for having treated some forms of congenital immunodeficiency with bone marrow transplantation. And Spira was CDC's Tom Spira.

Spira was born in Czechoslovakia and left with his parents when communists took over the country. After completing his medical training, he came to CDC to take a position in the immunology program of CDC's Bureau of Laboratories. During this time, he also volunteered as a care provider at the pediatric immunodeficiency clinic at Grady Memorial Hospital

Harold W. Jaffe, *Mothers and Infants* In: *Dispatches from the AIDS Pandemic*. Kevin M. De Cock, Harold W. Jaffe, and James W. Curran and Edited by: Robin Moseley, Oxford University Press. © Oxford University Press 2023. DOI: 10.1093/oso/9780197626528.003.0007

in Atlanta. There he met James (Jim) Oleske, who was training in pediatric infectious diseases and immunology before taking a faculty position at the University of Medicine and Dentistry of New Jersey in Newark. In 1981, Spira was doing a sabbatical at MSKCC in New York and, as he recalled, ". . . working with Robert Good. . . [who] was like the grandfather of immunodeficiency diseases here in the United States."[2] He further remembered that during that time "Jim [Oleske] was sending over some patients with possible Nezelof syndrome."* [1]

On September 29, 1982, Oleske called me from Newark to report a Haitian infant, born in November 1981, who developed PCP at four and a half months and died a few months later. Nothing was known about the health status of the parents. He had also seen an infant with "failure to thrive" (a term commonly used in pediatrics to describe a child who was not growing normally) and unexplained enlargement of the liver, spleen, and lymph nodes. The mother was an IV drug user.

Shortly after speaking with Oleske, I received a call from Jerry Friedland at Montefiore Medical Center in the Bronx. I had gotten to know Friedland from his investigations of the sex partners of AIDS patients (Chapter 5), and he asked me if I had heard about the immunodeficient children who had been seen by Arye Rubinstein—his pediatrician colleague at The Albert Einstein College of Medicine. When I said no, Friedland gave me Rubinstein's phone number. I called Rubinstein the next day, and he described seeing seven young children with failure to thrive, unexplained lymph node enlargement, and a severe immunodeficiency, resembling that seen in adults with AIDS. He said that all but one of the mothers were IV drug users and five were sex workers. The health status of the mothers was being investigated.

What was this pediatric immunodeficiency? Except for Nezelof syndrome, it didn't fit the description of any known congenital immunodeficiency. The findings that the mothers of these children either had AIDS or were in groups at increased risk for AIDS suggested that the putative "AIDS agent" could be transmitted from mother to child. Other STIs, including HBV and syphilis, were known to be transmitted from mothers to their unborn infants (syphilis) or from mothers to newborns (HBV). But before reaching the alarming conclusion that AIDS could occur in children, we needed to be sure

---

* Nezelof syndrome is a rare, poorly characterized form of pediatric immunodeficiency that was thought by some not to be a specific entity but a group of syndromes for which more precise diagnoses were lacking.

of the facts. The Task Force agreed that Spira and I should visit Newark and New York City to review the reported cases. We would be accompanied by Isabel Guerrero (Chapter 5) in New Jersey and Polly Thomas in New York City on visits to their respective jurisdictions.

Given that the reporting physicians were also academic competitors, I was a bit worried that they would be unwilling to share more of their findings with CDC. Fortunately, my worries proved unfounded. We met first with Oleske, who was very friendly and clearly cared deeply for the children under his care. He confirmed the details of the patients that he had reported and told us about other patients who were under investigation. Rubinstein agreed to provide us with the confirmatory data that we needed and told us about other possible cases. And Richard O'Reilly also reviewed his patient data with us.

As a side note, the visit not only improved my understanding of pediatric immunology but also expanded my culinary horizons. As an Orthodox Jew, Spira ate only kosher meals. This led us to sample the kosher cuisine of New York City, ranging from Moshe Peking, a kosher Chinese restaurant, to the entirely kosher cafeteria at the Albert Einstein College of Medicine. The food at Moshe Peking was better.

After returning to Atlanta, I received a call from Arthur (Art) Ammann, a well-known pediatric immunologist at the University of California, San Francisco. Ammann had studied the children of a woman with a history of IV drug use and prostitution. The woman had given birth to a son in 1973 and subsequently had three female children. Each of the four children had a different father. While the son remained healthy, two of the daughters developed PCP and the third was immunodeficient. The mother was also immunodeficient and had an oral candida infection but had not developed a serious OI. The occurrence of immunodeficiency in three half-sisters raised the possibility of some sort of inherited immunologic disorder, but the inheritance theory was problematic. In an interview, Ammann described the problem:

> So, we couldn't figure out genetically how you could have a disease where the mother would be partially immunodeficient and only the females inherit the immunodeficiency, and the male normal. I actually talked to a number of geneticists and, believe it or not, some of them came up with some theories as to how that could happen, none of which seemed sound to me.[3]

In a report published in the *MMWR* on December 17, 1982, we summarized what we had learned from our visit and ongoing investigations in New York, New Jersey, and California.[4] Detailed information was provided on four infants diagnosed with serious OIs—three with PCP and one with disseminated *M. avium* infection. The report noted that six other young children with OIs were under investigation and twelve more young children with unexplained immunodeficiency had been reported. Clinical features in these twelve children included failure to thrive; oral candida infections; enlarged liver, spleen, and lymph nodes; and chronic pneumonia without a demonstrable infection. Of the nine mothers for whom information was available, seven were IV drug users. The report's editorial note stated, "Transmission of an 'AIDS agent' from mother to child either in utero [before birth] or shortly after birth could account for the early onset of immunodeficiency in these infants."[3] Not stated, but implicit in the case reports was the possibility that transmission could occur from infected mothers who had not yet developed AIDS.

Following the *MMWR* publication, the academic investigators from New York, New Jersey, and California published more detailed descriptions of the children they had reported to CDC.[5,6,7] Although the publications largely focused on characterizing the immune deficiency in these children, they also contained important clinical and epidemiologic findings. Both Oleske and Rubinstein reported that lung biopsies from children with chronic pneumonia revealed a rare condition called lymphocytic interstitial pneumonia (LIP).[†] Oleske also reported that one of the immunodeficient children in his case series had an identical twin whose immune function was normal, a finding not consistent with an inherited disorder. This observation also implied that if an infectious agent were causing immunodeficiency, it did not necessarily infect both twins.

Although we were aware that infants with unexplained immunodeficiency were also being seen at the University of Miami, the Miami investigators did not share their initial findings with CDC. In early 1984, they published a report of fourteen infants "with clinical and laboratory features of the acquired immunodeficiency syndrome."[8] Two pairs of these infants were siblings. At autopsy, two of the infants were found to have disseminated KS. For eleven of the fourteen infants, both parents were Haitian, as was the father of another

---

[†] In the subsequent development of a case definition for pediatric AIDS, LIP was included as an AIDS-defining condition.

infant. The mothers of the two infants with non-Haitian parents had histories of IV drug use. The authors reported that the mothers of the patients were under investigation, and one of them was already known to have AIDS.

Despite the growing evidence, skepticism about the existence of pediatric AIDS persisted. In a recent communication with me, Ammann wrote that he "felt the need to address [the skeptics] . . . primarily because of accusations that the pediatric and pediatric immunology community were trying to jump on the bandwagon of the AIDS epidemic. The doubt came primarily from the community of physicians caring for adults as well as some of the activists" (Personal communication October 11, 2020).

In an article published in the September 1983 issue of the journal *Pediatrics*, Ammann asked the question, "Is there an acquired immune deficiency syndrome in infants and children?"[9] After describing the epidemiologic and immunologic evidence, he wrote that the recently reported cases of pediatric immunodeficiency were not Nezelof syndrome but an entity similar to AIDS in adults. Further, he felt the evidence suggested the disease was the result of mother-to-child transmission of an infectious agent. He concluded that "I believe that AIDS in infants and children does exist and that increasing numbers of cases will be diagnosed in the pediatric population as the problem increases in the adult population."[8] He went on to call for "an infant and childhood AIDS registry to document and evaluate as many cases as possible."[8]

Under the leadership of Thomas in New York City and Martha Rogers (Chapter 4) in Atlanta, CDC developed a case definition for pediatric AIDS and implemented a national surveillance system for the disease.[10] Analysis of surveillance data from New York City revealed that the earliest birth of a child who developed AIDS had occurred in 1977.[11] By April 1985, eighty-one pediatric AIDS patients had been reported as having one or both parents with AIDS or at increased risk for AIDS.[12]

Ammann's prediction was proving to be correct.

Notes

1. Author's personal records.
2. "SPIRA, THOMAS," *The Global Health Chronicles*, accessed January 29, 2023, https://globalhealthchronicles.org/items/show/5396.
3. Ammann AJ. Online archive of California. (https://oac.cdlib.org/view?docId=kt1n39n4z1;NAAN=13030&doc.view=frames&chunk.id=d0e937&toc.depth=1&toc.id=d0e937&brand=oac4)

4. CDC. Unexplained immunodeficiency and opportunistic infections in infants—New York, New Jersey, California. MMWR Morb Mortal Wkly Rep 1982;31:665–667.
5. Oleske J, Minnefor A, Cooper R Jr., et al. Immune deficiency syndrome in children. JAMA 1983;249:2345–2349.
6. Rubinstein A, Sicklick M, Gupta A, et al. Acquired immunodeficiency with reversed T4/ T8 ratios in infants born to promiscuous and drug-addicted mothers. JAMA 1983;249:2350–2356.
7. Cowan MJ, Hellmann D, Chudwin D, Wara DW, Chang RS, Ammann AJ. Maternal transmission of acquired immune deficiency syndrome. Pediatrics 1984;73:382–386.
8. Scott GB, Buck BE, Leterman JG, Bloom FL, Parks WP. Acquired immunodeficiency syndrome in infants. N Engl J Med 1984;310:76–81.
9. Ammann AJ. Is there an acquired immunodeficiency syndrome in infants and children? Pediatrics 1983;72:430–432.
10. Rogers MF, Thomas PA, Starcher ET, Noa MC, Bush TJ, Jaffe HW. Acquired immunodeficiency syndrome in children. Report of the Centers for Disease Control National Surveillance, 1982 to 1985. Pediatrics 1987;79:1008–1014.
11. Thomas P, O'Donnell R, Williams R, Chiasson MA. HIV infection in heterosexual female intravenous drug users in New York City, 1977–1980. N Engl J Med 1988; 319:374.
12. CDC. Update: Acquired immunodeficiency syndrome—United States. MMWR Morb Mortal Wkly Rep 1985;34:245–248.

8

Blood and Blood Products

Harold W. Jaffe

The identification of cases of the new disease in persons whose only known risk factor was drug injection indicated the likelihood of bloodborne transmission of an "AIDS agent" and raised concerns about the nation's blood supply. Access to safe blood and blood products is a critical healthcare need for many individuals. Transfusions of whole blood or red blood cells are needed to replace excessive blood loss resulting from surgery, trauma, or medical conditions, while transfused white blood cells and platelets are used to prevent infection and bleeding in patients receiving intensive cancer chemotherapy. In addition, plasma (the liquid portion of blood) collected from thousands of individual donors can be pooled and fractionated (i.e., divided into components) to make a variety of products, including clotting factor concentrates.

Clotting factor concentrates are lifesaving for patients with hemophilia, an inherited bleeding disorder.[*] These individuals experience severe spontaneous or trauma-induced bleeding episodes. Bleeding into joints is common and may be disabling, while bleeding into the brain can be fatal. Hemophilia patients bleed because they have abnormally low levels of blood clotting factor VIII (hemophilia A, the most common form) or factor IX (hemophilia B).[†] The lower the level of the clotting factor, the more severe the disease. Treatment with factor VIII and factor IX concentrates greatly reduces bleeding episodes in hemophilia A and B patients, respectively, and improves both the quality and duration of their lives.

---

[*] The genes for factors VIII and IX are on the X chromosome. At least one normal gene for each factor is needed for the body to produce enough factor to prevent severe bleeding. Males inherit an X chromosome from their mother and a Y chromosome from their father, while females inherit an X chromosome from each parent. Almost all patients with hemophilia are male because they inherited a defective X chromosome gene from their mother. For a female to have hemophilia, she would have to inherit the defect from both parents, an exceedingly rare occurrence.

[†] In addition to hemophilia A and B, there are rarer forms of hemophilia that result from deficiencies of other clotting factors.

Harold W. Jaffe, *Blood and Blood Products* In: *Dispatches from the AIDS Pandemic*. Kevin M. De Cock, Harold W. Jaffe, and James W. Curran and Edited by: Robin Moseley, Oxford University Press. © Oxford University Press 2023. DOI: 10.1093/oso/9780197626528.003.0008

But along with the benefits of blood transfusions and blood products come risks, including the risk of infection. A variety of infections, including parasitic (e.g., malaria), bacterial (e.g., syphilis), and viral (e.g., HBV), are potentially transmitted through transfusion. The risk of infection with blood-borne viruses was particularly high for recipients of pooled plasma products, such as persons with hemophilia, because these products were derived from the blood of thousands of donors.

The blood-borne infection of most concern in the 1970s was HBV.[‡] Screening of blood donors for markers of HBV beginning in 1973, along with the elimination of paid blood donors, greatly reduced the risk of posttransfusion hepatitis.[§] [1] However, because of their need for frequent transfusions and heavy use of clotting factor concentrates, about 85 percent of patients with severe hemophilia had been infected with HBV by the early 1980s.[2] If, as suspected, the AIDS agent and HBV were transmitted similarly, the occurrence of AIDS in hemophilia patients and transfusion recipients might be expected.

On January 7, 1982, that expectation became a reality when N. Joel Ehrenkrantz, a physician at Cedars of Lebanon Hospital in Miami, Florida, called Michael Mallison, the EIS officer assigned to the Florida Department of Health, to report a hemophilia patient who had developed biopsy-proven PCP. In turn, Mallison forwarded the information to Bruce Evatt (Chapter 3).[3] Evatt had trained in hematology at Johns Hopkins University, served as an EIS officer in cancer epidemiology at CDC, returned to a faculty position at Hopkins, and was then recruited back to CDC to supervise its immunology, hematology, and pathology laboratories. His own research interests were in the field of blood coagulation, including hemophilia. Regarding the information received from Ehrenkrantz, Evatt recalled:

> We got a call. . . from a physician in Florida who said that he had a man, an elderly man, who was a hemophilia patient who had died with *Pneumocystis carinii* pneumonia. He was wondering whether or not the *Pneumocystis* could have been transmitted in a vial of [clotting factor] concentrate. The processing of concentrate would have eliminated *Pneumocystis*, and

---

[‡] In adults, most HBV infections resolve spontaneously. In 5 percent to 10 percent of cases, however, HBV becomes a chronic infection. Chronically infected persons who donated blood or plasma were the main source of HBV for transfusion recipients and persons with hemophilia.
[§] The residual risk of posttransfusion hepatitis was attributed to "non-A, non-B" hepatitis, which was subsequently found to result from hepatitis C virus.

I assured him [of] that. But it raised my curiosity because . . . hemophilia patients were sensitive to blood-borne diseases.[4]

Although this case was concerning, it was not clear that the patient had AIDS. He had received a brief course of steroids, which might have predisposed him to develop PCP. And the patient had died before he could be interviewed for potential risk factors or have laboratory studies done to characterize his presumed immune deficiency. I recall CDC Director Bill Foege saying that if this hemophilia patient had AIDS, there would be others. There were.

To ascertain whether additional cases were occurring, Evatt turned to CDC's Parasitic Disease Drug Service. As described in Chapter 2, the Drug Service was the only US source for pentamidine, the drug used to treat PCP. Evatt spoke to Sandy Ford, the CDC technician who ran the Drug Service and who early on had noticed an increase in pentamidine requests. He asked her to find out if the drug was being requested to treat PCP in hemophilia patients. She reported to Evatt that individual requests for use with hemophilia patients had been received in June and July 1982 from Colorado and Ohio, respectively.

Evatt asked Dale Lawrence[5] to investigate these newly recognized patients. Lawrence, a former EIS officer who had studied the genetics of immunity during a sabbatical at the University of Oxford, recalled that "Bruce called me and said, 'You've got to go to Colorado. We've got a case in the ICU [intensive care unit] there. They've called for pentamidine. He may not be alive much longer. Please try, if he's not on a respirator, interviewing him and talking to his wife.' I raced out there, and that became an intense week-long investigation."[5]

Lawrence, known as a meticulous researcher, further stated, "[I] got all the factor concentrate records from that person and 60 others. I put them on a giant spreadsheet: all the blood work, clinical studies, and factor concentrates."[5] Three weeks later, on the July 4 weekend, Lawrence traveled to northern Ohio to conduct a similarly detailed investigation of the third hemophilia patient with PCP.

On July 9, 1982, Foege sent a letter to all US hemophilia treatment centers to inform them that "three cases of *Pneumocystis carinii* pneumonia among patients with severe hemophilia A have recently been reported to the Centers for Disease Control."[6] He noted that "Although the cause of this immune dysfunction [described in patients with PCP] is unknown, the possibility of a transmissible agent has been suggested, and concerns about possible transmission through blood products has [sic] been raised."[6] Foege requested that similar cases be reported through state health departments to CDC.

A week later, more details about the three patients were published in the *MMWR*.[7] By this time, the Colorado patient had died. The three patients were described as heterosexual males with no history of IV drug use. Immunologic findings in the Colorado and Ohio patients were similar to those previously reported in homosexual men with PCP. None of the patients was known to have received factor VIII concentrates from the same lot. The editorial note accompanying the article stated that there were an estimated 20,000 Americans with hemophilia A, of whom about 60 percent were classified as having severe disease. The note also announced, "A Public Health Service advisory committee is being formed to consider the implications of these findings."[7]

On the same day the *MMWR* was published, July 16, 1982, FDA's Bureau of Biologics convened a meeting to discuss the CDC findings.[8] In addition to CDC and FDA attendees, the meeting included representatives of NIH, the National Hemophilia Foundation (NHF), the American Red Cross (ARC), and the American Blood Resources Association (ABRA), which represented the plasma fractionation companies that produced clotting factor concentrates. After reviewing the CDC data, the group decided to establish a "Committee on Opportunistic Infections in Patients with Hemophilia"[8] to share information and increase surveillance for OIs in hemophilia patients.

The Committee held a meeting, chaired by Foege, on July 27, 1982. Evatt described the meeting as very frustrating:

> Well, we presented that information [about the three cases], but we received somewhat of a cold shoulder. The blood banking industry is a very stable industry. . . The blood banking community wasn't interested at all in raising any kind of hassle about the fact that some of their donors may be donating and may be causing this disease. And three patients with hemophilia they felt was no proof at all. The hemophilia community was interested, but. . . they saw this drug [clotting factor concentrate] as being a major life-changing event for patients with hemophilia. And to raise the possibility that maybe it was transmitting this new disease, when there were only three cases, it was so rare that they didn't want patients stopping the medicine. . . The FDA didn't believe it was a disease. They were not particularly interested.[4]

One accomplishment of the meeting was agreement on a name for the new disease. At CDC, we were still calling it KS/OI, while some in the media used the term GRID (gay-related immune deficiency), an inaccurate and offensive label. Different accounts of the origin of the name AIDS (first acquired immune deficiency syndrome and then acquired immunodeficiency syndrome) have been given by meeting attendees.[9] Regardless of the origin, the meeting participants voted to call the disease AIDS—the name that continues today.**

Over the next four months, CDC received case reports of four additional hemophilia A patients that met the AIDS case definition. Three were heterosexual men, and the fourth was a ten-year-old boy. Two of the men had died. A seven-year-old boy with severe hemophilia A was also reported with suspected AIDS, although he had not yet met the case definition. The editorial note of the December 10, 1982, *MMWR* article describing these patients concluded that "[C]hildren with hemophilia must now be considered at risk for the disease. In addition, the number of cases continues to increase, and the illness may pose a significant risk for patients with hemophilia."[10]

In late November 1982, I received a call from Art Ammann. He first gave me an update on the family he had reported earlier (Chapter 7) then described another patient he had recently seen in San Francisco (Figure 8.1). The patient was a twenty-month-old boy born to a mother with Rh disease.†† Treatment of the infant's anemia and jaundice required administration of six exchange transfusions, a procedure in which the infant's entire blood volume is replaced by donor blood shortly after birth. The transfused blood had come from nineteen donors. On follow-up, the infant was noted to have an enlarged liver and spleen at four months of age. At age seven months, he was hospitalized with a severe ear infection, and at fourteen months he was found to have blood abnormalities and impaired immune function typical of AIDS. Culture of his bone marrow grew *Mycobacterium avium*, an AIDS-defining OI in adults. All the blood received by the infant had been collected from donors at the Irwin Memorial Blood Bank in San Francisco.

The firsthand accounts of the next steps in the investigation vary, but all agree that the list of blood donors, maintained by the Irwin Memorial Blood Bank, had to be compared with the list of reported AIDS patients,

---

** The first recorded use of "AIDS" at CDC was in a Task Force briefing document dated August 13, 1982 (Author's personal records).

†† Rh disease is a disorder that occurs in pregnancy when a mother and her unborn child have incompatible blood types. The mother's immune system forms antibodies against the baby's blood type, which then cross the placenta and begin to destroy the baby's red blood cells. Infants are born with severe anemia and jaundice, a serious condition called erythroblastosis fetalis.

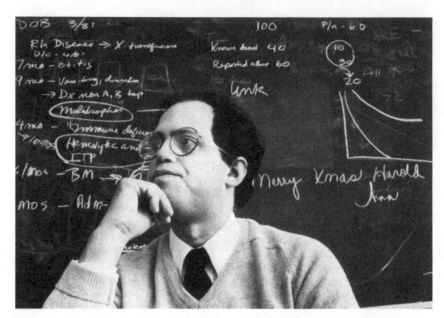

Figure 8.1. Harold Jaffe in his CDC office, late 1982. Notes on left side of blackboard refer to the San Francisco infant with transfusion-associated AIDS. (Science 83)

maintained by the San Francisco Department of Public Health. After confidentiality issues were addressed, the comparison took place. I remember receiving a call from Selma Dritz, the Assistant Director of Disease Control at the Health Department, telling me, "You're not going to believe this, but one of the blood donors is on our AIDS case list."

The donor was a male resident of San Francisco, who was in good health when he donated blood on March 10, 1981. The next day, platelets derived from the donation were administered to the infant. Eight months later the donor began feeling ill, and he was hospitalized with PCP in December 1981. He died of disseminated cytomegalovirus infection and a brain infection of unknown etiology in August 1982. The donor's risk factors for AIDS were unknown.

At the time, virtually all reported AIDS patients in San Francisco were gay men, so the blood donor stood out as very unusual. In fact, he was so unusual that he had been previously interviewed by CDC's Los Angeles-based EIS officer, David Auerbach, as part of an investigation of "no identified risk" patients. Auerbach remembered:

I met this man at his office. He was a very well-educated, sophisticated man. He understood the importance of what we were doing. I went through the whole questionnaire. He seemed to be very forthcoming. I should explain he was perhaps in his, I'll say, mid- to late-forties, I think. He was single. He'd never been married.[11]

Auerbach believed that the man was heterosexual. But when he discussed his interview with the CDC research sociologist, Bill Darrow, he recalled Darrow saying, "This man is gay, David—what don't you understand here?"[11] Darrow was right. After the donor's death, his brother went through his papers and found bills from a physician who was not the donor's physician of record. I asked Dave to contact this physician the next time he was in San Francisco. The San Francisco Health Department arranged a visit, and Auerbach found that the doctor had treated the man several times for rectal gonorrhea. The donor was gay.

The case report of the San Francisco infant was published in the December 10, 1982, issue of the *MMWR*.[12] The editorial note stated, "If the platelet transfusion contained an etiologic agent for AIDS, one must assume that the agent can be present in the blood of a donor before onset of symptomatic illness and that the incubation period for such illness can be relatively long."[12] The note also mentioned that two other cases of possible transfusion-associated AIDS were under investigation and ended by announcing that the Assistant Secretary for Health would be convening an advisory committee to address the possibility that the etiologic agent of AIDS could be blood borne.

Until this time, the mainstream media had paid little attention to AIDS. But that changed abruptly with the December 10th *MMWR* publication. I recall television crews from the then three major US networks lined up in the corridor outside my sub-basement CDC office, waiting to interview me about the San Francisco baby. I was glad that they were interested, but I wondered where they had been for the last eighteen months. I think the answer relates to the perception of AIDS that was held at the time by most Americans. As long as AIDS was seen as a problem of marginalized groups such as gay men, IV drug users, and Haitian immigrants, it was easy to ignore. But anyone might need a blood transfusion, and anyone was potentially at risk for the disease.

On the same day the *MMWR* article was published, a copy of an announcement of "The Second Open Meeting of the PHS Committee on Opportunistic Infections in Patients with Hemophilia" was sent to senior CDC staff.[13] The announcement stated that the purpose of the meeting was to "formulate recommendations for the prevention of AIDS with special emphasis on possible transmission through blood and blood products."[13] The meeting would take place in Atlanta on January 4, 1983, and would be chaired by CDC's Assistant Director for Public Health Practice, Jeffrey (Jeff) Koplan.[14] ‡‡

Although I have been unable to find a transcript of the meeting, I can provide an account of the meeting based on interviews with CDC participants, the contemporary reporting of the *Philadelphia Inquirer's* Donald Drake,[15] and my own recollections. In addition to CDC, FDA, and NIH, meeting participants included representatives of the nation's three major blood banking organizations—the ARC, the American Association of Blood Banks (AABB), and the Council of Community Blood Centers (CCBC)—as well as the NHF and plasma fractionation companies. Other attendees included representatives of two gay advocacy groups—the American Association of Physicians for Human Rights and the National Gay Task Force—several expert clinicians, and officials from the New York City and San Francisco health departments.

The meeting was structured to begin with an overview of the AIDS epidemic, followed by presentations of the CDC case investigations of AIDS in hemophilia patients and transfusion recipients, followed by a discussion of options for improving the safety of blood and blood products. I was expecting that the case presentations would be straightforward, with the real debate not starting until the discussion of prevention approaches. But I was wrong. The case presentations were immediately attacked for being inconclusive, with some attendees stating their doubts the patients even had AIDS. As Evatt recalled, "[W]e were met with a wall of criticism... we were jumping the gun, we didn't have an agent... we were jumping to conclusions... we were bad scientists."[4] I recall that at some point during this debate, Donald Armstrong, the highly respected Chief of Infectious Diseases at Memorial Sloan-Kettering Cancer Center, stood up and said that he couldn't believe what he was hearing. He said he had no doubts that the patients had AIDS and didn't understand why this was even being discussed. Armstrong was ignored and the debate continued.

The discussion of prevention options was no less contentious. Jim Curran began by presenting the two major prevention options: blood banks and commercial plasma fractionators could stop accepting donations from

‡‡ Koplan was to become CDC Director in 1998.

"high-risk" individuals, mainly homosexual men, or they could test the donation for a "surrogate marker" of the AIDS agent and discard donations that tested positive. The options were not mutually exclusive. Curran also pointed out the long incubation period between infection with the agent and the development of AIDS. Even if prevention measures were adopted immediately, their impact would not be seen for at least a year.

Roger Enlow and Bruce Voeller, representatives of the gay advocacy groups, spoke up immediately. They made the point that the homosexual community was a diverse group. Many gay men were not in the "fast lane" of men with multiple sex partners and frequent visits to bathhouses, the men at highest risk for AIDS. Banning gay men from donating blood would be highly stigmatizing. Enlow and Voeller advocated for the surrogate testing approach.

Because the AIDS agent had not yet been identified, testing of donors would require identifying a marker that would likely predict the presence of the agent. But what was the best surrogate marker? The Stanford University blood bank was already screening blood using a test for CD4 T-lymphocytes, cells that are depleted in AIDS. But this approach was considered impractical because it required sophisticated instruments not available to the great majority of blood banks. A more feasible approach would be to test blood for antibody to the hepatitis B core antigen, a marker of prior HBV infection. CDC immunologist Tom Spira (Chapter 7) presented data showing that the great majority of sexually active gay men would have a positive antibody test compared with about 5 percent of the general population. But the blood banking representatives opposed testing. Aaron Kellner of the New York Blood Center pointed out that such testing would cost the Blood Center more than $5 million to implement and would result in discarding 5 percent of donated blood. Given that blood banks struggled to keep up with demand, a 5 percent cut in supply would result in blood shortages.

As the arguments continued, CDC representatives became increasingly frustrated. Finally, Donald (Don) Francis ([16]) (Figure 8.2), a CDC epidemiologist/virologist, banged his fist on the table and said, "[T]his is so straightforward. You can't walk out of this room saying we need more research, that we need more studies of this."[16] In reflecting on the meeting that he had chaired, Koplan recalled, "It was a hell of a meeting. . . The outcome of the meeting was that we did not reach consensus. . . I think it's denial behavior [of the NHF and blood bankers]. It's like, I don't want to hear about those cases, we've got to do what we've got to do, don't tell me about that stuff."[14]

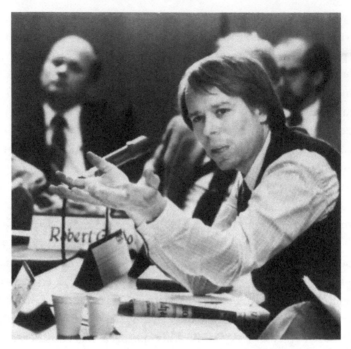

Figure 8.2. Don Francis at the January 4, 1983, blood safety meeting.
(Science 83)

Although the meeting participants failed to reach a consensus, the
meeting did result in actions by the participating organizations. On January
13, 1983, the three major blood banking organizations (ARC, AABB, and
CCBC) issued a joint statement to urge their members to extend educational
campaigns to physicians on balancing the risks and benefits of transfusions
and to encourage the use of autologous donations[§§] before elective surgeries.[8]
They further advised not targeting groups at increased risk for AIDS in donor
recruitment efforts but stopped short of recommending that blood banks exclude donations by members of these groups.

The next day, NHF published recommendations to prevent AIDS
in patients with hemophilia.[8] They advised using cryoprecipitate[***] instead of clotting factor concentrates in young children, patients who had

---

[§§] Autologous donation refers to collecting and banking blood from an individual and transfusing
the blood back to the same individual when required, such as during elective surgery.
[***] Cryoprecipitate is prepared from the plasma of an individual blood donor and was used to treat
hemophilia A before clotting factor concentrates became available.

never received concentrates, and patients with mild hemophilia. NHF also recommended that manufacturers of concentrate, who had historically relied heavily on paid donors, not collect plasma from high-risk populations and exclude (by direct questioning) donors at increased risk for AIDS. ABRA, representing companies involved in collecting plasma for production of clotting factor concentrates, also supported high-risk donor exclusion in its recommendations to members on January 28.[8] None of the three organizations advocated for the use of surrogate laboratory testing without further study.

Following the January 4 meeting, CDC also began drafting recommendations for the prevention of AIDS transmission through both sexual contact and transfusion. With input by FDA, NIH, and the Office of the Assistant Secretary for Health, the guidelines were published under the authorship of PHS in the March 4, 1983, issue of the *MMWR*.[17] Persons considered at increased risk for AIDS included those with signs or symptoms of the disease, sexual partners of AIDS patients, homosexual or bisexual men with multiple partners, Haitian entrants to the United States, past or present IV drug users, patients with hemophilia, and sexual partners of persons at increased risk. The prevention recommendations now included avoidance of sexual contact with persons with known or suspected AIDS and exclusion of persons at increased risk from blood donation. Persons in known risk groups were advised that having multiple sexual partners increased their probability of developing AIDS. Also included was a recommendation for further studies on procedures to identify blood donations at high risk of transmitting AIDS, including laboratory testing.

Looking back at these recommendations, Foege recalled:

[L]ess than two years after the first cases had been reported, the *MMWR* was able to provide an article on prevention of AIDS that is so good you can still use it today, and this was before we knew there was a virus. So, this is work we should look back on and understand the power of epidemiology to define something even before the science can define it.[18]

Subsequent CDC investigations further established proof of transfusion-associated AIDS. A 1984 article in the *New England Journal of Medicine* reported on eighteen patients whose only known risk factor was receipt of transfused blood within five years of their AIDS diagnosis.[19] Donor investigations, completed for seven of these patients, found one or more "high-risk" donors (a person with behavioral risk factors for AIDS and/or laboratory evidence of immunodeficiency) for each of the AIDS patients. None of these identified donors had AIDS or severe symptoms of immunodeficiency—evidence that the AIDS agent could be transmitted by infected individuals early in the course of their infection.

Soon after reports from the Institut Pasteur and the National Cancer Institute indicated that a novel retrovirus, now known as HIV, was likely the AIDS agent (Chapter 9), Paul Feorino,[20] a virologist who had been with CDC since 1957, reported isolating the virus from a blood donor-recipient pair.[21] The recipient had required transfusion with two units of packed red blood cells during surgery. PCP was diagnosed thirteen months after transfusion in the recipient and two months after donation in one of the donors, a homosexual man. Feorino and colleagues wrote that their findings offered further proof that the virus was the etiologic agent of AIDS.

After the discovery of HIV, major advances were made in reducing the risk of AIDS in transfusion recipients and persons with hemophilia. As described in Chapter 9, screening donated blood for antibodies to HIV made the blood supply much safer. The development of methods to inactivate HIV in clotting factor concentrates, as exemplified by the work of CDC scientists Steve McDougal and Linda Martin, also greatly reduced the threat of AIDS for persons with hemophilia.[22]

But before these interventions became available, many Americans became infected with HIV through receipt of infectious blood and blood products. In 1987, CDC estimated that approximately 12,000 persons living in the United States, excluding patients with hemophilia, had acquired HIV through blood transfusion between 1978 and 1984.[23] The overall prevalence of HIV in hemophilia A and B patients was estimated to be approximately 70 percent and 35 percent, respectively.[24] From 1988 through 1995, deaths due to AIDS in patients with hemophilia A exceeded all other causes of death combined for this population.[25]

Notes

1. Epstein JS, Jaffe HW, Alter HJ, Klein FG. Blood system changes since recognition of transfusion-associated AIDS. Transfusion 2013;58:2365–2374.
2. White GC II, Lesesne HR. Hemophilia, hepatitis, and the acquired immunodeficiency syndrome (Editorial). Ann Intern Med 1983;98:404.

3. Memorandum from Dale Lawrence to James Curran, June 29, 1982, (Author's personal records).

4. "EVATT, BRUCE," *The Global Health Chronicles*, accessed January 29, 2023, https://www.globalhealthchronicles.org/items/show/6479.

5. "LAWRENCE, DALE," *The Global Health Chronicles*, accessed January 29, 2023, https://www.globalhealthchronicles.org/items/show/7975.

6. Letter from William Foege to Hemophilia Treatment Centers, July 9, 1982, (Author's archives).

7. CDC. *Pneumocystis carinii* pneumonia among persons with hemophilia A. MMWR Morb Mortal Wkly Rep 1982;31:365–367.

8. Leveton LB, Sox HC Jr, Stoto MA (eds). HIV and the blood supply. An analysis of crisis decision making. Washington DC: National Academy Press; 1995.

9. J. Curran, J. Koplan, personal communications.

10. CDC. Update on acquired immune deficiency syndrome (AIDS) among patients with hemophilia A. MMWR Morb Mortal Wkly Rep 1982;31:644–652.

11. "AUERBACH, DAVID," *The Global Health Chronicles*, accessed January 29, 2023, https://www.globalhealthchronicles.org/items/show/8135

12. CDC. Possible transfusion-associated acquired immune deficiency syndrome (AIDS)—California. MMWR Morb Mortal Wkly Rep 1982;31:652–654.

13. "BLOOD BANKING," *The Global Health Chronicles*, accessed January 29, 2023, https://globalhealthchronicles.org/items/show/6579.

14. "KOPLAN, JEFFREY," *The Global Health Chronicles*, accessed January 29, 2023, https://www.globalhealthchronicles.org/items/show/5386.

15. Drake DC. The disease detectives puzzle over methods of control. Philadelphia Inquirer. January 9, 1983.

16. "FRANCIS, DON," *The Global Health Chronicles*, accessed January 29, 2023, https://www.globalhealthchronicles.org/items/show/6874.

17. CDC. Prevention of acquired immune deficiency syndrome (AIDS): report of inter agency recommendations. MMWR Morb Mortal Wkly Rep 1983;32:101–104.

18. "FOEGE, WILLIAM H," *The Global Health Chronicles*, accessed January 29, 2023, https://www.globalhealthchronicles.org/items/show/6480.

19. Curran JW, Lawrence DL, Jaffe HW, et al. Acquired immune deficiency syndrome (AIDS) associated with transfusions. N Engl J Med 1984;310:68–75.

20. "FEORINO, PAUL," *The Global Health Chronicles*, accessed January 29, 2023, https://www.globalhealthchronicles.org/items/show/7951.

21. Feorino PM, Kalyanaraman VS, Haverkos HW, et al. Lymphadenopathy-associated virus (LAV) infection of a blood donor-recipient pair with acquired immunedeficiency syndrome. Science 1984;225: 69–74.

22. McDougal JS, Martin LS, Cort SP, Mozen M, Heldebrant CM, Evatt BL. Thermal inactivation of the acquired immunodeficiency syndrome virus, human T lymphotropic virus–III/lymphadenopathy-associated virus, with special reference to antihemophilic factor. J Clin Invest 1985;76:875–877.

23. CDC. Human immunodeficiency virus infection in transfusion recipients and their family members. MMWR Morb Mortal Wkly Rep 1987;36:137–140.

24. CDC. Human immunodeficiency virus infection in the United States. MMWR Morb Mortal Wkly Rep 1987;36:801–804.
25. Chorba TL, Holman RC, Clarke MJ, Evatt BL. Effects of HIV infection on age and cause of death for persons with hemophilia A in the United States. Am J Hematol 2001;66:229–240.

9

HIV

Discovery, Diagnosis, and Disease

Harold W. Jaffe

As the epidemiologic evidence for an infectious cause of AIDS increased, so did the efforts of laboratory scientists to identify the causative agent. The working assumption of most investigators was that they were looking for a virus. Given that AIDS appeared to be a newly emerging disease, the virus would presumably be a new variant of a known human virus or a virus that had been newly introduced into humans. Further, the virus would have the capacity to cause progressive and presumably irreversible loss of CD4+ T-lymphocytes leading to immunodeficiency.

In a guest editorial in the *Journal of the National Cancer Institute* that was accepted for publication on March 10, 1983, Don Francis and Jim Curran from CDC and Myron (Max) Essex from the Harvard School of Public Health reviewed the epidemiology of AIDS and concluded that three groups of viruses should be studied further to find the etiologic agent.[1] As previously described, the epidemiology of HBV infection was like that of AIDS, and thus a related virus might be considered. However, AIDS patients did not typically have the liver dysfunction that would be characteristic of hepatitis virus infections. Herpes viruses, such as cytomegalovirus (CMV), also deserved study, but, as noted in Chapter 4, earlier studies did not identify a CMV strain that was specific to AIDS patients. The third group of viruses that merited special attention were retroviruses, RNA viruses that use the enzyme reverse transcriptase to make a DNA copy of their genome. This copy can then integrate into the genome of the infected host cell ("proviral DNA"), leading to lifelong infection. The authors noted two potential retroviral models for the AIDS virus: feline leukemia virus (FeLV) and human T-cell leukemia virus type I (HTLV-I).

FeLV was of special interest to Francis and Essex. Francis had served as an EIS officer in the 1970s and had participated in the smallpox eradication

Harold W. Jaffe, *HIV* In: *Dispatches from the AIDS Pandemic.* Kevin M. De Cock, Harold W. Jaffe, and James W. Curran and Edited by: Robin Moseley, Oxford University Press. © Oxford University Press 2023.
DOI: 10.1093/oso/9780197626528.003.0009

program and in the response to an Ebola virus outbreak in South Sudan. During a CDC-sponsored infectious diseases fellowship at Harvard, he became interested in the work on FeLV being done by Essex, a veterinarian and virologist. Francis became a doctoral student of Essex's, studying the epidemiology and virology of FeLV in domestic cats in Boston. Francis recalled, "Here we had a disease transmissible by close contact in cats that produced immunosuppression and cancer. When I finished [his doctoral research], there was no similar disease in humans. The closest were the hepatitis viruses in terms of their transmission pattern."[2] Because CDC had no program in retrovirology, Francis decided to join the agency's hepatitis program upon completion of his studies in Boston. At the time, the program was located in Phoenix, Arizona.

HTLV-I, the first known human retrovirus, was discovered in 1980 in the laboratory of Robert (Bob) Gallo at the National Cancer Institute (NCI)[3] and was then independently isolated by Japanese investigators.[4] The virus had the potential to "transform" normal T-lymphocytes into immortalized cells, leading to T-cell leukemia/lymphoma. Although initially thought to be limited to Japan and the Caribbean, HTLV-I was subsequently found to have a much wider geographic distribution and a broader spectrum of disease including a neurologic disorder—HTLV-I-associated myelopathy/tropical spastic paraparesis. Two years later, Gallo's laboratory isolated a second human retrovirus, HTLV-II, from a patient with hairy cell leukemia.[5] To date, however, HTLV-II has not been definitively linked to any human disease.

The May 20, 1983, issue of *Science* included four reports on retroviral infection and AIDS. Three of the reports suggested an association between AIDS and HTLV-I infection. Essex and colleagues, including Francis, reported that at least 25 percent of AIDS patients had antibodies against HTLV-I or a closely related virus.[6] Gallo's laboratory had two of the publications: the first described detection of proviral HTLV-I DNA in two of thirty-three AIDS patients,[7] and the second reported isolation of HTLV-I from the T-lymphocytes of another AIDS patient.[8] But the fourth report was different. Investigators from the laboratory of Luc Montagnier at the Institut Pasteur in Paris, led by Françoise Barré-Sinoussi, had isolated a novel retrovirus from a lymph node biopsy taken from a homosexual man with generalized lymph node enlargement, often a precursor to AIDS.[9] The virus grew in T-lymphocytes and appeared to be distinct from HTLV-I. Unlike HTLV-I, the virus killed, rather than transformed, infected lymphocytes. The authors wrote, "The role of this virus in the etiology of AIDS remains to be determined."[9]

CDC laboratories were also searching for the cause of AIDS. Walter Dowdle,[10] a distinguished virologist who was serving as Director of the agency's Center for Infectious Diseases recalled the scenario:

> The lab, of course, in the early days you didn't know exactly what you were looking for, so it was pretty well a shotgun approach to what it might be. But then it didn't take too long before it was very clear it was a retrovirus . . . . The only retrovirologist we had in CDC was actually working in hepatitis in Phoenix, and that was Don Francis. Don came to Atlanta and was actually actively involved in the lab work and starting it in earnest.[10]

In Atlanta, Francis faced the daunting task of establishing a new laboratory at a time when the Reagan administration was reducing federal spending. As Francis described the situation, "And so when I came and saw the laboratory that I was supposed to build in Atlanta, it was just a shock because compared to what we had. . . in Phoenix, it was nothing. So, it had to be built from the bottom up."[2] Nonetheless, he was able to hire several experienced retrovirologists, including V.S. Kalyanaraman who had been a member of Gallo's laboratory group at NCI. Francis and his team worked through the summer and fall of 1983, trying to find a retrovirus in clinical material from AIDS patients by cell culture, electron microscopy, and animal inoculation studies. Although some of their studies were suggestive of a retroviral infection, nothing definitive was found.

In early February 1984, Curran and Francis attended a retrovirology meeting in Park City, Utah, where they heard a talk by Jean-Claude Chermann, a member of Montagnier's laboratory group in Paris. Chermann described progress they had made in studies of the retrovirus that the laboratory had reported the previous May, now called lymphadenopathy-associated virus (LAV). He described obtaining multiple isolates of LAV from patients with generalized lymphadenopathy and with AIDS and developing an LAV antibody test, which was positive in many of these patients. Shortly after the Park City meeting, Chermann visited CDC, where he gave a seminar on the new findings. I remember walking out at the end of the seminar and thinking to myself that the Institut Pasteur group had done it. They had found the AIDS virus.

CDC virologist Paul Feorino (Chapter 8) was working in parallel with Don Francis's team. Most recently he was studying the role of Epstein-Barr virus, a herpesvirus, in lymphomas and was familiar with the techniques used to grow lymphocytes in culture. Feorino had received a blood sample from a patient with transfusion-associated AIDS and thought he had isolated a virus with characteristics similar to those that Chermann had observed for LAV. As he recalled,

> It was killing them, killing the white blood cells, which is consistent with the disease. It looked like LAV virus, and I'd seen pictures by that time from Montagnier. . . When Chermann was at CDC, and he came over to my lab. We were all excited because we said, "It killed the goddamn white cells."[11]

Subsequently, the isolate was sent to Paris where, according to Feorino, "Luc [Montagnier] tested the virus we found, and it was indeed LAV."[11]

In an April 7, 1984, article in *The Lancet*, the Montagnier laboratory reported isolating LAV from two brothers with hemophilia B.[12] One of the brothers had AIDS, while the other appeared to be healthy. The virus specifically infected CD4+ T-lymphocytes, the cells that are depleted in AIDS. In the *Discussion* section of the article, the authors noted that they had also isolated LAV from several additional AIDS patients, including a homosexual man with KS, a Haitian man, and a woman from Zaire. They also stated that antibodies against LAV were "widely distributed in the population at risk for AIDS"[12] but did not present supporting data.

While Montagnier and colleagues were characterizing LAV and its association with AIDS, Gallo's laboratory had changed the focus of its work from conducting additional studies on HTLV-I to a broader search for a retrovirus as the cause of AIDS. CDC had been providing Gallo with clinical specimens for his studies, and we were aware that he had isolated a novel retrovirus from AIDS patients. But we were unaware of the details of his findings until we saw drafts of papers about to be published in the May 4, 1984, issue of *Science*, where Gallo and colleagues reported the discovery of a new member of the HTLV virus family, HTLV-III. Antibodies to the virus were detected in almost 90 percent of patients with AIDS,[13] and the virus could be isolated from patients with AIDS and "pre-AIDS" (unexplained lymph node enlargement) as well as from the apparently well mothers of infants and children with AIDS.[14] A total of forty-seven HTLV-III isolates were reported. Moreover, the Gallo laboratory was able to grow the virus continuously in immortalized T-cells, allowing for production of large amounts of virus. The authors suggested that HTLV-III and LAV were different viruses but noted that "[I]t is possible that this is due to insufficient characterization of LAV."[15]

In recalling the situation, James (Jim) Mason ([16]), who followed Bill Foege as CDC Director in 1983, stated,

> NCI scientists weren't sharing information with us. CDC didn't know about their research findings. We only knew about the French accomplishments. A *New York Times* medical reporter [Lawrence Altman] visited CDC a week before Secretary Heckler's [Margaret Heckler, the Secretary of the US Department of Health and Human Services] announcement [regarding Gallo's discovery]. I knew him [Altman] personally, and he asked me when I thought the virus causing AIDS would be discovered. I responded that the French had probably already isolated the virus. . . A week later the *New York Times* heard about the planned press conference in Washington about the [Gallo] virus causing AIDS. . . The *New York Times* went back to my conversation a week earlier with their reporter. They published an article on Sunday [April 22, 1984] with my picture on the front page, reporting the French had isolated the AIDS virus. This was the day before Margaret Heckler, Ed Brandt [the Assistant Secretary for Health], and Bob Gallo's planned press conference.[16]

Mason was asked to attend the April 23 press conference. As he recalled, when he arrived in Washington, he was informed that

> [T]hey were going to announce that NIH had isolated the AIDS virus, and NIH would have developed an AIDS vaccine within a year or two. I advised them that making either statement would be a mistake. I suggested they announce that both NIH and French scientists had isolated the virus responsible for AIDS and warned them not to promise an AIDS vaccine in a year or two.[16]

But at the press conference, Heckler stated that "the probable cause of AIDS has been found—a variant of a known human cancer virus, called HTLV-III. . . credit must go to our eminent Dr. Robert Gallo"[17] (Figure 9.1). When later asked if he thought he might be fired for asserting that Montagnier's laboratory had discovered that LAV was the cause of AIDS, Mason replied, "I

1-231127U114007 04/23/84 ICS WA12139   NYAA
01233 MLTN VA 04/23/84

JOHN MILES
AIDS PROGRAM OFC.
NY STATE HLTH DEPT.
125 WORTH ST., RM. 608
NEW YORK, NY 10013

TO ALL STATE & TERRITORIAL EPIDEMIOLOGISTS & STATE HEALTH
OFFICERS AND SELECTED BIG CITY AND COUNTY HEALTH OFFICERS:
ON APRIL 23, 1984, SECRETARY MARGARET HECKLER OF THE DEPARTMENT
OF HEALTH AND HUMAN SERVICES ANNOUNCED RECENT FINDINGS FROM THE
NATIONAL CANCER INSTITUTE RELATED TO RETROVIRUSES AS THE PROBABLE
CAUSE OF AIDS. BECAUSE OF THE PUBLIC HEALTH IMPORTANCE OF THE AIDS
PROBLEM IN MANY PARTS OF THE COUNTRY, AND BECAUSE OF THE ATTEN-
TION BEING GIVEN TO IT BY THE MEDIA, THIS LETTER IS BEING
PROVIDED TO SUMMARIZE OUR PRESENT UNDERSTANDING OF THE ROLE
HUMAN RETROVIRUSES PLAY IN THIS DISEASE.
FOR SOME TIME EPIDEMIOLOGIC EVIDENCE HAS INDICATED THAT AIDS IS
CAUSED BY A TRANSMISSIBLE INFECTIOUS AGENT MOST LIKELY A VIRUS.
OF THE MANY DIFFERENT TYPES OF VIRUSES, THE RETROVIRUSES HAVE
BEEN CONSIDERED THE BEST CANDIDATES. INFECTIONS CAUSED BY
PARTICULAR RETROVIRUSES IN ANIMALS INCLUDES FELINE LEUKEMIA,
BOVINE LEUKEMIA, AND EQUINE INFECTIOUS ANEMIA. SUCH ANIMAL
INFECTIONS ALSO SHARE IMMUNOLOGIC AND PATHOLOGIC CHARACTER-
ISTICS WITH AIDS IN MAN. PARTICULAR ANIMAL RETROVIRUSES ALSO
EXHIBIT AN AFFINITY FOR LYMPHOCYTES, AGAIN A CHARACTERISTIC
WHICH WOULD BE EXPECTED OF THE ETIOLOGIC AGENT OF AIDS.
THE FIRST HUMAN RETROVIRUS WAS ISOLATED AT THE NATIONAL CANCER
INSTITUTE; IT WAS DESIGNATED HUMAN T-CELL LEUKEMIA VIRUS
(HTLV-I). IT WAS IDENTIFIED AS THE CAUSE OF ADULT T-CELL
LEUKEMIA, A NEOPLASTIC DISEASE COMMON IN SOUTHERN JAPAN BUT
RARE IN THE UNITED STATES. IN THE MAY 20, 1983 ISSUE OF SCI-
ENCE, SEROLOGIC, VIROLOGIC AND EPIDEMIOLOGIC EVIDENCE OF AN
ASSOCIATION OF THIS VIRUS WITH AIDS WAS PRESENTED, IN
THIS VIRUS AIDS WAS PRESENTED, IN THIS SAME ISSUE OF SCIENCE.
WORKERS AT THE PASTEUR INSTITUTE IN PARIS REPORTED ANOTHER
RETROVIRUS, NOW TERMED LYMPHADENOPATHY-ASSOCIATED VIRUS (LAV.)
THE PASTEUR INSTITUTE SHOWED HTLV-I AND LAV TO DIFFER BIOCH-
EMICALLY AND SEROLOGICALLY. ANTIBODIES TO LAV WERE ALSO FOUND
TO BE PRESENT IN A SIGNIGICATLY HIHER PROPORTION OF LYMPHADEN
OPATHY SYNDROME (LAS) AND AIDS PATIENTS THAN IN CONTROLS
(TO BE PUBLISHED). THE GROUP FROM PASTEUR INSTITUTE REPORTED IN
THE APRIL 7TH ISSUES OF LANCET THAT A VIRUS, POSSIBLY IDENTICAL
TO LAV WAS ISOLATED FROM 2 SIBLINGS WITH HEMOPHILLIS B.
AS SECRETARY HECKLER HAS PERFORMED STUDIES THAT IMPLICATE A

TO REPLY BY MAILGRAM MESSAGE, SEE REVERSE SIDE FOR

Figure 9.1. Western Union Mailgram from Jim Mason to state health departments concerning Margaret Heckler's announcement. (Mary Chamberland, personal collection)

thought I might and didn't care."[16] Mason was not fired and became a trusted advisor to Secretary Heckler.

The story of the ensuing controversy over which laboratory discovered the cause of AIDS is complex and beyond the scope of this chapter.* In summary, LAV and HTLV-III were eventually found to be the same virus.[18] The virus was also independently isolated by Jay Levy and colleagues from the University of California, San Francisco, and named AIDS-associated retrovirus (ARV).[19] In May 1986, the International Committee on Taxonomy of Viruses proposed that the virus causing AIDS be named human immunodeficiency virus.[20] The current scientific consensus is that the Montagnier laboratory was the first to isolate the virus, and the Gallo laboratory established that the virus was the cause of AIDS. Françoise Barré-Sinoussi and Luc Montagnier were awarded the 2008 Nobel Prize for Medicine "for their discovery of human immunodeficiency virus."†

Once HIV had been found to be the cause of AIDS, the highest public health priority became the development of a diagnostic test for the virus. Viral isolation in cell culture was far too complex and time consuming to be used outside of a few research laboratories, so attention turned to creating an HIV antibody test. For most viral infections, the immune system recognizes the virus and eliminates it from the body. A positive test for antibodies in blood indicates past viral infection or immunization against the virus. But HIV was different. Because it is a retrovirus whose genetic material integrates into host cell DNA, infection persists for the life of the host. A positive antibody test for HIV would indicate that an individual had been infected with the virus and was potentially infectious to others. In her remarks at the April 23 press conference, Secretary Heckler announced that an antibody test for HIV would be widely available within approximately six months. To facilitate commercial development of a test, NCI made bulk quantities of HIV available to interested companies. In the meanwhile, research laboratories worked with their own in-house antibody tests to gain a better understanding of the prevalence of HIV infection in populations at increased risk for AIDS, the potential use of antibody tests to screen blood donors, and disease progression in persons found to be infected.

---

* See Reference 18 for an account of this controversy.
† Barré-Sinoussi and Montagnier shared the Prize with Harald zur Hausen, a German virologist who discovered that human papilloma viruses caused cervical cancer.

Most of the research antibody tests for HIV were enzyme-linked immunosorbent assays (ELISAs). The technology of ELISA (also known as EIA, enzyme immunoassay) was well established and could easily be scaled to test large numbers of samples. Early studies using ELISA tests found detectable HIV antibody in 22 percent to 65 percent of homosexual men, 87 percent of IDUs seen at a detoxification center in New York City, 56 percent to 72 percent of persons with hemophilia A, and 35 percent of women who were the sexual partners of men with AIDS.[21] In contrast, less than 1 percent of persons with no known risk factors for AIDS were seropositive.

At CDC, Paul Feorino used an ELISA, developed by Kalyanaraman and fellow CDC laboratorian Jane Getchell, to investigate twenty-four patients with transfusion-associated AIDS and the persons who had donated the transfused blood.[22] The ELISA was positive in the six patients with transfusion-associated AIDS who were available for testing; all six were also culture positive for HIV. Of twenty-three seropositive donors with evaluable culture results, twenty-two were culture positive an average of two years after their donations. Most of the donors had remained asymptomatic. The authors concluded that "The persistence of infection with HTLV-III/LAV [HIV] in asymptomatic donors supports the use of serologic screening to supplement current procedures for the identification of blood donors from populations with an increased incidence of AIDS."[22]

We also used the CDC ELISA to examine the outcomes of HIV infection in a large cohort of gay men who had been treated for STDs at the San Francisco City Clinic.[23] The cohort, which was established to study the epidemiology of HBV in gay men, began enrolling patients in 1978 and had followed the patients prospectively for six years. As of December 1984, 2.4 percent of the 6,875 cohort members had been reported to have AIDS. Physical examination of a representative sample of cohort members conducted in 1984 found that another 21 percent of these men had generalized lymph node enlargement. Antibody testing of both stored and recently collected blood specimens found that the HIV infection rate in the cohort had increased from 4.5 percent in 1978 to 67.4 percent in 1984. Thus, the epidemic of AIDS and related conditions in these men was preceded by an epidemic of HIV infection (Figure 9.2) with an average interval of forty-three months between the first positive antibody test and the diagnosis of AIDS. We concluded that the 8,000 AIDS cases reported in the United States at the end of 1984 could indicate that about 240,000 Americans were already infected with the virus, writing that "[E]ven if all transmission of the virus were to stop immediately,

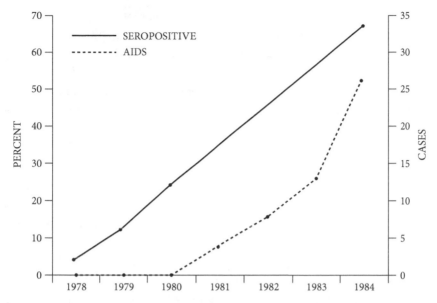

Figure 9.2. Percent of men seropositive for HTLV(HIV) antibody and number with AIDS by year of diagnosis. (Jaffe HW, Darrow WW, Echenberg DF, et al. AIDS in a cohort of homosexual men. A six-year follow-up study. Ann Intern Med 1985;103:210–214).

the acquired immunodeficiency syndrome would continue to be a major health problem for the foreseeable future."[23]

Anticipating the licensure of commercial HIV antibody tests, PHS issued provisional guidelines for their use on January 11, 1985.[21] The guidelines stated that all potential blood donors should be informed that their donated blood or plasma would be tested for HIV antibodies. If individuals did not want their blood or plasma tested, they would not be accepted as donors. Blood or plasma testing positive would not be used for transfusion or manufacturing into blood products. Before donors were notified of a positive test result, the test would have to be repeated. Donors found to be repeatedly positive by EIA would be referred for medical evaluation, which could include the use of other tests to confirm the infection. The most widely used confirmatory test was the Western blot, an assay that used electrophoresis to separate and identify viral proteins by their molecular weight. The guidelines also emphasized the importance of maintaining the confidentiality of positive test results and provided information and advice for seropositive individuals.

On March 1, 1985, FDA licensed Abbott Laboratories to sell the first commercially available EIA for HIV antibody detection. This test and tests of other manufacturers that would soon follow enabled HIV antibody screening of donated blood and plasma and were also approved for medical diagnostic use. Blood banks quickly implemented donor testing, with 155 collection centers testing more than 1.1 million units of blood through mid-June 1985.[24] This screening was estimated to have removed as many as 1,000 potentially infectious units of blood from the US blood supply.

Because of a concern that high-risk individuals might seek to determine whether they were HIV infected by volunteering to be blood donors, CDC proposed establishing a network of "alternate" testing sites. These sites would also ensure that individuals seeking HIV testing receive pre- and post-test counseling along with referral for medical evaluation, if needed. Patients had the option of being tested anonymously. Although the rationale for these testing sites seemed sound, the proposal was opposed by several large city health departments, including the Philadelphia Department of Public Health. In a strongly worded letter to Secretary Heckler, Philadelphia health officials and academic physicians urged her to "immediately reconsider" the plan for alternative testing sites. ([25]). The authors argued that "[T]he test is not clinically useful, and it does not currently enable physicians to either predict or change the patient's outcome."[25] Further, they wrote that a positive test result "[M]ay have a significant negative impact on a person's emotional status."[25] Despite these dissenting views, CDC funded fifty-five state and local health departments to establish alternate sites for HIV antibody testing.[26] By the end of 1985, almost 80,000 persons had been tested at these sites, with 17.3 percent of these individuals testing repeatedly positive by EIA.[‡]

Some gay advocacy groups also voiced their opposition to HIV testing other than by blood banks, maintaining that testing would lead to harms without benefits.[27] They argued that without stronger confidentiality requirements, persons whose HIV infection became known to others could be subject to stigma and discrimination, loss of insurance, and, potentially, loss of housing and employment. Given that no treatment for HIV existed, they saw no clinical benefits for testing and believed that all gay men needed to reduce their risk behaviors, regardless of their infection status. The accuracy of testing was also challenged. In his book *How to Survive a Plague,* David

---

[‡] In 1985, CDC established a proficiency testing program to assure the accuracy of HIV antibody testing done by these laboratories.

France quotes Dr. Stephen Caiazza, President of the New York Physicians for Human Rights, as saying, "To put it simply, this test helps no one. . . The test is so primitive that we cannot know who is who [who is infected and who is uninfected]."[28] The perspective of some gay activists was captured by their slogan, "No Test is Best."

Over the ensuing years, attitudes about testing gradually changed. Health departments established an excellent record of maintaining the confidentiality of test results. Legal protections from discrimination against HIV-infected individuals were strengthened,[§] and the accuracy of antibody testing improved. But most importantly, the introduction of prophylaxis for OIs and the subsequent development of effective treatment for HIV, including its use in reducing mother-to-child transmission, meant that individuals could gain life-saving benefits by knowing that they were infected. Voluntary counseling and testing became a critically important component in efforts to control the AIDS epidemic, both in the United States and around the world.

Notes

1. Francis DP, Curran JW, Essex M. Epidemic acquired immune deficiency syndrome: epidemiologic evidence for a transmissible agent. J Natl Cancer Inst 1983;71:1–4.
2. "FRANCIS, DON," The Global Health Chronicles, accessed January 29, 2023, https://www.globalhealthchronicles.org/items/show/6874.
3. Poiesz BJ, Ruscetti FW, Gazdar AF, Bunn PA, Minna JD, Gallo RC. Detection and isolation of type C retrovirus particles from fresh and cultured lymphocytes of a patient with cutaneous T-cell lymphoma. Proc Natl Acad Sci USA 1980;77:7415–7419.
4. Yoshida M, Miyoshi I, Hinuma Y. Isolation and characterization of retrovirus from cell lines of human adult T-cell leukemia and its implication in the disease. Proc Natl Acad Sci USA 1982;79:2031–2035.
5. Kalyanaraman VS, Sarngadharan MG, Robert-Guroff M, Miyoshi I, Golde D, Gallo RC. A new subtype of human T-cell leukemia virus (HTLV-II) associated with a T-cell variant of hairy cell leukemia. Science 1982;218:571–573.
6. Essex M, McLane MF, Lee TH, et al. Antibodies to cell membrane antigens associated with human T-cell leukemia virus in patients with AIDS. Science 1983;220:859–862.
7. Gelman EP, Popovic M, Blayney D, et al. Proviral DNA of a retrovirus, human T-cell leukemia virus, in two patients with AIDS. Science 1983;220:862–865.

§ The 1990 Americans with Disabilities Act, which guarantees equal opportunities for individuals with disabilities, also protects persons with HIV infection.

8. Gallo RC, Sarin PS, Gelman EP, et al. Isolation of human T-cell leukemia virus in ac-quired immune deficiency syndrome. Science 1983;220:865–867.

9. Barré-Sinoussi F, Chermann J-C, Rey F, et al. Isolation of a T-lymphotropic retrovirus from a patient at risk for acquired immune deficiency syndrome (AIDS). Science 1983;220:868–871.

10. "DOWDLE, WALTER," The Global Health Chronicles, accessed January 29, 2023, https://www.globalhealthchronicles.org/items/show/5394.

11. "FEORINO, PAUL," The Global Health Chronicles, accessed January 29, 2023, https://www.globalhealthchronicles.org/items/show/7951.

12. Vilmer E, Barre-Sinoussi F, Rouzioux C, et al. Isolation of new lymphotropic retrovirus from two siblings with haemophilia B, one with AIDS. Lancet 1984;1(8380):753–757.

13. Sarngadharan MG, Popovic M, Bruch L, Schüpbach J, Gallo RC. Antibodies reactive with human T-lymphotropic retroviruses (HTLV-III) in the serum of patients with AIDS. Science 1984;224:506–508.

14. Gallo RC, Salahuddin SZ, Popovic M, et al. Frequent detection and isolation of cyto-pathic retroviruses (HTLV-III) in patients with AIDS and at risk for AIDS. Science 1984;224:500–503.

15. Popovic M, Sarngadharan MG, Read E, Gallo RC. Detection, isolation, and contin-uous production of cytopathic retroviruses (HTLV-III) from patients with AIDS and pre-AIDS. Science 1984;224:497–500.

16. "MASON, JAMES," The Global Health Chronicles, accessed January 29, 2023, https://www.globalhealthchronicles.org/items/show/8047.

17. Press conference, Secretary Margaret Heckler, April 23, 1984. https://quod.lib.umich.edu/c/cohenaids/5571095.0488.004?rgn=main;view=fulltext

18. Vahlne A. A historical reflection on the discovery of human retroviruses. Retrovirology 2009;6:40.

19. Levy JA, Hoffman AD, Kramer SM, Landis JA, Shimabukuro JM, Oshiro LS. Isolation of lymphocytopathic retroviruses from San Francisco patients with AIDS. Science 1984;225:840–842.

20. Coffin J, Haase A, Levy JA, et al. Human immunodeficiency viruses. Science 1986;232:697.

21. CDC. Provisional Public Health Service inter-agency recommendations for screening donated blood and plasma for antibody to the virus causing acquired immunodefi-ciency syndrome. MMWR Morb Mortal Wkly Rep 1985;34:1–5.

22. Feorino PM, Jaffe HW, Palmer E, et al. Transfusion-associated acquired immunode-ficiency syndrome—evidence for persistent infection in blood donors. N Engl J Med 1985;312:1293–1296.

23. Jaffe HW, Darrow WW, Echenberg DF, et al. The acquired immunodeficiency syn-drome in a cohort of homosexual men. A six-year follow-up study. Ann Intern Med 1985;103:210–214.

24. CDC. Update: Public Health Service workshop on human T-lymphotropic virus type III antibody testing—United States. MMWR Morb Mortal Wkly Rep 1985;34:477–478.

25. "HTLV-III ANTIBODY TEST: Alternative Testing Sites," *The Global Health Chronicles*, accessed January 29, 2023, https://www.globalhealthchronicles.org/items/show/6576.

26. CDC. Human T-lymphotropic virus type III /lymphadenopathyassociated virus antibody testing at alternate sites. MMWR Morb Mortal Wkly Rep 1986;35:284–287.

27. Bayer R, Edington C. HIV testing, human rights, and global AIDS policy: exceptionalism and its discontents. J Health Polit Policy Law 2009;34:301–323.

28. France D. How to survive a plague: The story of how activists and scientists tamed AIDS. New York: Random House; 2017.

10

Responding to Fears

Real and Imagined Threats

Harold W. Jaffe

In the early days of the epidemic, AIDS was a terrifying disease. Once AIDS had developed in adults, their average survival time was about six to eighteen months[1]—less than the average patient survival time for all but the most aggressive cancers. The threat of AIDS was all too real for MSM in the United States, the population first recognized with the disease, and their fears were well justified. Fear then spread to healthcare workers (HCWs), including both clinical and laboratory staff, who risked acquiring the disease through occupational exposures to blood and other body fluids of HIV-infected patients. When cases were identified in partners of bisexual men and IDUs, sexually active heterosexuals became worried that the epidemic might sweep through the heterosexual population, as it had done in MSM. And the public developed unfounded fears that HIV might be spread by other routes, such as through everyday "casual" contact or insect bites. Responding to these fears required studies to determine risks and then effective communication of study findings by trusted figures and organizations.

Although PHS had published early AIDS prevention recommendations for MSM that emphasized the risk associated with having multiple sexual partners,[2] CDC lacked funding for communication efforts to promote behavioral change in MSM. Much of the educational efforts came from national organizations, including the American Association of Physicians for Human Rights, and local organizations such as the Gay Men's Health Crisis in New York City.[3] Once the threat of AIDS was recognized by MSM, reported rates of both gonorrhea and syphilis for this population fell—surrogate indicators of sexual behavior change.[3,4]

Also at clear risk were HCWs, who had a long and unfortunate history of acquiring infections with bloodborne pathogens through occupational exposure. For example, a 1985 CDC study of over 5,000 hospital employees

Harold W. Jaffe, *Responding to Fears* In: *Dispatches from the AIDS Pandemic.* Kevin M. De Cock, Harold W. Jaffe, and James W. Curran and Edited by: Robin Moseley, Oxford University Press. © Oxford University Press 2023. DOI: 10.1093/oso/9780197626528.003.0010

found that 14 percent had serologic evidence of past or present infection with HBV.[5] Infection rates were highest in workers with frequent occupational exposure to blood and were independently associated with frequency of needlestick accidents. CDC first published AIDS precautions for clinical and laboratory workers in the November 5, 1982, issue of the *MMWR*,[6] noting the similarities in the risk factors for HBV infections and AIDS. The article stated that no hospital personnel had been reported with AIDS resulting from contact with AIDS patients or clinical specimens. Nonetheless, these workers were urged to take steps to reduce exposure to blood and advised that "Extraordinary care must be taken to avoid accidental wounds from sharp instruments contaminated with infectious material. . . from AIDS patients."[6]

Over the ensuing eight months, four HCWs with AIDS were reported as not having behavioral risk factors for the disease.[7] My CDC colleague Allyn Nakashima and I participated in the investigation of one of these patients, a man who worked in the housekeeping department of a Baltimore hospital. The patient had died before Allyn and I could interview him, but he had denied known risk factors for AIDS when questioned by his physicians. We determined that his duties could have exposed him to blood and that he had sustained a needlestick injury while disposing of a box containing used needles. However, no direct contact with the blood of an AIDS patient could be documented. The other three HCW cases were judged less likely to have had blood exposures than the Baltimore patient, and no conclusions were reached regarding their sources of infection.

In October 1984, I received a call from a colleague, a British virologist whom I had met the previous year in London. He wanted to let me know about a nurse in a London hospital who appeared to have been infected with HIV as the result of a needlestick injury that had involved exposure to the blood of an AIDS patient. To maintain confidentiality, the case report was to be published anonymously in *The Lancet,* but my colleague felt that CDC should be aware of the report before the publication date. In the pre-fax, pre-email era, the only way we could devise to transmit the report quickly was to have his personal assistant read it to my secretary, who dutifully recorded the details with her electric typewriter. On December 12, 1984, CDC's head of infectious diseases, Walter Dowdle, sent a memo to all the country's state and territorial epidemiologists, alerting them to the upcoming *Lancet* report and requesting that all HCWs with AIDS be reported so that appropriate investigations could be initiated.[8]

The case report, published on December 15, 1984, was described by *The Lancet* as "news of worrying events in a British hospital."[9] The needlestick sustained by the nurse was unusual in that a small amount of the AIDS patient's blood may have been injected into the nurse. Several weeks later, the nurse developed a severe "flu-like" illness, now recognized as evidence of acute HIV infection. A blood sample drawn two weeks after the onset of illness was negative for HIV antibodies, but samples obtained several months later were antibody positive. The report concluded that "The utmost care should be taken to avoid self-inoculation when handling blood and blood-products from a patient with HTLV-III [HIV]-related disease."[9]

Although the British case report established that HCWs could acquire HIV following exposure to the blood of an AIDS patient, other studies were needed to determine the frequency and risk factors for occupational transmission. Under the leadership of Steven Solomon and Eugene McCray[10] of CDC's Hospital Infections Program, a prospective surveillance system had been started in August 1983, more than a year before the *Lancet* publication. Through this system, HCWs with documented exposure to blood and other body fluids of patients with definite or confirmed AIDS were followed for the development of signs or symptoms suggestive of AIDS; HIV antibody testing was added when it became available.

McCray had completed a residency in internal medicine at the University of North Carolina in Chapel Hill before joining CDC as an EIS officer earlier in 1983. As McCray recalled,

> I took care of several people who were dying from this disease. Of course, we didn't know what it was, and there was a lot of fear in Chapel Hill at the time. Nurses were actually refusing to take care of patients who were living with HIV, so, as a resident and intern, we did a lot of the nursing care... When I came to CDC and, more involved, I spent a huge amount of time traveling and giving educational seminars to nurses, to prison guards, to a number of different folks in healthcare settings about risk related to transmission of this disease.[10]

Fear of caring for AIDS patients extended beyond hospital settings to dental offices. The AIDS clinic at Grady Memorial Hospital in Atlanta, where I volunteered as a physician provider, established its own dental clinic to serve clients who were denied care elsewhere. Ironically, many dentists were not practicing basic infection control measures. In the late 1980s, I asked my own dentist, who wore neither masks nor gloves, if he was worried about HIV infection. He replied that he wasn't worried because, "We don't see those kinds of patients in this practice." I thought to myself: Would you like to bet on that?

CDC published updated results from the HCW surveillance system in 1984, 1986, and 1988.[11,12,13] By the time of the last report, three infections had been documented in HCWs who had experienced needlestick exposures to the blood of an HIV-infected patient. Two of the three exposures occurred when the worker sustained an accidental injury from a needle used by a co-worker during attempted resuscitation of an AIDS patient. The rate of HIV seroconversion for 860 exposed workers was 0.35 percent.[13] The authors noted that although only one additional seroconversion had been reported in other prospective studies of about seven hundred HCWs, thirteen case reports of well-documented HIV acquisition in healthcare settings had been published. Nine of the thirteen infections occurred following injuries with needles or other sharp instruments, while four involved other types of blood exposure.

To reinforce the message that the risk of HIV infection in the workplace could be reduced by taking precautions to avoid blood exposures, CDC published additional prevention recommendations in November 1985.[14] These recommendations, made in consultation with multiple public health and professional organizations, went beyond risk reduction for clinical and laboratory personnel in hospitals to include precautions for homecare of AIDS patients, as well as guidelines for sterilization, disinfection, house-keeping, and waste disposal.* The broad input to these guidelines added to their credibility. Respected authorities in hospital infection control, such as Julie Gerberding at San Francisco General Hospital (who later became CDC Director) and David Henderson at the NIH Clinical Center, were also effective spokespersons in addressing HCW concerns.

Nonetheless, some individuals, such as Lorraine Day, Chief of Orthopedic Surgery at San Francisco General Hospital, continued to spread fear among HCWs and received considerable media attention. Day insisted that the risk of HIV infection for surgeons was much greater than the estimates from

---

* CDC later issued "universal precautions" guidelines, under which blood and certain body fluids of *all* patients are considered potentially infectious for HIV, HBV, and other bloodborne pathogens. (CDC. Perspectives in disease prevention and health promotion update: universal precautions for prevention of transmission of human immunodeficiency virus, hepatitis B virus, and other bloodborne pathogens in health-care settings. MMWR Morb Mortal Wkly Rep 1988; 37;377–388).

CDC or her hospital colleague, Gerberding. The risk, according to Day, was particularly high during orthopedic procedures, in which the use of surgical power instruments, such as bone drills and saws, might generate aerosols containing HIV. As reported by the *Los Angeles Times*, "Day spoke out for mandatory HIV testing of all hospital patients, and, finally, she donned a full-body 'space suit' while operating on patients classified as high-risk for the disease."[15] She was also quoted as saying, "the virus goes through them [surgical masks] like BBs through a tennis net."[15] Fearing for her safety, Day left her hospital job and wrote a book, *AIDS: What the Government Isn't Telling You.*

To examine the occupational risk of HIV infection for orthopedic surgeons like Lorraine Day, CDC collaborated with the American Academy of Orthopedic Surgeons to conduct a voluntary HIV serosurvey (Figure 10.1) of attendees at the Academy's annual meeting in March 1991.[16] Participants completed self-administered questionnaires, which included information about their surgical practices, exposures to blood, and non-occupational risk factors for HIV infection. Although surgeons were not asked specifically about their use of power instruments, it was assumed that many used them. Results of HIV antibody testing were available within forty-eight hours and

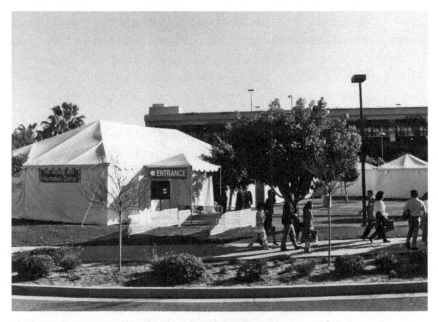

Figure 10.1. Testing tent for the 1991 American Academy of Orthopedic Surgeons' HIV serosurvey. (Mary Chamberland, personal collection)

were provided anonymously to participants. Although almost 40 percent of 3,420 participants reported a percutaneous (skin-penetrating) injury with a sharp object contaminated with a patient's blood in the previous month, only two (0.06%) were found to be HIV infected—both of whom reported nonoccupational risk factors. While the findings of the study were very reassuring with respect to HIV infection risk, the high rates of blood exposure were concerning and reinforced the need to comply with recommended precautions for preventing these exposures.

From 1985 to 2013, CDC received reports of fifty-eight HCWs with documented, occupationally acquired HIV infection.[17] Of these HCWs, only one was infected after 1999: a laboratory worker who sustained a needlestick injury while working with a culture of HIV. The editorial note of the *MMWR* describing these findings stated that acquisition of HIV in HCWs had become rare in the United States. The reduction in risk could be attributed to better infection control practices and the use of antiretroviral therapy to reduce infectiousness of patients' blood as well as postexposure prophylaxis with antiretroviral drugs in exposed HCWs.[18]

As described earlier (Chapter 5), heterosexual transmission of the "AIDS agent" was reported early in the epidemic, but the magnitude of the risk of infection for Americans was unknown. Lacking this information, both the perception of risk and fear of infection rapidly grew. CDC's Mary Chamberland (Chapter 3), who had worked on studies of heterosexual transmission, recalled, "There was a growing sort of drumbeat among the so-called 'general population' about what their risk of AIDS might be, and this almost hysteria that was beginning to percolate along about the risk of AIDS to all heterosexuals."[19] Fears were stoked by publications such as *Life* magazine's cover story of July 1985, titled, "Now No One is Safe from AIDS," and the book *Crisis: Heterosexual Behavior in the Age of AIDS* by the well-known sex researchers, William Masters, Virginia Johnson, and Robert Kolodny. Some religious conservatives serving in the Reagan Administration also saw these fears as supportive of their abstinence-until-marriage agenda.

Of 2,259 persons reported to have AIDS as of September 2, 1983, 1 percent were described as "heterosexual partners of persons with AIDS or persons at increased risk of AIDS."[20] By the time of the third international conference on AIDS in 1987, data presented by Chamberland showed a small but statistically significant increase in this proportion to 2 percent.[21] Most of the heterosexual contact patients were black or Hispanic (71%) and female (79%). The "source patients" for infection of these heterosexual contacts were mainly

IDUs (60%); in addition, 12 percent of the female patients had bisexual male partners. When interviewed about her presentation, Chamberland noted that it had taken only five months for the first five hundred homosexual male AIDS patients to be reported versus five years for reporting the same number of heterosexual contact cases.[22]

Shortly after the international conference, I was contacted by an editorial writer for the *New York Times*, who had been given approval from the CDC Office of Public Affairs to interview me about the threat of heterosexual spread of HIV in the United States. I spoke with the writer and gave what I thought were cautious answers to his questions. I wasn't worried about what I had said until I opened my copy of the *Times* on June 15, 1987, and read the following in the editorial,

> Administration officials liken the disease to the Black Death, and now the President himself [Ronald Reagan] declares that 'AIDS is surreptitiously spreading throughout our population.' By contrast, here is the judgment of Harold Jaffe, chief AIDS epidemiologist at the Federal Centers for Disease Control: "We really have not seen much evidence for the spread of the virus [outside] risk groups. For most people, the risk of AIDS is essentially zero . . . Why it isn't getting out beyond the immediate sexual partners of the risk group members, I don't know. Is the disease going to sweep into the heterosexual population, like Africa? I don't see it."[23]

Now I was worried! When I went to work that morning, no one spoke to me about the editorial. But their expressions seemed to convey messages ranging from "I can't believe you said that" to "Well, it's been nice working with you." I thought I was going to be fired, but somehow was not.

Over time, the proportion of AIDS cases attributed to heterosexual transmission of HIV gradually increased. In 1991, ten years into the American epidemic, 6 percent of cases were reported to be in this category.[24][†] But the much-feared spread of AIDS into the "general population" of heterosexuals never materialized. Several factors likely reduced the risk of infection for heterosexual Americans compared with MSM. As shown in subsequent studies, the estimated risk of HIV transmission per sex act with an infected person was much greater for anal intercourse than for vaginal intercourse.[25]

[†] By 1991, persons from Haiti had been placed in the "heterosexual transmission" category. To be consistent with earlier data, the 6 percent figure excludes Haitians.

Because the prevalence of HIV was considerably higher in MSM than in heterosexuals, the likelihood of having an infected partner was also higher for MSM. On average, heterosexuals also had fewer sex partners than MSM and lower rates of the other STIs that facilitated HIV transmission.

As AIDS fears grew in the general population, so did the belief that HIV might be spread through "casual contact," such as might occur in a household, office, or school setting. In New York City, as recalled by EIS officer Polly Thomas, "There was a lot of fear... people were being evicted from their apartments and fired from jobs."[26] To protest a decision that allowed an HIV-infected second grade student to attend school in Queens, New York, parents organized a boycott that kept 11,000 elementary and junior high school students out of classes. The *New York Times* quoted a parent as saying, "They send children home if they have lice or chicken pox, but they want to let them in if they have AIDS. Now what kind reasoning is that?"[27]

Perhaps the most disturbing examples of fear of HIV transmission in schools involved HIV-infected children with hemophilia. In 1985, Ryan White,[‡] an Indiana teenager with hemophilia-related AIDS, was barred from attending school by his local school district. His family filed a lawsuit seeking to overturn the decision, which was later reversed by Indiana's State Board of Education. As the debate about his school attendance took place, a bullet was fired through a window of his home. In Florida, the family of three HIV-infected brothers with hemophilia—Ricky, Robert, and Randy Ray—filed a federal lawsuit to allow the children to attend public school. The court ruled in favor of the Rays, and shortly after their house was burned down.

The first study to examine the possibility of HIV transmission in close, but nonsexual, contacts of HIV-infected persons was done by Gerald Friedland and colleagues in the Bronx, New York.[28] Martha Rogers was a CDC collaborator in the study and recalled, "We [CDC] funded his group... because he was at Montefiore Hospital where they were seeing a lot of the families from the Bronx that were getting HIV. We were looking to see if they transmitted to other members of their family."[29] The investigators studied 101 nonsexual contacts of forty-one patients with AIDS or AIDS-related complex with oral candida infection. As would be expected, there was substantial contact between the patients and their family members. Over an average of twenty-two months during which the patients were presumed to be infectious,

‡ Named in honor of the Indiana teenager, the Ryan White Care Act was enacted by Congress in 1990 to fund care for HIV-infected patients when no other resources are available.

90 percent to 93 percent of household members shared toilet, bath or shower, and kitchen facilities with a patient, and about 80 percent reported hugging or kissing the cheek of a patient. Only one household member was found to be HIV-infected: a five-year-old child born to a mother with AIDS and most probably infected before or during birth.

The results of the Montefiore study and several additional studies, which confirmed its findings, enabled CDC and national public health and educational organizations to publish guidelines for the education and foster care of HIV-infected children.[30] The publication noted that no instances of HIV transmission had been reported in school, day-care, or foster-care settings and stated, "Based on current evidence, casual person-to-person contact as would occur among schoolchildren appears to pose no risk."[30] The guidelines further stated that most infected children "should be allowed to attend school and after-school day-care and to be placed in a foster home in an unrestricted setting."[30] More restricted settings would be considered for children who lacked control of their body secretions or displayed behaviors such as biting. In addition to these guidelines, photographs of celebrities including Diana, Princess of Wales, hugging children with AIDS did much to dispel the fear of casual contact.

Another fear that required a CDC response was that HIV could be transmitted by biting insects, such as mosquitoes. As I was reviewing abstracts submitted to the first international conference on AIDS, which was being organized by CDC to be held in Atlanta in April 1985, a submission caught my attention. The abstract, "Outbreak of No Identifiable Risk Acquired Immunodeficiency Syndrome (AIDS) in Belle Glade, Florida," was authored by two South Florida physicians, Mark Whiteside and Caroline MacLeod, and several local collaborators.[31] They described an unusually high proportion of AIDS patients without documented risk factors living in this agricultural town. The authors suggested that "environmental factors contribute to the development of AIDS in this region."[31] Given that no specific environmental factor had been reported to increase the risk of AIDS, I thought the abstract was worthy of a poster presentation at the meeting. Little did I realize the impact the presentation would have on Belle Glade.

Whiteside and MacLeod's theories about AIDS in Belle Glade soon began to receive coverage in the popular press. For example, the *Los Angeles Times* noted that the two physicians "contend that mosquitoes also are playing a role, either by transmitting the AIDS virus from one person to another by bites, or by carrying certain other viruses that act as co-factors to activate the

AIDS virus in bitten individuals."[32] This coverage brought attention to a community, which already had a history of unwanted media interest. In 1960, the television series *CBS Reports* broadcast an episode, "Harvest of Shame," in which the legendary journalist Edward R. Murrow explored the plight of the migrant farm workers who harvested the crops of Belle Glade. Agriculture continued to dominate the economy of Belle Glade and surrounding areas in the 1980s, when the main cash crop was sugar cane. Harvesting sugar cane required manual labor, which was largely provided by African American workers as well as laborers from the Caribbean, who were permitted to enter the country for this specific task.

CDC was invited by the State of Florida and the Palm Beach County Health Departments to help assess the HIV problem in Belle Glade. With local officials, we visited the impoverished neighborhoods in which most of the AIDS patients resided. We heard anecdotes about the impact of the AIDS publicity on the town. High school football teams from other communities forfeited games rather than playing in Belle Glade. Relatives were fearful of visiting family members in the town. We agreed that CDC would assist in conducting a community-wide survey to determine the prevalence of HIV and risk factors for infection. Ken Castro, who had overseen CDC's study on AIDS in Haitian Americans (Chapter 6), and John Narkunas, a PHA, would take the lead for CDC.

The Belle Glade study posed several challenges. The first challenge was assuring adequate study participation. As Castro recalled,

Think of this: you have a government official showing up at your door, inviting you to participate in a survey that's going to ask about your sexual practices, drug-using habits, etc. Not something that most people would be willing to participate in. We. . . went to the media to announce our plans to do the survey, to encourage people to participate. Interestingly, I believe that about seventy seven percent of households that we knocked on doors agreed to participate in this type of survey, which is very unusual. . . Fortunately for us, in the sampling scheme [a random survey of households] it turns out that the mayor's household was part of the sampling scheme, and the mayor also publicly agreed to be interviewed and be tested, and that I think also helped encourage others to participate in this survey.[33]

Other challenges were logistical. As Castro explained,

We did a community-based survey using a twenty-four-footer Winnebago*
camper to enable us to conduct private interviews, do physical exams in the
field, and draw bloods. I was able to check for lymphadenopathy, any presence of skin lesions that would be consistent with Kaposi' [sarcoma] and
draw blood specimens to bring back to CDC.[33]

Unsurprisingly, the camper attracted considerable attention when parked in
the Belle Glade neighborhoods.

Of approximately 16,500 Belle Glade residents, 877 adults were enrolled
in the study. [34] Of these adults, twenty-eight (3.2%) were found to be HIV
infected—fifteen Haitian and thirteen African American. No infections
were found in adults over age sixty or in 138 children aged two to ten who
lived in the households of the adult study participants. The only instances
of clustering of infected persons in households occurred in sex partners.
The risk factors for infections in adults were all related to sexual behavior.
In contrast, HIV infections were not significantly related to either measures
of potential mosquito exposure, such as farm work or hours spent outdoors,
or the presence of antibodies to five mosquito-borne viruses found in South
Florida or the Caribbean, such as dengue 2 virus. The authors concluded
that "the evidence does not suggest transmission of HIV through insects."[34]
The Belle Glade findings were also considered in a comprehensive review,
"Do Insects Transmit AIDS," conducted by The United States Office of
Technology Assessment.[35] The review concluded, "In sum, there is no evidence that insect transmission causes HIV infections in temperate zones or
even in tropical climates."[35]

CDC Director Jim Mason felt strongly that the American public needed to
be better informed about the risks of AIDS. As he recalled, "Everyone needed
to understand how AIDS is and isn't spread. Too many people in the United
States believed that AIDS was spread through casual contact. They heard
AIDS could be mosquito-borne."[36] As part of an ongoing CDC public information campaign, "America Responds to AIDS," Mason proposed developing a brochure, *Understanding AIDS,* to be mailed to every US household.
Ogilvy and Mather, a well-known advertising agency, would be tasked with
creating the brochure. Although the White House Domestic Policy Council
showed little enthusiasm for the proposal, Congress passed a $25 million ap-
propriation to support it. Mason stated, "Congressional intent language with
that appropriation spelled out that the content of the mailed-out brochure
would be the responsibility of the CDC Director."[36]

Mason asked Surgeon General C. Everett Koop to be the "lead person in the brochure." Prior to serving as Surgeon General, Koop was a famed pediatric surgeon. His biblical looks and PHS uniform added to the impact of his statements as Surgeon General. Koop had strong personal antiabortion

Understanding AIDS

A Message From The Surgeon General

T his brochure has been sent to you by the Government of the United States. In preparing it, we have consulted with the top health experts in the country.

I feel it is important that you have the best information now available for fighting the AIDS virus, a health problem that the President has called "Public Enemy Number One."

Stopping AIDS is up to you, your family and your loved ones.

Some of the issues involved in this brochure may not be things you are used to discussing openly. I can easily understand that. But now you must discuss them. We all must know about AIDS. Read this brochure and talk about it with those you love. Get involved. Many schools, churches, synagogues, and community groups offer AIDS education activities.

I encourage you to practice responsible behavior based on understanding and strong personal values. This is what you can do to stop AIDS.

C. Everett Koop, M.D., Sc.D.
Surgeon General

Este folleto sobre el SIDA se publica en Español.
Para solicitar una copia, llame al 1-800-344-SIDA.

U.S. Department of Health
& Human Services
Public Health Service
Centers for Disease Control
P.O. Box 6003
Rockville, MD 20850

BULK RATE
CARRIER ROUTE PRESORT
POSTAGE & FEES PAID
PHS/CDC
Permit No. G-284

Official Business

POSTAL CUSTOMER

HHS Publication No. (CDC) HHS-88-8404. Reproduction of the contents of this brochure is encouraged.

Figure 10.2. *Understanding AIDS* brochure, 1988. (Harold Jaffe, personal collection)

views, which were consistent with those of the Reagan Administration. But on AIDS, his views were much more progressive. Koop agreed to have his picture featured in the brochure and to serve as its primary spokesperson.

Between May 26 and June 30, 1988, 107 million copies of *Understanding AIDS* (Figure 10.2) were mailed to every home and residential post office box in the United States.[37] Another four million copies of a Spanish-language version were sent to Puerto Rico. *Understanding AIDS* described the risks for AIDS in clear and simple language. The brochure specifically stated that HIV was not transmitted by everyday contact with infected persons, through kissing, or through mosquito bites. In comparing responses from the National Health Interview Survey conducted before (August 1987) and after (August 1988) the distribution of *Understanding AIDS*, CDC concluded that

> [T]he most substantial increase in knowledge was related to transmission of HIV. The increases in the percentages of adults who considered it "very unlikely" or "definitely not possible" to transmit HIV through various forms of casual contact represent important gains in knowledge. The overall gain in levels of knowledge about HIV and AIDS coincided with the national multimedia public awareness campaign.[38]

No single study or spokesperson can be credited with changing the knowledge and attitudes of Americans regarding AIDS. But the combined effects of good science and trusted communicators went a long way in addressing unwarranted fears.

Notes

1. Collaborative Group on AIDS Incubation and HIV Survival including the CASCADE EU Concerted Action. Concerted Action on SeroConversion to AIDS and Death in Europe. Time from HIV-1 seroconversion and death before widespread use of highly-active antiretroviral therapy: a collaborative re-analysis. Lancet 2000;355:1131–1137.
2. CDC. Prevention of acquired immune deficiency syndrome (AIDS): report of inter-agency recommendations. MMWR Morb Mortal Wkly Rep 1983:32:101–104.
3. CDC. Declining rates of rectal and pharyngeal gonorrhea among males—New York City. MMWR Morb Mortal Wkly Rep 1984;33:295–297.
4. CDC. Syphilis—United States, 1983. MMWR Morb Mortal Wkly Rep 1984;33:433–436,441.
5. Hadler SC, Doto IL, Maynard JE, et al. Occupational risk of hepatitis B infection in hospital workers. Infect Control 1985;6:24–31.

6. CDC. Acquired immune deficiency syndrome (AIDS): precautions for clinical and laboratory staffs. MMWR Morb Mortal Wkly Rep 1982;31:577–580.

7. CDC. An evaluation of acquired immunodeficiency syndrome (AIDS) reported in health-care personnel—United States. MMWR Morb Mortal Wkly Rep 1983;32:358–360.

8. "HEALTH CARE WORKERS: Risk Assessment," *The Global Health Chronicles*, accessed January 29, 2023, https://www.globalhealthchronicles.org/items/show/6643.

9. Anonymous. Needlestick transmission of HTLV-III from a patient infected in Africa. Lancet 1984;2:1376–1377.

10. "MCCRAY, EUGENE," *The Global Health Chronicles*, accessed January 29, 2023, https://www.globalhealthchronicles.org/items/show/6470.

11. CDC. Prospective evaluation of health-care workers exposed via parenteral or mucous-membrane routes to blood and body fluids of patients with acquired immunodeficiency syndrome. MMWR Morb Mortal Wkly Rep 1984;33:181–182.

12. McCray E, The Cooperative Needlestick Surveillance Group. Special report. Occupational risk of the acquired immunodeficiency syndrome among health care workers. N Engl J Med 1986 314:1127–1132.

13. Marcus R, CDC Cooperative Needlestick Surveillance Group. Surveillance of health care workers exposed to blood from patients infected with the human immunodeficiency virus. N Engl J Med 1988;319;1118–11123.

14. CDC. Recommendations for preventing transmission of infection with human T-lymphotropic virus type III/lymphadenopathy-associated virus in the workplace. MMWR Morb Mortal Wkly Rep 1985;34:691–696.

15. Rogers M. Doctor doom: Lorraine Day keeps asking life-or-death questions about the dangers of AIDS. Some say she's an alarmist. Some say she's just ahead of her time. Los Angeles Times. April 21, 1991.

16. Tokars JI, Chamberland ME, Schable CA, et al. A survey of occupational blood contact and HIV infection among orthopedic surgeons. JAMA 1992;268;489–494.

17. Joyce MP, Kuhar D. Brooks JT. Notes from the field: occupationally acquired HIV infection among health care workers—United States, 1985–2013. MMWR Morb Mortal Wkly Rep 2015;63:1245–1246.

18. Cardo DM, Culver DH, Ciesielski CA, et al. A case-control study of HIV seroconversion in health care workers after percutaneous exposure. N Engl J Med 1997;337:1485–1490.

19. "CHAMBERLAND, MARY," *The Global Health Chronicles*, accessed January 29, 2023, https://www.globalhealthchronicles.org/items/show/7728.

20. CDC. Update: acquired immunodeficiency syndrome (AIDS) —United States. MMWR Morb Mortal Wkly Rep 1983;32:465–467.

21. Chamberland ME, Dondero TJ Jr. Heterosexually acquired infection with human immunodeficiency virus (HIV). A view from the III International Conference on AIDS (Editorial). Ann Intern Med 1987;107:763–766.

22. Jemison T, Burke M. U.S. Medicine—AIDS Conference Report. US Medicine 1987;23:2,10–12.

23. Editorial. AIDS: good news and bad news. New York Times. June 15, 1987.
24. CDC. Update: Acquired immunodeficiency syndrome—United States, 1991. MMWR Morb Mortal Wkly Rep 1992;41:69–73.
25. Patel P, Borkowf CB, Brooks JT, Lasry A, Lansky A, Mermin J. Estimating per-act HIV transmission risk: a systematic review. AIDS 2014; 28:1509–1519.
26. "THOMAS, PAULINE," The Global Health Chronicles, accessed January 29, 2023, https://www.globalhealthchronicles.org/items/show/7792.
27. Rohter L. 11,000 boycott start of class of classes in AIDS protest. New York Times. September 10, 1985.
28. Friedland GH, Saltzman BR, Rogers MF, et al. Lack of transmission of HTLV-III/LAV infection to household contacts of patients with AIDS or AIDS-related complex with oral candidiasis. N Engl J Med 1986;314:344–349.
29. ROGERS, MARTHA," The Global Health Chronicles, accessed January 29, 2023, https://www.globalhealthchronicles.org/items/show/5395.
30. CDC. Education and foster care of children infected with human T-lymphotropic virus type III/lymphadenopathy-associated virus. MMWR Morb Mortal Wkly Rep 1985;34:517–521.
31. Whiteside ME, Withum D, Tavris D, MacLeod C. Abstract W 73 in the Official Program of the International Conference on Acquired Immunodeficiency Syndrome (AIDS), April 14–17, 1985, Atlanta, Georgia.
32. Nelson H. Epidemic of AIDS defies pattern in south Florida city. Los Angeles Times. January 27, 1986.
33. "CASTRO, KENNETH," The Global Health Chronicles, accessed January 29, 2023, https://www.globalhealthchronicles.org/items/show/6478.
34. Castro KG, Lieb S, Jaffe HW, et al. Transmission of HIV in Belle Glade, Florida: lessons for other communities in the United States. Science 1988;239:193–197.
35. Office of Technology Assessment. Do Insects Transmit AIDS? September 1987. UNT Digital Library (https://digital.library.unt.edu/ark:/67531/metadc39877/m1/1/).
36. "MASON, JAMES," The Global Health Chronicles, accessed January 29, 2023, https://www.globalhealthchronicles.org/items/show/8047.
37. "Understanding AIDS," The Global Health Chronicles, accessed January 29, 2023, https://www.globalhealthchronicles.org/items/show/8156.
38. CDC. Current trends HIV epidemic and AIDS: trends in Knowledge—United States, 1987 and 1988. MMWR Morb Mortal Wkly Rep. 1989;38:353–354,357–388,363.

11

Making Predictions

Harold W. Jaffe

Among the many quotations attributed to the New York Yankees' baseball player Yogi Berra is "It's tough to make predictions, especially about the future." Whether or not he actually said this (He is also credited with saying, "I never said most of the things I said."), making predictions about the magnitude and trajectory of the epidemic was important in America's early response to AIDS. How big would the epidemic become? What medical personnel and facilities would be needed to care for AIDS patients? What would be the cost of providing such care?

The key person in CDC's efforts to predict the course of the epidemic was Task Force statistician Meade Morgan (Chapter 3). Morgan's first efforts to model the epidemic were published in 1985, at a time when approximately 13,000 cases of AIDS in the United States had been reported to CDC.[1] Using data from the San Francisco City Clinic Cohort (SFCCC) (Chapter 4), which indicated that the ratio of HIV infections to AIDS cases was between 50:1 and 100:1, Morgan estimated that there were between 500,000 and one million Americans already infected with HIV. He then used a two-step process, referred to as the "extrapolation approach," to project future AIDS cases. First, AIDS case counts were adjusted for delays in reporting. Second, an equation was fitted to the adjusted case counts and used to estimate future cases. Based on this approach, Morgan projected that the cumulative number of AIDS cases would double over the next year.*

Epidemic projections were next considered by PHS at a meeting convened at the Coolfont Conference Center in Berkeley Springs, West Virginia, in June 1986.[2] This meeting was attended by representatives of virtually all the US government agencies involved in AIDS and was viewed as extremely

---

* From December 1985 through December 1986, cumulative reported cases increased from about 16,000 to about 29,000 (https://www.cdc.gov/hiv/pdf/library/reports/surveillance/cdc-hiv-surveillance-report-1986.pdf)

Harold W. Jaffe, *Making Predictions* In: *Dispatches from the AIDS Pandemic.* Kevin M. De Cock, Harold W. Jaffe, and James W. Curran and Edited by: Robin Moseley, Oxford University Press. © Oxford University Press 2023. DOI: 10.1093/oso/9780197626528.003.0011

important in planning a response to the epidemic. Morgan's extrapolation approach was again used to make projections.[3] At the time of the meeting, the estimated number of HIV-infected Americans had increased to between 1.0 and 1.5 million with 20 percent to 30 percent expected to develop AIDS by the end of 1991. If the model proved correct, the cumulative US case count by the end of 1991 would total more than 270,000 with more than 179,000 deaths due to AIDS. The direct healthcare costs of persons with AIDS were estimated to be between $8 billion and $16 billion in 1991. These estimates were shocking to many of the attendees. A *New York Times* article stated that Donald Ian Macdonald, Acting Assistant Secretary of Health and Human Services, had "described as 'staggering' and 'devastating' the 'huge problem' caused by 'the escalating AIDS epidemic.'"[4]

Two years after the Coolfont conference, a second PHS meeting to examine the AIDS epidemic was held in Charlottesville, Virginia.[5] At this 1988 meeting, the Coolfont case projections were examined and found to be reasonably accurate for the years 1986 and 1987. The number of projected cases for these years were 15,800 and 23,000 cases, respectively, while the actual number of cases, adjusted for reporting delays, were 17,100 for 1986 and 25,200 for 1987. However, the utility of the extrapolation method for making longer-term projections was less clear. The approach assumed that past trends in reported AIDS cases would predict future trends, and it could not incorporate changes in HIV infection rates.

To address the limitations of the extrapolation approach, a second method for AIDS case projection, namely "back-calculation," had been developed by Ron Brookmeyer from Johns Hopkins University and Mitchell Gail from NIH's National Cancer Institute.[6]) This method estimated trends in HIV incidence by applying an incubation time distribution (the proportion of people developing AIDS each year after infection) to reported AIDS cases and "back calculating" the number of persons infected each year. The incubation time distribution was then applied to estimate the number of infected persons who would develop AIDS in future years. The limitation of this approach was that it required accurate estimates of the incubation time.

Brookmeyer and Gail used an average incubation period of 4.3 years in their initial work, a figure derived from studies of persons with transfusion-associated AIDS. But there were biases in this estimate. The incubation period for infected persons developing AIDS early in the epidemic would be skewed toward those with short incubation periods. Those with longer incubation periods would not yet have developed AIDS. Although not known at the time, another bias was that transfusion recipients were often older adults who tend to have short incubation periods.[7] Robert (Bob) Byers, a statistician recruited from Emory University to CDC by Morgan, worked on estimating the incubation period and concluded, "Everybody who was doing incubation estimation was coming up with different answers ."[8] Regarding meetings held with other statisticians to discuss this problem, Byers recalled, "Basically, each one would stand up and explain what he or she had done, and then people would throw bricks at them. Then everybody would go home, unfortunately."[8]

Investigators in San Francisco developed a "convolution" model for their city's epidemic.[9] The model, described as a variation on the back-calculation method, made projections for the MSM epidemic by first using data from an HIV seroprevalence survey, conducted using randomly selected households in high-risk census tracts. The size of the MSM population was then estimated from a previously conducted random-digit telephone survey and the census-tract survey. These two estimates allowed for the calculation of the number of infected MSM in the city. The rate of progression from the time of infection of these MSM to AIDS was modeled using data from a subset of men in the SFCCC. The median incubation period estimate used in the San Francisco study, eleven years, was remarkably like currently used estimates.[7]

Although each statistical method had strengths and weaknesses, the Charlottesville report noted that both the extrapolation and back-calculation methods generated relatively similar estimates of AIDS cases that would occur over the next several years.[5] The report also concluded that, "Despite current uncertainty about the incidence of new infection and the ultimate magnitude of the problem, HIV-related disease remains a growing threat to the public health of the Nation and will continue to have a significant impact on health care and social service delivery systems."[5]

Estimates of HIV prevalence and projected AIDS cases were updated at a CDC-sponsored workshop held in Atlanta in the fall of 1989.[10] Workshop participants concluded that the Coolfont estimate of 1 million to 1.5 million HIV-infected Americans in 1986 was likely too high and that around one million Americans were currently infected. Of these infected persons, about 10 percent had been diagnosed with AIDS. CDC surveillance data showed yearly increases in reported AIDS cases, with a slowing of the rate of increase starting in mid-1987. Projections presented at the meeting suggested than the number of persons diagnosed with AIDS would continue to increase each year through 1993, albeit at a lower rate of increase than in previous years.

The epidemic projections made by CDC and others were not universally accepted, with the most pointed criticism coming from an unexpected source: Alexander Langmuir. In 1949, Langmuir headed the Epidemiology Division of the then newly formed CDC and subsequently became the "father" of EIS.[11] His formidable persona and belief in the power of epidemiology made him a legendary figure at CDC. Although retired, he paid close attention to CDC activities.

Langmuir's contention, as stated in the letters to CDC and in a 1990 journal article coauthored with a former CDC statistician, Dennis Bregman, was that the AIDS epidemic was subject to Farr's Law of Epidemics.[12] According to Bregman and Langmuir, the "Law," as developed by William Farr in 1840, stated that "in large epidemics, the incidence of new cases tends to rise to a crest and then fall in a manner so that the entire curve forms a shape approximately described by the normal [bell-shaped] curve."[12] Using CDC data on AIDS cases reported from 1982 through 1987, Bregman and Langmuir believed that the epidemic would "crest" in late 1988 and then decline to a low point in the mid-1990s, resulting in a total epidemic size "in the range of 200,000 cases."[12] But contrary to their prediction, a cumulative total of 200,000 AIDS cases had been reported to CDC by December 1991 and cases were continuing to increase each year.[13] What Bregman and Langmuir did not appreciate was that Farr's Law was valid only in "closed" populations, that is, populations with a fixed number of susceptible individuals. In contrast to epidemics studied by Farr, the number of persons susceptible to HIV infection continuously increased, primarily as additional MSM became sexually active and increasing numbers of IDUs shared injection equipment.

Disbelief in CDC's epidemic projections also came from other surprising sources: Stirling Colgate, a famed nuclear weapons physicist (and heir to the Colgate toothpaste family fortune), and Carl Sagan, the well-known astronomer and popular author. In contrast to Langmuir, Colgate and Sagan maintained that CDC was seriously underestimating the potential magnitude of the American AIDS epidemic. Morgan and I met with Colgate and Sagan on their individual visits to CDC (Figure 11.1) and heard each of them express the view that it was only a matter of time before all sexually active Americans would become HIV infected.

Our response to Colgate and Sagan was based on the concept of R_0, the basic reproductive rate of an infection. As described by the mathematical modelers Robert May and Roy Anderson, R_0 (pronounced "R naught") is "the average number of secondary infections produced by one infected

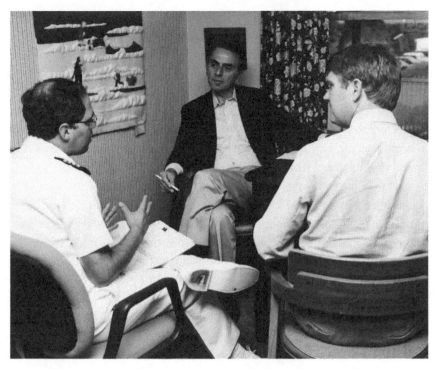

Figure 11.1. Harold Jaffe (left) and Meade Morgan (right) meeting with Carl Sagan (center) at CDC headquarters in Atlanta, circa 1988. (CDC Photo Archives)

individual in the early stages of an epidemic (when essentially all contacts are susceptible); clearly the infection can maintain itself within the population only if R_0 exceeds unity."[14] They further noted that for STIs such as HIV, R_0 depends on the average rate of acquisition of new partners, the average rate of transmission of the infection to a partner per sexual contact, and the average duration of infectiousness. Although not all these variables were precisely known at this stage of the epidemic, we could say with certainty that the rate of partner change was much higher for MSM than for heterosexuals and that anal intercourse appeared to be more efficient for transmitting HIV than vaginal intercourse. Based on the relatively low number of cases attributed to heterosexual contact, we felt confident that R_0 was well below 1.0 for heterosexual Americans.

I don't know if either Colgate or Sagan believed us. Nonetheless, Colgate and his colleagues from Los Alamos National Laboratory (LANL) developed a "risk-based" model, extending earlier work done by May and Anderson. The LANL researchers suggested that the decreasing rate of growth of the epidemic through 1988 was not the result of behavioral change; rather, they postulated "a saturation wave of infection moving from high- to low-risk groups."[15] They further suggested that population groups, such as MSM, "were infected by a few high-risk individuals early in the epidemic, and only highly isolated groups may remain untouched by the epidemic."[15] The high-risk individuals who were infected early in the epidemic may also have died, thus removing them from the "pool" of transmitters.

However, as a surrogate for decreasing sexual risk behavior, rates of infectious syphilis in MSM had fallen from 1982 to 1987.[16] Models of the San Francisco epidemic, developed by Herb Hethcote from the University of Iowa and collaborators, including Ira Longini from Emory University and John Karon from CDC, were also consistent with both a saturation effect and behavioral change contributing to a plateau of HIV incidence in MSM during the late 1980s.[17,18]

In 1991, Ron Brookmeyer updated his back-calculation estimates to provide a reconstruction of the AIDS epidemic in the United States.[19] He calculated that "The cumulative number of [HIV] infections from 1977 to the beginning of 1981, 1983, and 1986 were 50,000, 250,000, and 715,000, respectively."[19] In addition, he wrote that the infection rate probably peaked in 1984 at about 160,000 infections per year. Based on these figures and an estimated median incubation period of ten years, he projected that annual AIDS cases would reach a plateau over the next five years. Consistent with Brookmeyer's estimates, CDC's AIDS surveillance data showed that reported cases peaked in 1995,[†] the year that highly active antiretroviral therapy (HAART, or just ART) was becoming widely available in the United States.

What insights were gained through efforts to model the early epidemics of HIV and AIDS? Perhaps the most important and tragic insight was that large numbers of AIDS cases and deaths were unavoidable. Even if behavioral interventions had been widely deployed and adopted in those early years, many individuals had already been infected well before the disease was recognized and would progress to AIDS. Modeling also correctly predicted that after the

---

† The CDC case definition for AIDS was expanded in 1993 to include additional clinical illnesses (Chapter 3), creating an artificial peak in cases that year. When reported cases were adjusted for this change, the peak shifted to 1995, when the adjusted case total was about 61,500 cases (CDC HIV/AIDS Surveillance Report December 1997). https://www.cdc.gov/hiv/pdf/library/reports/surveillance/cdc-hiv-surveillance-report-1997-vol-9-2.pdf

highest-risk individuals became infected, AIDS incidence would peak and gradually fall. But given that newly susceptible individuals would enter the at-risk population each year, the epidemic would not spontaneously disappear.

Yogi Berra was right; it is difficult to predict the future. As Bob Byers concluded about modeling, "You start to think this is reality. But it's not."[8]

Notes

1. Curran JW, Morgan WM, Hardy AM, Jaffe HW, Darrow WW, Dowdle WR. The epidemiology of AIDS: current status and future prospects. Science 1985;229:1352–1357.
2. Coolfont report: a PHS plan for prevention and control of AIDS and the AIDS virus. Public Health Rep 1986;101:341–348.
3. Morgan WM, Curran JW. Acquired immunodeficiency syndrome: current and future trends. Public Health Rep 1986;101:459–465.
4. Pear R. Tenfold increase in AIDS death toll is expected by '91. New York Times. June 13, 1986.
5. Report of the Second Public Health Service AIDS prevention and control conference. Public Health Rep 1988;103 (Suppl 1):10–18.
6. Brookmeyer R, Gail MH. Minimum size of the acquired immunodeficiency syndrome (AIDS) epidemic in the United States. Lancet 1986;8519:1320–1322.
7. Collaborative Group on AIDS Incubation and HIV Survival including the CASCADE EU Concerted Action. Time from HIV-1 seroconversion to AIDS and death before widespread use of highly-active antiretroviral therapy: a collaborative re-analysis. Lancet 2000;355:1131–1137.
8. "BYERS, ROBERT," The Global Health Chronicles, accessed January 29, 2023, https://www.globalhealthchronicles.org/items/show/7974
9. Lemp GF, Payne SF, Rutherford GF, et al. Projections of AIDS morbidity and mortality in San Francisco. JAMA 1990;263:1497–1501.
10. HIV prevalence, projected AIDS case estimates: workshop, October 31–November 1, 1989. JAMA 1990;263:1477–1480.
11. Etheridge EW. Sentinel for Health. A History of The Center for Disease Control. Berkeley, CA: University of California Press; 1991.
12. Bregman DJ, Langmuir AD. Farr's law applied to AIDS projections. JAMA 1990;263:1522–1524.
13. CDC. The second 100,000 cases of the acquired immunodeficiency syndrome—United States, June 1981–December 1991. MMWR Morb Mortal Wkly Rep 1992;41:28–29.
14. May RM, Anderson RM. Transmission dynamics of HIV infection. Nature 1987;326:137–142.
15. Colgate SA, Stanley EA, Hyman JM, Layne SP, Qualls C. Risk behavior-based model of the cubic growth of acquired immunodeficiency syndrome in the United States. Proc Natl Acad Sci USA 1989;86; 4793–4797.

16. CDC. Increases in primary and secondary syphilis—United States. MMWR Morbid Mortal Wkly Rep 1987;36:393–397.
17. Hethcote HW, Van Ark JW, Longini IM Jr. A simulation model of AIDS in San Francisco: I. model formulation and parameter estimation. Math Biosci 1991;106:203–222.
18. Hethcote HW, Van Ark JW, Karon JM. A simulation model of AIDS in San Francisco: II. simulations, therapy, and sensitivity analysis. Math Biosci 1991;106:223–247.
19. Brookmeyer R. Reconstruction and future trends of the AIDS epidemic in the United States. Science 1991;253;37–42.

SECTION II

CDC AND THE EARLY INTERNATIONAL RESPONSE TO AIDS

12

Working Internationally

Kevin M. De Cock

As described in this book's opening chapter, malaria control in the southern United States led to CDC's creation in 1946 and the choice of Atlanta for its location.[1] And although no disease is more emblematic than malaria of "tropical medicine" or "international health," the precursors of today's "global health,"[2,3] in the agency's first twenty years of existence little international work was done.

CDC's first intervention outside the United States was in Winnipeg, Canada, in 1950 and concerned not an infectious disease but a flood.[4] Despite its later global involvement, CDC's early EIS program was primarily domestic in its focus.[5] Stan Foster, a renowned CDC epidemiologist and internationalist, recounted that he found only three instances of international epidemiologic assistance by the agency over the course of the 1950s. A review of CDC's international epidemic assistance investigations ("Epi-Aids") conducted over its first sixty years (1946–2005) showed a steep increase in their number over time, but only two occurred during the period 1946–1955.[6] Overall, the great majority of these Epi-Aids were for acute infectious disease outbreaks. However, the issue that drew CDC into international operational involvement and expanded its outlook beyond American shores was not an acute emergency, but an ancient scourge—smallpox.[7,8]

The eradication of smallpox, formally declared in 1980 at the World Health Assembly, the governing body of WHO,[9] is one of the greatest public health achievements in history. Semantic discussions distinguish among infectious disease control, elimination, and eradication.[10] Eradication means a biologic agent no longer exists in nature. To date, this has only been accomplished for smallpox and rinderpest,[11] a measles-like illness of ruminants. Several eradication aspirations—such as for measles, yaws, yellow fever, or malaria—have foundered. Eradication of an infectious agent is the ultimate in social justice and health equity—once an infection is eradicated, it is gone forever, everywhere, and for everyone. Today, eradication programs continue for polio[12]

Kevin M. De Cock, *Working Internationally* In: *Dispatches from the AIDS Pandemic.* Kevin M. De Cock, Harold W. Jaffe, and James W. Curran and Edited by: Robin Moseley, Oxford University Press. © Oxford University Press 2023. DOI: 10.1093/oso/9780197626528.003.0012

and for dracunculiasis,[13] the parasitic disease referred to as guinea worm. CDC is a leading participant in both programs, which are close to but have not yet achieved their frustratingly elusive goals. And "almost eradicated" does not count.

The multiorganizational smallpox experience and CDC's involvement share many similarities to and lessons for later work. Foremost, public health is political. President Lyndon Johnson instructed the US delegation to the World Health Assembly in 1965 to commit to the eradication of smallpox within a decade.[7] The relevant resolution at the 1967 Assembly was supported by both the United States and the Soviet Union, despite Cold War tensions.

Three organizations merit the greatest credit for the success of smallpox eradication: CDC, WHO, and the United States Agency for International Development (USAID). And, although often overlooked in global health history, the contributions of the host countries in terms of infrastructure, staff, commodities, and other support are immeasurable. Accounts of the experience among the organizations describe the relative strengths and weaknesses of the partners, the frequent interagency tensions, and the diverse efforts to achieve supervision and control. Which international organization contributed the most in the various accounts was heavily influenced by which organization the author or speaker belonged to. As many who have experienced rivalries in global health will say, *plus ça change, plus c'est la même chose* (the more things change, the more they stay the same). What is most important, however, is how profoundly the smallpox experience and legacy changed CDC, both in the perception of the agency across the world and in its own self-identity. Suddenly, much more seemed possible.

Three conclusions were evident. First, the program convincingly vindicated the view of then CDC Director David Sencer (Chapter 3) that protection of the United States against certain diseases may require and even best be accomplished by their control in other countries.[7,14] Smallpox eradication champion Bill Foege (Chapter 2), who served as CDC director after Sencer, spoke of the need "to link the fears of the rich to the needs of the poor."[14] A second lesson was the importance of individuals, and the difference one person can make. And thirdly, CDC could be proactive internationally. Years later, on a visit to one of CDC's international sites, another CDC Director (and later Surgeon General), David Satcher, referred to the paradox of golden opportunities skillfully disguised as apparently irresolvable problems. Seeking out those opportunities was important in the smallpox program, as it has been throughout CDC's work in global health.

After smallpox eradication, CDC continued to work on public health programs internationally through its International Health Program Office, often supplying technical officers to other agencies, especially USAID and WHO. Focus areas included child survival, such as through USAID's Combatting Childhood Communicable Diseases project that operated in ten African countries,[15] and refugee health. CDC technical experts were also assigned to WHO headquarters or its regional offices for specific priorities such as malaria. Bill Foege strongly supported the agency's collaboration with WHO, emphasizing CDC influence and impact through "soft power" and quiet leadership.[14] Donald (DA) Henderson,[16] leader of the WHO Smallpox Eradication Program, had fulfilled that role for years while a full-time CDC employee. Many other CDC staff were seconded to WHO in senior capacities in programs such as immunization, diarrheal diseases, respiratory illness, and, as described in this book, HIV/AIDS.[17] CDC staff were also seconded to the United Nations Children's Fund (UNICEF), and later to other international organizations such as the Food and Agriculture Organization of the United Nations.

On a programmatic level, many CDC domestic groups expanded their international involvement through technical work of subject matter experts, collaborative projects, and provision of technical assistance upon request for outbreaks or other specific problems. Long-term presence overseas was unusual, but certain groups established small outposts. In 1976, Joseph (Joe) McCormick, working for the highly respected Karl Johnson who headed CDC's hemorrhagic fever group, established a site in Kenema, in southeastern Sierra Leone, to study Lassa fever.[18] That same year had marked the first-ever recognized epidemic of Ebola in Yambuku, Zaire.[19] Under the leadership of Harrison Spencer, CDC's malaria group established long-term research collaboration in Kenya in 1979—an initiative that continues today.[20]

These productive and specialized long-term assignments reflected the interests and drive of specific individuals or groups more than an agency-driven or congressional prioritization. A more unified vision, "One CDC" in global health, was to come much later[21] following the establishment of larger programs and activities by the United States for HIV/AIDS (the US President's Emergency Plan for AIDS Relief [PEPFAR]), malaria (The President's Malaria Initiative), and health security, all of which entailed the commitment of more resources and staff to work in the field. In 2010, CDC Director Thomas (Tom) Frieden gave an anchor to these large programs by creating CDC's newest center, the Center for Global Health, for which I[22] served as founding director.

For HIV/AIDS, international collaborations were instituted over the course of the 1980s under the overall direction of Jim Curran. It was evident to him that understanding AIDS internationally was important to the United States. AIDS had to be seen and understood in its global context, through different populations affected, and not just through the prism of New York or San Francisco. Investigations overseas could give insight into modes of transmission, natural history, or different disease manifestations more difficult to study domestically. HIV also epitomized the newly recognized challenge of emerging infectious diseases, a global issue that would become increasingly prominent in subsequent years.[23] And although CDC was not a development agency, it exerted influence and garnered respect through supporting and strengthening public health capacity internationally, prioritizing the technical over the political. In essence, CDC almost functioned as a global public good.

Helene Gayle,[24] who had joined CDC as an EIS officer in 1984 and rapidly risen through the ranks of global as well as domestic health programs at CDC, captured the justification for spending domestic funds on international AIDS work:

> [W]e broadly used. . . authority to do research that had a bidirectional purpose to it. Yes, it helped globally, but because our mandate was a domestic mandate, we were able to do the research because it also had important precursor information, or leading-edge information, about things that we thought could become a problem in the United States. . . It was a bit challenging, because it probably threatened, to a certain extent, international agencies like USAID and others that had the real international role. . . Our justification was that it would help the American people.[24]

Between 1984 and 1990, CDC worked with host countries to develop three major collaborative sites for research on HIV/AIDS—in Kinshasa, Zaire (now the Democratic Republic of Congo [DRC]); in Abidjan, Cote d'Ivoire; and in Bangkok, Thailand—each with its own justifications and interests. Reminiscent of the smallpox program, the world and CDC benefitted from the cadre of people who participated in these efforts. These individuals made a difference locally and contributed to understanding of this new disease, often going on to other leadership positions in global health. The knowledge gained would alone have justified these investments, but equally important were less tangible issues—the solidarity and trust engendered, the local as well as CDC capacity developed, and the foundations laid for much larger programs later to address the HIV pandemic.

Notes

1. Etheridge EW. Sentinel for health. A history of the Centers for Disease Control. Berkeley and Los Angeles: University of California Press; 1992.
2. Koplan JP, Bond TC, Merson MH, et al. Towards a common definition of global health. Lancet 2009;373:1993–1995.
3. De Cock KM, Simone P, Davison V, Slutsker L. The new global health. Emerg Infect Dis 2013;19:1192–1197.
4. Thacker SB, Stroup DF, Sencer DJ. Epidemic assistance by the Centers for Disease Control and Prevention: role of the Epidemic Intelligence Service, 1946–2005. Am J Epidemiol 2011;174(Suppl):S4–S15.
5. Pendergrast M. Inside the outbreaks. The elite medical detectives of the Epidemic Intelligence Service. New York: Houghton Mifflin Harcourt; 2010.
6. Rolle IV, Pearson ML, Nsubuga P. Fifty-five years of international epidemic-assistance investigations conducted by CDC's disease detectives. Am J Epidemiol 2011;174(Suppl):S97–S112.
7. Ogden HG. CDC and the smallpox crusade. Washington, DC: US Department of Health and Human Services;1987, Publication No (CDC) 87-8400.
8. Foege WH. House on fire: the fight to eradicate smallpox. Berkeley, Los Angeles, London: University of California Press; 2011.
9. Resolution of the World Health Assembly. Declaration of Global Eradication of Smallpox. 33rd World Health Assembly, 8 May 1980. https://apps.who.int/iris/bitstr eam/handle/10665/155528/WHA33_R3_eng.pdf?sequence=1&isAllowed=y
10. Cochi SL, Dowdle WR, eds. Disease eradication in the 21st century. Implications for global health. Cambridge, MA: The MIT Press; 2011.
11. Resolution of the World Assembly of Delegates, World Organization for Animal Health (OIE). Declaration of Global Eradication of Rinderpest and Implementation of Follow-up Measures to Maintain World Freedom from Rinderpest. Resolution No. 18. 79th Session of the World Assembly of Delegates, Paris, 22–27 May 2011. https://www.oie.int/fileadmin/Home/eng/Media_Center/docs/pdf/RESO_18_EN.pdf
12. The Global Polio Eradication Initiative. https://polioeradication.org/
13. Roberts L. Exclusive: battle to wipe out debilitating Guinea worm parasite hits 10 year delay. Nature 2019;574:157–158.
14. Foege WH. The fears of the rich, the needs of the poor. My years at the CDC. Baltimore: Johns Hopkins University Press; 2018.
15. Foster SO, Shepperd J, Davis JH, et al. Working with African nations to improve the health of their children. Combatting childhood communicable diseases. JAMA 1990;263:3303–3305.

16. "HENDERSON, DA," *The Global Health Chronicles*, accessed December 4, 2022, https://globalhealthchronicles.org/items/show/3532.
17. Merson M, Inrig S. The AIDS pandemic. Searching for a global response. Cham, Switzerland: Springer International Publishing; 2018.
18. McCormick JB, Fisher-Hoch S. Level 4: virus hunters of the CDC. Atlanta, GA: Turner Publishing; 1996.
19. Report of an International Commission. Ebola haemorrhagic fever in Zaire, 1976. Bull WHO 1978;56:271–293.
20. CDC Kenya. Annual Report 2018. https://www.cdc.gov/globalhealth/countries/kenya/reports/pdf/kenya-annual-report-2018-508.pdf
21. De Cock KM. Trends in global health and CDC's international role, 1961–2011. In: Public health then and now: celebrating 50 years of MMWR at CDC. MMWR Morb Mortal Wkly Rep 2011;60(Suppl):104–111.
22. "De Cock, Kevin," *The Global Health Chronicles*, accessed January 29, 2023, https://globalhealthchronicles.org/items/show/6481.
23. Institute of Medicine Committee on Emerging Microbial Threats to Health. Emerging infections: microbial threats to health in the United States. Lederberg J, Shope RE, Oaks SC Jr, eds. Washington, DC: National Academies Press; 1992.
24. "GAYLE, HELENE," *The Global Health Chronicles*, accessed January 29, 2023. https://globalhealthchronicles.org/items/show/7957

13

Projet SIDA in the Democratic Republic of Congo

Kevin M. De Cock

As US epidemiologists were puzzling over the unexplained and growing reports of AIDS among Haitians in the United States (Chapter 6), researchers and health officials in Europe were perplexed by AIDS-like illnesses in Africans seeking care in European medical centers (Chapter 5). In late 1983, before continent-wide surveillance for the disease was instituted, 21 percent of documented AIDS patients in Europe were Africans.[1] A world literature review in 1984 found reports of eighty-five cases of AIDS in Africans, three fourths from the former Zaire and one fifth from Rwanda, both former Belgian colonies.[2]

In the early 1980s, Joe McCormick had become Chief of CDC's Viral Special Pathogens Branch, specializing in hemorrhagic fevers. Earlier in life, fresh from college, he had been sent to Belgium by the Methodist Church to learn French prior to embarking on three years of teaching science in Zaire.[3] Following medical training and specialization in pediatrics, he joined CDC as an EIS officer in 1973. In 1976 he helped investigate the first recognized outbreaks of Ebola in Zaire and Sudan, along with others who would feature in the history of AIDS, including Peter Piot from Belgium's Institute of Tropical Medicine (ITM) and CDC's David Heymann and Don Francis.[3,4,5]

McCormick's connections in the world of tropical virology alerted him in early 1983 to the reports from European medical centers of cases resembling AIDS in Africans who had none of the risk factors found in American AIDS patients. If enough patients were being seen there to cause discussion, even with the expense of travel and consultation, an unrecognized problem was probably unfolding on the African continent itself. With most of the European cases reported among Zaireans in Belgium,[2,6] the logical place to investigate was Kinshasa, Zaire's capital city. With support from Jim Curran,

Kevin M. De Cock, *Projet SIDA in the Democratic Republic of Congo* In: *Dispatches from the AIDS Pandemic.* Kevin M. De Cock, Harold W. Jaffe, and James W. Curran and Edited by: Robin Moseley, Oxford University Press.
© Oxford University Press 2023. DOI: 10.1093/oso/9780197626528.003.0013

McCormick began to plan a field study, which required diplomatic outreach through the US Embassy to Zaire's Ministry of Health.

Institutional competition played out in this scientific quest. In Belgium, rivalry existed between the francophone infectious disease group in Brussels headed by Nathan Clumeck[6] and the team at ITM in Antwerp—Flemish-speaking and headed by Piot.[4] In the United States, NIH, represented by Tom Quinn, was also planning a study in Zaire, in collaboration with ITM. Eventually, CDC, NIH, and ITM joined forces, and McCormick asked one of his senior technologists, Sheila Mitchell, to provide laboratory field support. Clumeck's group focused their efforts on Rwanda.[7]

The CDC team conducted their search for potential AIDS cases at Mama Yemo Hospital, Kinshasa's sprawling public facility named after Zairean President Mobutu Sese Seko's mother. They were fortunate in gaining support from Bila Kapita, the hospital's chief of medicine who had trained in Belgium as a cardiologist. A short, humble man with sharp intellect and political awareness, Kapita served as an advisor throughout CDC's subsequent work. CDC's Robin Ryder, described later in this narrative, spoke of Kapita in reverential terms, "this is a noble figure on the same level I would say as Kofi Annan. Just a presence. And when he speaks, charismatic. No one doubts him. The fact that Dr. Kapita was behind us every step of the way, who was coaching us, 'don't do this, do this,' he was really the godfather of the project."[8] Ryder painted a stark image of Mama Yemo, recalling "not a house of cure. This was a house of death."[8] According to Ryder, Kapita recounted how for several years the hospital had been seeing increasing cases of unexplained fatal wasting and of cryptococcal meningitis, a fungal infection of the brain. He is on record elsewhere as saying his clinical practice changed in 1975 when aggressive KS became increasingly common.[9]

In the fall of 1983, the diagnosis of AIDS was based on clinical findings, supported by, if possible, laboratory evidence of immune deficiency. While the team examined patients and documented their findings, Mitchell performed laborious lymphocyte subset analyses under the most rudimentary laboratory conditions, often working excessively long hours. Today, these tests are automated; in this early study, they were done by hand. These lymphocyte subset analyses served to prove immune deficiency, a surrogate for infection with the then still unrecognized AIDS agent.

Over a three-week period, the team found more than three dozen patients with clinical AIDS and characteristic immune deficiency. Males and females were equally affected, and all patients were heterosexual. The team also found some heterosexual cases linked by sexual contact in a cluster, suggestive of transmission of an infectious agent through a heterosexual network. CDC had long been convinced that the AIDS virus could be heterosexually transmitted, a concept that had taken time to be accepted but was now reinforced by this African field work. A paper from the Kinshasa study published in *The Lancet* in mid-1984,[10] along with results of an analogous investigation by Phillippe Van de Perre from Clumeck's group in Rwanda,[7] convincingly demonstrated an ongoing epidemic of heterosexually acquired AIDS.

The Kinshasa study also contributed to efforts to identify the causative agent. Collaborative work with Montagnier's group at the Institut Pasteur, published in *Science* in 1984, showed the presence of antibodies to the AIDS virus (which they still referred to as LAV [Chapter 9]) in the Zairean patients.[11] The Kinshasa study also yielded specimens from patients with AIDS and AIDS-related complex from which HIV was later isolated by CDC staff in Atlanta, providing some of the first isolates from the African continent.[12,13] The study offered early evidence of greater genetic diversity in the Zairean specimens than in isolates from North America,[12] suggesting HIV had been circulating longer in the African environment.

Upon his return to Atlanta in November 1983, McCormick briefed his colleagues including Curran and CDC Director Bill Foege.[3] These discussions led to the proposal to establish long-term collaboration with Zaire's Ministry of Health through a full-time field presence. Curran immediately recognized that allocating domestic funds to this overseas venture was a good investment for learning about HIV's diverse epidemiology and potential impact in the United States. The title of a much-cited article in the journal *Science* just three years later (NIH's Quinn, the first author) conveyed it well, "AIDS in Africa: An Epidemiologic Paradigm."[14]

In early 1984, Lyle Conrad, the director of CDC's domestic field services, alerted Curran that Jonathan Mann, State Epidemiologist in New Mexico for about a decade, was restless and open to a career change.[15] Mann was a former EIS officer and was fluent in French. McCormick was impressed with Mann's intellect and demeanor, and the pair travelled together to Kinshasa in March. By the summer of 1984, Mann had moved there full-time with his French-born wife and three young children. Curran, his direct supervisor in Atlanta, approved the appointment despite Mann's lack of international work experience. Although Mann was to stay in Kinshasa only two years, the impact of the science conducted during his tenure there and his subsequent public health trajectory were to have lasting influence on the history of AIDS and the global response (Chapter 14).

Projet SIDA

Projet SIDA was the name given to the nascent collaboration with Zaire's Ministry of Health, SIDA being the French name for AIDS (*syndrome d'immunodéficience acquise*). The project's leadership represented a triumvirate comprising CDC, NIH, and ITM. Mann was the director, Henry (Skip) Francis from the intramural program at NIH's National Institute of Allergy and Infectious Diseases (NIAID) directed laboratory work, and ITM's Robert (Bob) Colebunders led clinical investigations. By naming the project director and providing two thirds of the budget, CDC essentially had overall control, but institutional tensions in the field were nonetheless frequent, sometimes requiring resolution at higher levels of the agencies involved.

Mann astutely hired and empowered Zairean physicians and technologists who with time became the face of the project. Among these was N'Galy Bosenge, who essentially served as Projet SIDA's second in command and later headed Zaire's national AIDS control program. Tragically, he died in a car crash in 1989 at age 33. With investment in training of Zairean staff and study visits to the United States, the technical work of the Projet SIDA laboratory became state of the art, perhaps the best outside of South Africa, and highlighted the strength of interdisciplinary collaboration—linking epidemiology, clinical medicine, and laboratory science.

Early Research

Projet SIDA's early work showed yet again that when knowledge is limited, simple studies done well yield important information that becomes foundational for subsequent research and action. The ability to test for HIV in these early days when commercial assays were not available gave the collaboration a tremendous research advantage. Even viral nomenclature had not yet been agreed upon; some of the early research papers still referred to HTLV-III or LAV, rather than HIV.[11,16,17] Projet SIDA's initial research was largely descriptive and analytic in nature, aiming to gain understanding of the distribution of HIV infection, risk factors for different modes of transmission, and clinical presentations and natural history.

Worldwide, there remained a reluctance to accept heterosexual transmission as an important mode of spread. An early Projet SIDA study examined the prevalence of HIV infection in hospital workers, around 6 percent[18] but increasing to almost 9 percent over the subsequent two years.[19] Indirect evidence supported sexual transmission as dominant: HIV prevalence was similar in medical, administrative, and manual workers despite their different occupational exposures to blood or needles. This early study showed other findings persistent over the years in Africa, a higher prevalence in women than men and a younger age for infected females. Another observation that caused relentless debate was the association between HIV-positivity and receipt of injections. HIV-infected persons had received more injections than the uninfected, but a cross-sectional study such as this could not unravel the temporal nature of that association. Receipt of injections might have transmitted HIV to the study subjects, but symptoms from HIV might have led to medical consultation with subsequent injections.

Other theories about HIV's modes of transmission were circulating, such as suggestions that HIV could be transmitted by casual contact and insect vectors (Chapter 10). In the early days of AIDS, these alternative hypotheses had considerable influence. A definitive paper from Projet SIDA published in *JAMA* in 1986 showed that HIV prevalence in nonsexual household contacts of AIDS patients was similar to that among contacts in non-AIDS households and was no greater than expected in relation to the general population of Kinshasa.[17]

Early discussions by project staff and other experts prioritized surveillance for AIDS to give rapid insight into the extent and nature of HIV infection and disease in this African setting. By establishing a rudimentary surveillance system in Kinshasa's five major hospitals, applying a modified CDC case definition, and applying immunologic analysis of T-lymphocyte subsets, Mann and colleagues published shattering results.[20] Their estimate of AIDS incidence—the rate of new AIDS cases in the general population of Kinshasa in the mid-1980s—was 550 to 1,000 cases per million population per year. This first population-based incidence measurement on the continent showed AIDS incidence in Kinshasa to be similar to that in recent Haitian immigrants to the United States, and about one third of that in American MSM. Clearly, the magnitude of the epidemic in Zaire far exceeded that affecting the general population of the United States. Building on the initial case series from Kinshasa described in *The Lancet* in 1984,[10] these new estimates provided evidence of an unfolding public health crisis in Central Africa.

The age- and sex-specific estimates, with AIDS incidence equal overall in males and females but respectively higher in older men and younger women, were compatible with the epidemiology of an STI. A study of female sex workers in Kinshasa found their HIV prevalence to be 27 percent, with numbers of lifetime sex partners a significant risk factor.[21] This cross-sectional study showed male condoms were protective against infection [21,22] and found no increased risk of HIV infection from fellatio. Most importantly, these early data provided scientific support for the HIV educational and prevention programs that slowly began to be rolled out.

While at Projet SIDA, Colebunders led a series of clinical epidemiologic studies showing strong associations between HIV and specific conditions that seemed more common in this African setting than in Europe and North America. Most important was chronic diarrhea,[23,24] generally without fever but associated with extreme wasting*—even greater than that seen in persons suffering from cancer or TB. Other indicative conditions included parotid gland swelling[25] and varicella zoster ("shingles"),[26] the latter sometimes extensive, painful, disfiguring, and threatening to vision if involving the eyes. A novel entity of unknown etiology, but with a strong HIV association, was pruriginous dermatosis,[27] a skin condition with darkly pigmented, itchy, nodular plaques that indicated advanced immune deficiency. Colebunders and colleagues drew attention to the increased risk in HIV-infected persons for cutaneous reactions to certain drugs[28], including cotrimoxazole, commonly used as prophylaxis against PCP.

Clinical observations from Projet SIDA greatly influenced the formulation of a clinical case definition for AIDS surveillance that could be used in the absence of laboratory testing. The key meeting at which this definition was developed was held in Bangui, capital of the Central African Republic, in October 1985, and was attended by delegates from nine Central African countries, as well as from Europe and the United States.[29] The "Bangui definition," as it came to be called, was intended for AIDS surveillance in Africa at a time when testing for HIV was almost nonexistent. It was not meant to be a clinical tool, though its major and minor criteria became accepted as

---

* The term "slim disease" was introduced in Uganda in 1985 for this HIV wasting syndrome. (Serwadda D, Mugerwa RD, Sewankambo NK, et al. Slim disease: a new disease in Uganda and its association with HTLV-III infection. Lancet 1985;2:849–852).

highly predictive of HIV disease. Although later work showed the definition's limitations,[30,31] especially the fact that many ill, HIV-infected persons did not fulfill the required criteria (limited sensitivity), most of those who did were indeed suffering from AIDS (high specificity and predictive value). The Kinshasa group also contributed to the then very neglected issue of AIDS surveillance in children.[32]

Projet SIDA's descriptive studies were broad in scope. They included some of the first observations concerning use of routine vaccines in children with HIV,[33] and the first descriptions of HIV seroconversion illness in African adults and children.[34,35] Risk factors for HIV in hospitalized children were defined, providing the basis for later studies of both mother-to-child transmission and the association between malaria and blood transfusions,[36,37] and insights were gained into HIV's natural history in Africa.[38,39,40] Over the course of these early studies, HIV testing capacity was expanding internationally but predominantly for public health purposes such as blood screening and surveillance. Projet SIDA contributed to international discussions and operational implementation of testing through different laboratory evaluations and experiences.[41,42,43,44]

Mann and colleagues were probably the first in Africa to report an association between HIV and TB and to highlight the difficulties of diagnosis and management of patients without HIV testing.[16,45,46] Despite the brevity in their initial letter to JAMA,[16] their conclusions were prescient: "Infections with HTLV-III/LAV may substantially complicate both management of individual patients with tuberculosis and public health strategies for tuberculosis control in developing countries."[16] The association between HIV infection and increased incidence of TB, and the impact on TB epidemiology globally, have been among the most important consequences of the HIV pandemic. It is notable that Projet SIDA raised the alarm.

Projet SIDA and the Epidemic Intelligence Service

Over the years, numerous EIS officers passed through Kinshasa to assist with diverse research studies. One of the first (and repeated) visitors was Alan Greenberg[47] from CDC's Malaria Branch. Greenberg trained in internal medicine in New York City at the beginning of the American AIDS epidemic and turned down a chief residency and infectious disease fellowship after interviewing for EIS at CDC, excitedly telling his mother, "I found my people."[47] Eager to work in Africa, malaria offered Greenberg the opportunity. Early in his time at CDC, the Branch was approached for assistance to a foreign military serviceman in Texas with severe malaria who also was infected with HIV. Greenberg and his supervisor, Kent Campbell, wondered whether the severity of the soldier's malaria could be related to his HIV infection. Mann and colleagues had described an HIV prevalence of 11 percent in children hospitalized at Mama Yemo compared with only 1 percent in their siblings, as well as an association with malaria.[37] Greenberg and Campbell, along with an experienced clinical parasitologist named Phuc Nguyen Dinh, approached Curran and Mann to propose a series of malaria studies in Kinshasa.

Greenberg described arriving late at night, relieved to be met by Mann at Kinshasa's menacing airport. Mann took him straight to Mama Yemo Hospital's pediatric pavilion where children filled mosquito-infested, crowded rooms, lying on the floor with their mothers who provided nursing care and comfort. Mann impressed on Greenberg that this was the problem he was here to address, high rates of malaria and HIV in children. "One of the issues," Greenberg said, "was, were mosquitoes transmitting HIV? I remember getting bit up, and, I said, 'I certainly hope what we find is that they're not.'"[47]

Greenberg and Nguyen-Dinh systematically showed that children with severe malarial anemia, likely worsened by the parasite's increasing resistance to chloroquine, were entering the hospital HIV-negative but often acquiring HIV through unscreened blood transfusions.[48,49,50] This investigation received widespread scientific and media attention, including for me a memorably engaging interview that Greenberg held with National Public Radio in the United States. The study findings led to rapid change in local transfusion practices and became part of the later extensive literature on malaria and HIV. Many subsequent years of research have been necessary to reach current understanding of the complex interaction between these two epidemic diseases, including in adults (and especially pregnant women) in whom HIV does increase susceptibility to and severity of malaria.

In 1985, McCormick proposed a study that was an epidemiologic version of looking for a needle in a haystack. As described earlier (Chapter 12), he had been one of the investigators of the famous Ebola outbreak that struck the Belgian-staffed mission hospital of Yambuku in the Equateur Province of Zaire in 1976.[3,4,5,51] During that outbreak, hundreds of blood samples were collected from people in the villages surrounding Yambuku and shipped back to Atlanta for long-term storage. Aware in 1985 of the serious AIDS situation in Kinshasa and suspecting that HIV might have been circulating considerably earlier, McCormick pulled these specimens from 1976 from the freezers and tested them for HIV. His hunch was correct: five out of 659 (0.8%) specimens were HIV-positive. He instructed his then EIS officer, Don Forthal, to travel to Yambuku and find the five positive individuals or determine what had happened to them. When I joined his branch as an EIS officer in 1986, McCormick sent me to Zaire to now look for the people who had been HIV-negative in 1976 and to determine if any had become infected over the intervening decade.

The journey to Yambuku, ten years after the Ebola epidemic, and the associated field work were colorful experiences. Phones did not work, Internet and e-mail obviously did not exist, and letters took weeks or months to arrive, if they arrived at all. Memories include a suitcase filled with tattered, devalued bank notes to pay for fuel; overloaded Land Rovers® crossing rickety bridges; the majestic River Congo; and resilient as well as broken, much-loved Belgian missionaries.

Forthal succeeded in finding two of the original five people who had been HIV-infected in 1976; both remained HIV-positive. CDC's Jane Getchell and colleagues successfully isolated HIV from a serum specimen taken in 1976 from a twenty-six-year-old unmarried woman who had died of AIDS-like illness in 1978.[52] This virus remains the earliest HIV isolate available and has served as a temporal reference in the study of viral evolution.[53] Three of the five HIV-positive individuals had died of illnesses compatible with AIDS. No HIV infections had occurred after ten years in the ninety people I located. The study found that the overall prevalence in the rural villages around Yambuku in 1986 was exactly the same as ten years before (0.8%). However, HIV was now slowly spreading in the area, with 11 percent of casual sex workers in small towns infected. AIDS cases were seen in the hospitals, and 2 percent of pregnant women were HIV-positive.

This study showed that HIV was not a new infection but had existed in Congo well before AIDS was described in the United States. In addition, while an epidemic of HIV had emerged in Kinshasa over this time, in the rural area around Yambuku viral prevalence had remained stable showing that the mere presence of the virus is not enough to cause an epidemic. Our paper was published in the *New England Journal of Medicine* in 1988[54] and was highlighted in the *New York Times* by Larry Altman. McCormick's imaginative thinking had paid off.

Expanding Research and Response

Robin Ryder, who had entered EIS in 1974, was selected to replace Mann when the latter moved to Geneva to lead WHO's first AIDS program (Chapter 14). Ryder had trained in medicine but never practiced, and he was a strongly committed, academic epidemiologist. By the time he took over the reins of Projet SIDA in 1986 he already had extensive international experience, having spent time in Bangladesh, the Gambia, Panama, and at the London School of Hygiene and Tropical Medicine. He was committed to using his epidemiologic skills in environments where those were rare. If Mann laid the philosophic and practical foundations for Projet SIDA and conducted essential descriptive science, Ryder sharpened the academic focus. Capitalizing on the infrastructure and relations developed through Projet SIDA, Ryder implemented longer-term and more complex cohort studies, especially relating to maternal and child health, all the while strengthening the project's international reputation (Figure 13.1).

Ryder emphasized how fortunate he felt working on practical problems the world was eager to hear about. "[F]or me, for CDC, this was an epidemiologic heaven. We were able to do large studies answering important epidemiologic (questions)—just a dream for an epidemiologist. I had all sorts of clever people back in Atlanta guiding me. We were an epidemiologic freight train."[8] He credited Curran with providing the necessary protection to allow local decision-making and avoid distraction from institutional rivalries. He emphasized that research addressed real-life questions:

"Our studies were never esoteric. . . We were trying to define how to protect [discordant] heterosexual couples. We were trying to define. . . which risk factors did the mother have to either infect or protect her baby. . . the consumers of our data were the local medical and public health authorities. . . I think that's why we had pretty much of a free rein."[8]

Projet SIDA provided short-term experience for many other CDC staff, mostly former EIS officers, to help increase the body of knowledge on HIV infection and its impact, particularly for infected women and children.[55] The project's study to determine the rate of mother-to-child transmission from women with HIV was emblematic of the high-impact research conducted. Mama Yemo Hospital had dozens of deliveries per day, and the prevalence of HIV infection in pregnant women was 6 percent. Including deliveries at

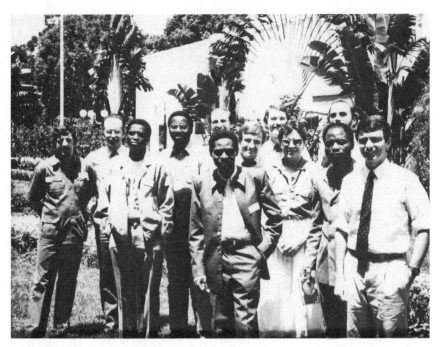

Figure 13.1. Projet SIDA site visit, circa 1986. Pictured (l–r): Joe McCormick, Jonathan Mann, Michel Lubaki, Skip Francis, Bila Kapita, Bob Colebunders, Jim Curran, Tom Quinn, Ann Nelson, N'Galy Bosenge, Peter Piot, Robin Ryder. (Jim Curran, personal collection)

Kinshasa's largest private hospital, Ngaliema, some five to ten HIV-infected women were delivering daily, and most were willing to be enrolled in studies, numbers not possible elsewhere. This study entailed testing over eight thousand women for HIV and following almost five hundred infected women and their infants, as well as a similar number of matched controls, for a year. The project staffed the delivery rooms twenty-four hours per day and provided basic maternal and child health services to all participants for the year of follow-up.

Projet SIDA and CDC staff recognized the potential ethical pitfalls of offering care to recruited pregnant women. Special attention might be considered coercive, yet this had to be balanced with the moral obligation to do the best for study subjects. Rigid follow-up had to be assured for study integrity and valid results, but also to avoid unjustifiable impositions on study participants in case of a failed or inconclusive study. Researchers had to be prepared for the possible criticism that the study was being done in Kinshasa only because of convenience and cost. The collective conclusion was that this study would provide locally as well as globally relevant findings essential for public health action. Still, complex questions such as these would persist and were a harbinger of angry exchanges years later concerning clinical trials of interventions to prevent perinatal HIV transmission in low-income settings (Chapters 15 and 16).

At the time of the study, molecular diagnosis of infection in infants was not possible. Outcomes studied were mainly clinical, including mortality, although a small number of infants had HIV cultures performed. Over 20 percent of tested infants of infected mothers were themselves infected, and almost one third had died or had AIDS at one year of age. Immunodeficiency in the mother was a risk factor for infection in the infant, and infants of infected women were more likely to be premature, have low birth weight, and die in the first twenty-eight days of life. Results from this study[56,57] provided basic information important for subsequent global research on preventing vertical transmission of HIV, which in breastfeeding populations could result in infection rates in surviving infants close to 45 percent.

The project also contributed to the understanding of basic HIV epidemiology that later was taken for granted. Veronique Batter, a Belgian statistician, analyzed the large data sets from sequential HIV testing of pregnant women and made two important observations.[58] First, new HIV infections were concentrated in the youngest women—those aged twenty to twenty-four years had an annual incidence in 1989 of 5.7 percent. Second, the apparently stable HIV prevalence in pregnant women, around 6 percent overall, gave a false sense of security. Unchanging overall prevalence masked the newly infected women who replaced those who dropped out of antenatal testing because of HIV-associated infertility, disease, or death.

In another study, over seven thousand employees of a bank and a factory were enrolled in follow-up to better understand the dynamics and impact of the virus.[59] The wealthier and better educated had higher levels of infection than more disadvantaged counterparts. Sexual behavior was the driver of HIV infection, and AIDS was the leading cause of death, responsible for one fifth to one quarter of deaths. Studies among heterosexual couples quickly showed the phenomenon of discordancy, where one partner was HIV-positive and the other HIV-negative, and studies of knowledge and attitudes were undertaken for later work on HIV counseling and support.[60]

A subsequent study led by William (Bill) Heyward (Figure 13.2), who would succeed Ryder as director, was one of the earliest attempts to introduce

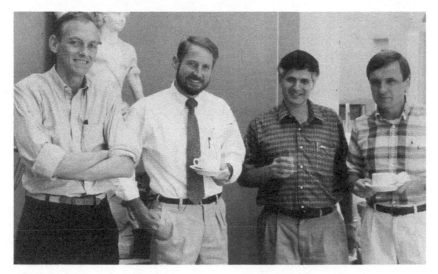

Figure 13.2. Pictured (l–r): Kevin De Cock, Bill Heyward, Bruce Weniger, Jim Curran; international AIDS conference, Florence, Italy, 1991. Heyward was the last Projet SIDA Director, and De Cock and Weniger were directors of CDC-supported field stations in Cote d'Ivoire and Thailand, respectively. (Kevin De Cock, personal collection)

and evaluate HIV testing and counseling in the African context, admittedly with limited impact initially.[61] HIV-infected women in the study who were followed after their last pregnancy were very reluctant to disclose their status to partners, and despite their being offered counseling and contraception, their fertility rates were actually higher than those of seronegative women.[62]

Nonetheless, work with discordant couples did not show high rates of abandonment, which Ryder attributed to cultural sensitivity as well as key project staff:

> "We emphasized. . . the importance of having a mother and father to raise these kids. It's a message that I, as a biomedical scientist, could never have gotten across, but Mama Mbuyi (the nurse counselor) with her wisdom and her knowledge and really philosophy and probably some psychology was able to pull on that, and as a result we had very little divorce."[8]

ITM had special expertise in STIs and established a clinic in Matonge, a crowded, vibrant *"quartier populaire"* (low-income district) in Kinshasa known for its active nightlife. Once again, expert laboratory work supported epidemiology. Prostitution was prevalent but, with clear exceptions such as the trade in upscale hotels, was difficult to define. The term *"femmes libres"* (free women) was used synonymously but incorrectly with sex workers. *Femmes libres* were women who did not necessarily have a steady male partner, might have many relationships that they used to varying transactional degrees, and lived in a context of considerable heterosexual freedom, devoid of stigma. Unsurprisingly, *femmes libres* were shown to have high rates of STIs and HIV. ITM's Marie Laga led important work showing the role of STIs as biological factors promoting HIV transmission and the impact of public health interventions in this vulnerable group.[63,64,65,66,67] The team also examined human papilloma virus (HPV) infection in HIV-infected women and showed an almost fifteenfold increase in lesions indicative of risk of later cervical cancer ("cervical intraepithelial neoplasia").[68,69] The association between HIV and HPV, and the likelihood of women developing cancer of the cervix, later became prominent topics of discussion internationally in relation to clinical management and AIDS surveillance.

Ann Nelson from the Armed Forces Institute of Pathology conducted early research on HIV-associated pathology.[70,71] Colebunders' Belgian replacement, Joseph (Jos) Perriëns, who also later took up a career at WHO, furthered the project's interest in TB and other clinical work.[72,73,74,75,76] A controlled trial examining duration of antituberculous therapy in relation to HIV status highlighted the increased risk of relapse after treatment completion in persons with HIV.[74] Other work explored the nature of diarrheal disease in children.[77,78]

Despite the NIH presence in the project, with Christopher (Chris) Brown succeeding the founding laboratory director, Skip Francis, it was a difficult environment in which to do basic science and the laboratory inevitably played a mostly supportive role. The highly skilled Zairian technicians benefited from training opportunities offered by NIH staff and contributed independently to the science, presentations, and papers. Frieda Behets, a Belgian technologist with extensive African experience, oversaw the day-to-day running of the laboratory and supervised useful evaluations of various diagnostics as well as more sophisticated work.[79,80,81,82,83,84,85,86] Tom Quinn provided overall supervision of the laboratory agenda but also participated in clinical and epidemiology research.

The project continued its work with the political protection Mann had ensured but with continuous attention to diplomacy. Zaire was a difficult and corruption-riddled country, with an autocratic President (Mobutu) who, faced with inability to pay his army, told soldiers, "*Débrouillez-vous*" ("sort yourselves out"), in effect, a license to loot. Projet SIDA did its work while keeping a low profile nationally and focusing on promoting Congolese scientists. People worked shoulder to shoulder, sharing the same working conditions and worker protection measures and facing the same uncertainties of where HIV was going. Among the approximately three hundred project staff, only five were expatriates. Study sections were all Congolese led, discussions were all in French, study priorities were decided in Kinshasa instead of Atlanta, and conference presentations were almost all delivered by the Congolese. At a time when some African countries were reticent to share data about their burgeoning AIDS epidemics, the government of Zaire was remarkably trusting of Projet SIDA, a trust that was both hard-earned and painstakingly maintained. Nonetheless, and paradoxically, the Zairean government did not report AIDS cases to WHO, despite the openness regarding scientific publications and presentations.

Ryder described how he and his counterparts established an ethical review board to evaluate study protocols, adhering to NIH guidance and standards, and how it succeeded despite societal dysfunction. Nonetheless, tensions between research and public health requirements were constant, such as the availability of HIV tests for research but not for screening blood for transfusion. Epidemiology dominated the agenda, funding for any clinical care was lacking, and the slowly developing donor agenda for HIV prevention was divorced from the research. All of this is explicable, but the always supportive Bila Kapita at Mama Yemo suffered and continually reminded colleagues of the needs of the patients.

Ryder ensured that the hierarchy established under Mann was maintained, with CDC the lead agency in the tripartite but unequal yet productive collaboration between Atlanta, Bethesda, and Antwerp. The term "health diplomacy" is widely used today, even if poorly defined. Projet SIDA was an example of health diplomacy ahead of its time, not only regarding international relations around AIDS but perhaps also concerning internal management and communications between partners.

The End of Projet SIDA

Heyward had been leading the International Activity in Curran's AIDS division at CDC in Atlanta and in 1990 wanted to return to field work. Strongly supported in Kinshasa by CDC epidemiologist Michael (Mike) St Louis, Heyward took over from Ryder when the latter returned to the United States, but political violence erupted in September 1991 with Zairean soldiers and mobs ransacking the city. St Louis recounted to me how his family fearfully sheltered in their compound, along with the Heywards, as looters broke into neighboring houses and stole anything removable, including electrical wiring and baby clothes. The US State Department ordered American employees to evacuate, and CDC staff were escorted across the River Congo by Belgian paratroopers to Brazzaville, capital of the adjacent Republic of Congo. In 1992, the sponsors of Projet SIDA assessed that the integrity of research could no longer be assured, and funding was stopped. The project had produced almost one hundred and fifty publications on AIDS in Africa, some of them seminal to the field, and probably close to one thousand presentations at scientific conferences.

NIH's Francis, who had left four years earlier, recounted to *Science* magazine's Jon Cohen how he was asked to return in 1992 to retrieve equipment and stored biologic specimens.[87] Difficult discussions ensued with Congolese staff who felt aggrieved they had been left in the lurch after CDC support had been discontinued because of conditions on the ground. Ultimately, the politics of Zaire and Mobutu's leadership were responsible for the end of this productive collaboration. For some years after the project collapsed, publications from work on saved specimens continued to appear in the literature and demonstrated the extensive molecular diversity of HIV strains in Zaire, indicative of HIV's longstanding circulation in the country.[88,89,90,91,92,93]

Musing on how he was affected personally by his Projet SIDA experience, Ryder commented that what gave him long-lasting satisfaction was the career progression of some of the Zairean colleagues.[8] The intensity of field work under conditions such as those in Kinshasa leaves indelible impressions and strong emotions. Bayende, a Congolese colleague from Projet SIDA who had taken an academic position in the United States, grew tired of Americans mispronouncing his name and decided to have it officially changed. He chose "Ryder," so now there are two "Dr Ryders" with experience of HIV research in the former Zaire.

CDC's Ryder commented that, after his departure, he spent many months writing up work from Projet SIDA but could marshal little enthusiasm for HIV research where he was working in New York. Several of these later papers concerned longer-term outcomes in HIV-infected families and the issue of orphanhood. Over a three-year period in Kinshasa, if a mother was HIV-infected, there was a five- to tenfold higher risk of maternal, paternal, and childhood death compared with families of HIV-negative mothers.[94] Annually, about 8 percent of children born to HIV-positive mothers became orphans, almost half of whom were themselves HIV-infected.[95]

"So, I moved on," he said. "I stayed in infectious diseases. . . but not HIV. It couldn't be recreated. I closed that chapter."[8] The melancholia that Ryder described was common among field workers returning to their countries of origin. Many sensed life was now mundane, so different from the chaotic vibrancy of the foreign environments to which they had given their all. And Ryder's last Kinshasa papers epitomized this period of the AIDS epidemic, a few years before the advent of effective treatment, when all looked desperately bleak.

Even after the demise of Projet SIDA, CDC has remained involved in the Democratic Republic of Congo (DRC). Important topics have included HIV under PEPFAR, monkeypox, polio, measles, Ebola (repeatedly), and now COVID-19. CDC and the world have not heard the last from or about the DRC, politically as well as medically.

Notes

1. Anonymous. The epidemiology of AIDS in Europe. Eur J Cancer Clin Oncol 1984;20:157–264.
2. De Cock KM. AIDS: An African Disease? In: Gupta S, ed., AIDS-associated syndromes. University of California, Irvine; 1984. Advances in Experimental Medicine and Biology, 1985;187:1–12.
3. McCormick JB, Fisher-Hoch S. Level 4: virus hunters of the CDC. Atlanta, GA: Turner Publishing; 1996.
4. Piot P. No time to lose. A life in pursuit of deadly viruses. New York: WW Norton and Co; 2012.
5. Report of an International Commission. Ebola haemorrhagic fever in Zaire, 1976. Bull WHO 1978;56: 271–293.
6. Clumeck N, Sonnet J, Taelman H, et al. Acquired immunodeficiency syndrome in African patients. N Engl J Med 1984;310:492–497.

7. Van de Perre P, Rouvroy D, Lepage P, et al. Acquired immunodeficiency syndrome in Rwanda. Lancet 1984;2:62–65.

8. "RYDER, ROBIN," *The Global Health Chronicles*, accessed January 25, 2023, https://www.globalhealthchronicles.org/items/show/7730

9. Garrett L. The coming plague. New York: Farrar, Strauss and Giroux; 1994:367.

10. Piot P, Quinn TC, Taelman H, et al. Acquired immunodeficiency syndrome in a heterosexual population in Zaire. Lancet 1984;2:65–69.

11. Brun-Vezinet F, Montagnier L, Chamaret S, et al. Prevalence of antibody to lymphadenopathy associated virus in African patients with AIDS. Science 1984;226:453–457.

12. Benn S, Rutledge R, Folks T, et al. Genomic heterogeneity of AIDS retroviral isolates from North America and Zaire. Science 1985;230:949–951.

13. McCormick JB, Krebs JW, Mitchell SW, et al. Isolation of human immune deficiency virus from African AIDS patients and from persons without AIDS or IgG antibody to human immune deficiency virus. Am J Trop Med Hyg 1987;36:102–106.

14. Quinn TC, Mann JM, Curran JW, Piot P. AIDS in Africa: an epidemiologic paradigm. Science 1986;234:955–963.

15. "CURRAN, JAMES," *The Global Health Chronicles*, accessed January 24, 2023, https://www.globalhealthchronicles.org/items/show/7743

16. Mann J, Snider DE Jr, Francis H, et al. Association between HTLV-III/LAV infection and tuberculosis in Zaire. JAMA 1986;256:346.

17. Mann JM, Quinn TC, Francis H, et al. Prevalence of HTLV-III/LAV in household contacts of patients with confirmed AIDS and controls in Kinshasa, Zaire. JAMA 1986;256:721–724.

18. Mann JM, Francis H, Quinn TC, et al. HIV seroprevalence among hospital workers in Kinshasa, Zaire: lack of association with occupational exposure. JAMA 1986;256:3099–3102.

19. N'Galy B, Ryder RW, Bila K, et al. Human immunodeficiency virus infection among employees in an African hospital. N Engl J Med 1988;319:1123–1127.

20. Mann JM, Francis II, Quinn T, et al. Surveillance for AIDS in a central African city. Kinshasa, Zaire. JAMA 1986;255:3255–3259.

21. Mann J, Quinn TC, Piot P, et al. Condom use and HIV infection among prostitutes in Zaire. N Engl J Med 1987;316:345.

22. Mann JM, Nzilambi N, Piot P, et al. HIV infection and associated risk factors in female prostitutes in Kinshasa, Zaire. AIDS 1998;2:249–254.

23. Colebunders R, Francis H, Mann JM, et al. Persistent diarrhea, strongly associated with HIV infection in Kinshasa, Zaire. Am J Gastroenterol 1987;82:859–864.

24. Colebunders R, Lusakumuni K, Nelson AM, et al. Persistent diarrhoea in Zairian AIDS patients: an endoscopic and histological study. Gut 1988;29:1687–1691. doi: 10.1136/gut.29.12.1687.

25. Colebunders R, Francis H, Mann JM, et al. Parotid swelling during human immunodeficiency virus infection. Arch Otolaryngol Head Neck Surg 1988;114:330–332. doi: 10.1001/archotol.1988.01860150112027.

26. Colebunders R, Mann JM, Francis H, et al. Herpes zoster in African patients: a clinical predictor of human immunodeficiency virus infection. J Infect Dis 1988;157:314–318. doi: 10.1093/infdis/157.2.314.

27. Colebunders R, Mann JM, Francis H, et al. Generalized papular pruritic eruption in African patients with human immunodeficiency virus infection. AIDS 1987;1:117–121.

28. Colebunders R, Izaley L, Bila K, et al. Cutaneous reactions to trimethoprim-sulfamethoxazole in African patients with the acquired immunodeficiency syndrome. Ann Intern Med 1987;107:599–600. doi: 10.7326/0003-4819-107-4-599_2.

29. Colebunders R, Mann JM, Francis H, et al. Evaluation of a clinical case-definition of acquired immunodeficiency syndrome in Africa. Lancet 1987;1:492–494. doi: 10.1016/s0140-6736(87)92099-x.

30. De Cock KM, Colebunders R, Francis H, et al. Evaluation of the WHO clinical case definition of AIDS in rural Zaire. AIDS 1988;2:219–221.

31. De Cock KM, Selik R, Soro B, Gayle H, Colebunders RL. AIDS surveillance in Africa: a re-appraisal of case definitions. BMJ 1991;303:1185–1188.

32. Colebunders RI, Greenberg A, Nguyen-Dinh P, et al. Evaluation of a clinical case definition of AIDS in African children. AIDS 1987;1:151–153.

33. Colebunders RL, Izaley L, Musampu M, Pauwels P, Francis H, Ryder R. BCG vaccine abscesses are unrelated to HIV infection. JAMA 1988;259:352.

34. Colebunders R, Greenberg AE, Francis H, et al. Acute HIV illness following blood transfusion in three African children. AIDS 1988;2:125–127. doi: 10.1097/00002030-198804000-00009.

35. Colebunders R, Ryder R, Francis H, et al. Seroconversion rate, mortality, and clinical manifestations associated with the receipt of a human immunodeficiency virus-infected blood transfusion in Kinshasa, Zaire. J Infect Dis 1991;164:450–456. doi: 10.1093/infdis/164.3.450.

36. Mann JM, Francis H, Davachi F, et al. Risk factors for human immunodeficiency virus seropositivity among children 1-24 months old in Kinshasa, Zaire. Lancet 1986;2:654–657. doi: 10.1016/s0140-6736(86)90167-4.

37. Mann JM, Francis H, Davachi F, et al. Human immunodeficiency virus seroprevalence in pediatric patients 2 to 14 years of age at Mama Yemo Hospital, Kinshasa, Zaire. Pediatrics 1986;78:673–677.

38. Mann JM, Bila K, Colebunders RL, et al. Natural history of human immunodeficiency virus infection in Zaire. Lancet 1986;2:707–709. doi: 10.1016/s0140-6736(86)90229-1.

39. Colebunders R, Francis H, Mann JM, et al. Slow progression of illness occasionally occurs in HIV infected Africans. AIDS 1987;1:65.

40. Colebunders RL, Lebughe I, Nzila N, et al. Cutaneous delayed-type hypersensitivity in patients with human immunodeficiency virus infection in Zaire. J Acquir Immune Defic Syndr 1989;2:576–578.

41. Mann JM, Francis H, Ndongala L, et al. ELISA readers and HIV antibody testing in developing countries. Lancet 1986;1:1504. doi: 10.1016/s0140-6736(86)91541-2.

42. Colebunders R, Francis H, Duma MM, et al. HIV-1 infection in HIV-1 enzyme-linked immunoassay seronegative patients in Kinshasa, Zaire. Int J STD AIDS 1990;1:330–334. doi: 10.1177/095646249000100505. PMID: 2098151.

43. Colebunders R, Ndumbe P. Priorities for HIV testing in developing countries? Lancet 1993;342:601–602. doi: 10.1016/0140-6736(93)91417-k.

44. Francis HL, Mann J, Colebunders RL, et al. Serodiagnosis of the acquired immune deficiency syndrome by enzyme-linked immunosorbent assay compared to cellular immunologicparameters in African AIDS patients and controls. Am J Trop Med Hyg 1988;38:641–646. doi: 10.4269/ajtmh.1988.38.641.

45. Colebunders RL, Braun MM, Nzila N, Dikilu K, Muepu K, Ryder R. Evaluation of the World Health Organization clinical case definition of AIDS among tuberculosis patients in Kinshasa, Zaire. J Infect Dis 1989;160:902–903. doi: 10.1093/infdis/160.5.902.

46. Colebunders RL, Ryder RW, Nzilambi N, et al. HIV infection in patients with tuberculosis in Kinshasa, Zaire. Am Rev Respir Dis 1989;139:1082–1085. doi: 10.1164/ajrccm/139.5.1082. PMID: 2496632.

47. "GREENBERG, ALAN," The Global Health Chronicles, accessed January 29, 2023. https://www.globalhealthchronicles.org/items/show/7907

48. Greenberg AE, Nguyen-Dinh P, Mann JM, et al. The association between malaria, blood transfusions, and HIV seropositivity in a pediatric population in Kinshasa, Zaire. JAMA 1988;259:545–549.

49. Nguyen-Dinh P, Greenberg AE, Mann JM, et al. Absence of association between Plasmodium falciparum malaria and human immunodeficiency virus infection in children in Kinshasa, Zaire. Bull World Health Organ 1987;65:607–613.

50. Greenberg AE, Nsa W, Ryder RW. Plasmodium falciparum malaria and perinatally acquired human immunodeficiency virus type 1 infection in Kinshasa, Zaire. A prospective, longitudinal cohort study of 587 children. N Engl J Med 1991;325:105–109. doi: 10.1056/NEJM199107113250206.

51. Close WT. Ebola. A novel of the first oubreak by a doctor who was there. New York: Ballantine Books; 1995.

52. Getchell JP, Hicks DR, Svinivasan A, et al. Human immunodeficiency virus isolated from a serum sample collected in 1976 in Central Africa. J Infect Dis 1987;156:833–836.

53. Srinivasan A, York D, Butler D Jr, et al. Molecular characterization of HIV-1 isolated from a serum collected in 1976: nucleotide sequence comparison to recent isolates and generation of hybrid HIV. AIDS Res Hum Retroviruses 1989;5:121–129. doi: 10.1089/aid.1989.5.121.

54. Nzilambi N, De Cock KM, Forthal DN, et al. The prevalence of infection with human immunodeficiency virus over a 10-year period in rural Zaire. N Engl J Med 1988;318:276–279. doi: 10.1056/NEJM198802043180503.

55. Ryder RW, Oxtoby MJ, Mvula M, et al. Safety and immunogenicity of bacille Calmette-Guérin, diphtheria-tetanus-pertussis, and oral polio vaccines in newborn children in Zaire infected with human immunodeficiency virus type 1. J Pediatr 1993;122:697–702. doi: 10.1016/s0022-3476(06)80007-7.

56. Ryder RW, Nsa W, Hassig SE, et al. Perinatal transmission of the human immunodeficiency virus type 1 to infants of seropositive women in Zaire. N Engl J Med 1989;320:1637–1642. doi: 10.1056/NEJM198906223202501.

57. St Louis ME, Kamenga M, Brown C, et al. Risk for perinatal HIV-1 transmission according to maternal immunologic, virologic, and placental factors. JAMA 1993;269:2853–2859.

58. Batter V, Matela B, Nsuami M, et al. High HIV-1 incidence in young women masked by stable overall seroprevalence among childbearing women in Kinshasa, Zaïre: estimating incidence from serial seroprevalence data. AIDS 1994;8:811–817. doi: 10.1097/00002030-199406000-00014.

59. Ryder RW, Ndilu M, Hassig SE, et al. Heterosexual transmission of HIV-1 among employees and their spouses at two large businesses in Zaire. AIDS 1990;4:725–732. doi: 10.1097/00002030-199008000-00002.

60. Irwin K, Bertrand J, Mibandumba N, et al. Knowledge, attitudes and beliefs about HIV infection and AIDS among healthy factory workers and their wives, Kinshasa, Zaire. Soc Sci Med 1991;32:917–930. doi:10.1016/0277-9536(91)90247-a.

61. Heyward WL, Batter VL, Malulu M, et al. Impact of HIV counseling and testing among child-bearing women in Kinshasa, Zaïre. AIDS 1993;7:1633–1637. doi:10.1097/00002030-199312000-00014.

62. Ryder RW, Batter VL, Nsuami M, et al. Fertility rates in 238 HIV-1-seropositive women in Zaire followed for 3 years post-partum. AIDS 1991;5:1521–1527. doi:10.1097/00002030-199112000-00016.

63. Goeman J, Kivuvu M, Nzila N, et al. Similar serological response to conventional therapy for syphilis among HIV-positive and HIV-negative women. Genitourin Med 1995;71:275–279. doi: 10.1136/sti.71.5.275.

64. Laga M. Interactions between STDs and HIV infection. STD Bull 1992;13:3–6.

65. Laga M, Alary M, Nzila N, et al. Condom promotion, sexually transmitted diseases treatment, and declining incidence of HIV-1 infection in female Zairian sex workers. Lancet 1994;344:246–248. doi: 10.1016/s0140-6736(94)93005-8.

66. Laga M, Manoka A, Kivuvu M, et al. Non-ulcerative sexually transmitted diseases as risk factors for HIV-1 transmission in women: results from a cohort study. AIDS 1993;7:95–102. doi: 10.1097/00002030-199301000-00015.

67. Nzila N, Laga M, Thiam MA, et al. HIV and other sexually transmitted diseases among female prostitutes in Kinshasa. AIDS 1991;5:715–721. doi: 10.1097/00002030-199106000-00011.

68. Laga M, Icenogle JP, Marsella R, et al. Genital papillomavirus infection and cervical dysplasia—opportunistic complications of HIV infection. Int J Cancer 1992;50:45–48. doi: 10.1002/ijc.2910500110.

69. St Louis ME, Icenogle JP, Manzila T, et al. Genital types of papillomavirus in children of women with HIV-1 infection in Kinshasa, Zaire. Int J Cancer 1993;54:181–184. doi:10.1002/ijc.2910540203.

70. Nelson AM, Firpo A, Kamenga M, Davachi F, Angritt P, Mullick FG. Pediatric AIDS and perinatal HIV infection in Zaire: epidemiologic and pathologic findings. Prog AIDS Pathol 1992;3:1–33.

71. Nelson AM, Perriëns JH, Kapita B, et al. A clinical and pathological comparison of the WHO and CDC case definitions for AIDS in Kinshasa, Zaïre: is passive surveillance valid? AIDS 1993;7:1241–1245. doi: 10.1097/00002030-199309000-00014.

72. Mugaruka Z, Perriëns JH, Kapita B, Piot P. Oral manifestations of HIV-1 infection in Zairian patients. AIDS 1991;5:237–238. doi: 10.1097/00002030-199102000-00025.

73. Perriëns JH, Mussa M, Luabeya MK, et al. Neurological complications of HIV-1-seropositive internal medicine inpatients in Kinshasa, Zaire. J Acquir Immune Defic Syndr. 1992;5:333–340.

74. Perriëns JH, Colebunders RL, Karahunga C, Willame JC, Jeugmans J, Kaboto M. Tuberculosis treatment failure rate among human immunodeficiency virus (HIV) seropositive compared with HIV seronegative patients with pulmonary tuberculosis treated with "standard" chemotherapy in Kinshasa, Zaire. Am Rev Respir Dis 1991;144:750–755. doi: 10.1164/ajrccm/144.4.750.

75. Mukadi Y, Perriens JH, St Louis ME, et al. Spectrum of immunodeficiency in HIV-1-infected patients with pulmonary tuberculosis in Zaire. Lancet 1993;342:143–146.

76. Klausner JD, Ryder RW, Baende E, et al. Mycobacterium tuberculosis in household contacts of human immunodeficiency virus type 1-seropositive patients with active pulmonary tuberculosis in Kinshasa, Zaire. J Infect Dis. 1993;168:106–111. doi: 10.1093/infdis/168.1.106. Erratum in: J Infect Dis 1993;168:802.

77. Pavia AT, Long EG, Ryder RW, et al. Diarrhea among African children born to human immunodeficiency virus 1-infected mothers: clinical, microbiologic and epidemiologic features. Pediatr Infect Dis J 1992;11:996–1003. doi: 10.1097/00006454-199211120-00002.

78. Thea DM, St Louis ME, Atido U, et al. A prospective study of diarrhea and HIV-1 infection among 429 Zairian infants. N Engl J Med 1993;329:1696–1702. doi: 10.1056/NEJM199312023292304.

79. Behets FM, Edidi B, Quinn TC, et al. Detection of salivary HIV-1-specific IgG antibodies in high-risk populations in Zaire. J Acquir Immune Defic Syndr 1991;4:183–187.

80. Behets F, Bertozzi S, Kasali M, et al. Successful use of pooled sera to determine HIV-1 seroprevalence in Zaire with development of cost-efficiency models. AIDS 1990;4:737–741. doi: 10.1097/00002030-199008000-00004.

81. Behets F, Bishagara K, Disasi A, Likin S, Ryder RW, Brown C, Quinn TC. Diagnosis of HIV infection with instrument-free assays as an alternative to the ELISA and western blot testing strategy: an evaluation in Central Africa. J Acquir Immune Defic Syndr. 1992;5:878–882.

82. Behets F, Kashamuka M, Pappaioanou M, et al. Stability of human immunodeficiency virus type 1 antibodies in whole blood dried on filter paper and stored under various tropical conditions in Kinshasa, Zaire. J Clin Microbiol. 1992;30:1179–1182.

83. Kashala O, Kayembe K, Kanki P, et al. Humoral aspects of anti-HIV immune responses in Zairians with AIDS: lower antigenemia does not correlate with immune complex levels. AIDS Res Hum Retroviruses 1993;9:251–258. doi: 10.1089/aid.1993.9.251.

84. Kashamuka M, Nzila N, Mussey L, et al. Short report: analysis of anti-malaria immune response during human immunodeficiency virus infection in adults in Kinshasa, Democratic Republic of the Congo. Am J Trop Med Hyg 2003;68:376–378.

85. Pappaioanou M, Kashamuka M, Behets F, et al. Accurate detection of maternal antibodies to HIV in newborn whole blood dried on filter paper. AIDS 1993;7:483–488. doi: 10.1097/00002030-199304000-00005.
86. Perriëns JH, Magazani K, Kapila N, et al. Use of a rapid test and an ELISA for HIV antibody screening of pooled serum samples in Lubumbashi, Zaire. J Virol Methods 1993;41:213–221. doi:10.1016/0166-0934(93)90128-e.
87. Cohen J. The rise and fall of Projet SIDA. Science 1997;278:1565–1568.
88. Kalish ML, Robbins KE, Pieniazek D. Recombinant viruses and early global HIV-1 epidemic. Emerg Infect Dis 2004;10:1227–1234. doi:10.3201/eid1007.030904.
89. Peeters M, Nkengasong J, Willems B, et al. Antibodies to V3 loop peptides derived from chimpanzee lentiviruses and the divergent HIV-1ANT-70 isolate in human sera from different geographic regions. AIDS 1994;8:1657–1661. doi: 10.1097/00002030-199412000-00003.
90. Yang C, Li M, Mokili JL, et al. Genetic diversification and recombination of HIV type 1 group M in Kinshasa, Democratic Republic of Congo. AIDS Res Hum Retroviruses 2005;21:661–666. doi: 10.1089/aid.2005.21.661.
91. Louwagie J, McCutchan F, Van der Groen G, et al. Genetic comparison of HIV-1 isolates from Africa, Europe, and North America. AIDS Res Hum Retroviruses 1992;8:1467–1469. doi: 0.1089/aid.1992.8.1467.
92. Potts KE, Kalish ML, Bandea CI, et al. Genetic diversity of human immunodeficiency virus type 1 strains in Kinshasa, Zaire. AIDS Res Hum Retroviruses 1993;9:613–618. doi: 10.1089/aid.1993.9.613.
93. Schaefer A, Robbins KE, Nzilambi EN, et al. Divergent HIV and simian immunodeficiency virus surveillance, Zaire. Emerg Infect Dis 2005;11(9):1446–1148. doi. 10.3201/eid1109.050179.
94. Ryder RW, Nsuami M, Nsa W, et al. Mortality in HIV-1-seropositive women, their spouses and their newly born children during 36 months of follow-up in Kinshasa, Zaïre. AIDS 1994;8:667–672. doi: 10.1097/00002030-199405000-00014.
95. Ryder RW, Kamenga M, Nkusu M, Batter V, Heyward WL. AIDS orphans in Kinshasa, Zaïre: incidence and socioeconomic consequences. AIDS 1994;8:673–679. doi: 10.1097/00002030-199405000-00015.

14

Jonathan Mann

Past as Prologue

Kevin M. De Cock

Perhaps what is most surprising about Jonathan Mann's career is that as promising and productive as it always was, nothing would have predicted in the earliest days of AIDS that he would come to personify the world's struggle against this new disease. Mann was born in 1947 in Boston, a city important in his training and career.[1,2] He studied history as an undergraduate at Harvard, graduating *magna cum laude* in 1969, and must have been deeply influenced by time spent in his third year, in 1967–68, at the famed *Institut d'études politiques de Paris* ('*Sciences Po*'), the Paris school of political science.

Those were heady days politically and socially in Paris. It was where he met his first wife, Marie-Paule Bondat, and it allowed him to perfect his French.[3] The couple was married in 1970 and went on to have nonidentical twin daughters (Lydia and Naomi) and a son (Aaron).

Mann studied medicine at Washington University in St Louis, graduated in 1974, and completed his internship at Beth Israel Hospital in Boston. He intended to pursue training in ophthalmology, but to pay back a PHS loan he joined CDC in 1975 for the two-year EIS program and was assigned to the New Mexico Health and Social Services Department.[4] After EIS, he became New Mexico's State Epidemiologist and Deputy Director of the Health Services Division, remaining there until 1984 when he rejoined CDC to move to Kinshasa. His responsibilities in New Mexico were broad and he published on a variety of infectious diseases, including bubonic plague. Canadian physician Jacques Pepin devoted several pages to reviewing Mann's life in his book on the origins of AIDS,[5] commenting that Mann had been influenced early on by Camus's *The Plague*.

Mann's time in Kinshasa, barely two years from 1984 to 1986, was short in relation to what was achieved. Describing Mann's productivity, his CDC colleague Alan Greenberg remarked, "He was prolific. He understood

Kevin M. De Cock, *Jonathan Mann* In: *Dispatches from the AIDS Pandemic*. Kevin M. De Cock, Harold W. Jaffe, and James W. Curran and Edited by: Robin Moseley, Oxford University Press. © Oxford University Press 2023. DOI: 10.1093/oso/9780197626528.003.0014

the importance of publishing. . . he set the standard for writing. He used the published literature. . . to get the message out about how severe a crisis this was."[6] Jim Curran, Mann's CDC supervisor, said, "He was controversial throughout his career and quite autocratic in Zaire but nothing close to Projet SIDA' s accomplishments would have occurred without his energy, ingenuity, and leadership."[7]

Mann's first substantive contacts with WHO concerning AIDS occurred in 1985.[8] Two meetings were critical: the first international conference on AIDS in Atlanta in April 1985, cosponsored by CDC and WHO; and the WHO-sponsored case definition meeting in Bangui, Central African Republic, in October (Chapter 13).[8,9] At the Atlanta meeting, Mann spoke on behalf of Projet SIDA and Zaire and indeed for the African continent itself. He was even more prominent at the international conference in Paris a year later. Robin Ryder, who would succeed Mann in Kinshasa, recalled how Mann "sparkled" at these meetings.[10] There was intense interest from the media in all he said. "His talks at the international AIDS conferences would bring thousands of people, literally thousands of people, cheering and to tears," Greenberg recalled later.[6]

At the 1985 Bangui meeting, Mann spent time with the head of WHO's Division of Communicable Diseases, the Egyptian Fakhry Assaad. The predominant attitude within WHO had been that AIDS was primarily a problem for wealthy countries, was largely restricted to homosexual men, and was not an area in which WHO could usefully engage. WHO's Director General, the charismatic, highly respected Halfdan Mahler, initially considered AIDS a distraction from the pressing problems of low-income countries, such as malaria and diarrheal diseases. Mahler was committed to the organization's vision at that time of "Health for All by the Year 2000," promoting the agenda defined at the seminal meeting on primary health care held in Alma Ata in 1978.[11]

WHO's attitudes on AIDS, however, were to change rapidly following pressure from multiple sides, including advice from CDC, as well as the disease's evolving epidemiology. CDC's Walt Dowdle (Chapter 9), Joe McCormick (Chapter 13), and William (Bill) Parra,[12] a CDC PHA seconded to Geneva, were particularly influential through their friendship with Assaad. WHO leadership became convinced that an AIDS program was needed, and in late 1985 Assaad, who was to die from leukemia just over a year later, began to look for a potential director. In early 1986, Mahler formally offered Mann the position of what initially would be called WHO's Control Programme on AIDS, after CDC had strongly recommended him. Greenberg later remarked, "I remember the day that he got the call asking him to go to Geneva... he actually asked me, 'Do you think this is a good idea'? I said 'Jon, if anyone can do this, you can.'... You know these certain people who have that aura and that glow."[6]

Mann became increasingly involved in WHO's AIDS efforts from early 1986 as a special consultant, but it was not until June of that year that he officially took up the WHO post full time. Notably, he remained a CDC staff member throughout his time at WHO, reporting to Curran in Atlanta. That arrangement, in which a US government employee was not only overseeing WHO fiscal resources and staff but also driving WHO's global policy, would be unlikely today. Mann's relative independence and autonomy were captured in comments by Ryder, reflecting on his own situation in Kinshasa: "There was a golden window there when we [Projet SIDA] were able to exploit our isolation... I think that being let loose [like that] will not happen again."[13]

Early strategies evolved as countries increasingly recognized the gravity of the epidemic. At the May 1986 meeting of the World Health Assembly, the Uganda representative spoke openly about his country's escalating AIDS problem, leading to unanimous approval of an AIDS resolution. Mann quickly learned the complicated structure and politics of WHO headquarters and its regional and country offices, as well as the functioning and rivalries of various United Nations (UN) agencies. Parra recalled the frenetic pace of work and the unceasing and diverse inquiries from countries for technical guidance.[12]

Mann found his feet and benefited from a close relationship with Mahler. The program underwent several changes in nomenclature, eventually being called the Global Programme on AIDS (GPA)—perhaps the first time the term "global" entered the public health lexicon. More importantly, GPA was moved into the office of the Director General which gave it unrivalled prominence. Crucially, Mann had managerial and budgetary independence and could navigate the WHO bureaucracy and bypass the WHO regional offices as he felt necessary.

Raising unparalleled resources in unparalleled time, GPA eventually expanded to over two hundred staff and a budget of more than $100 million, all under Mann's control. Key senior staff joining Mann in the program were Daniel Tarantola, responsible for program development; Manuel Carballo, leading behavioral science; and James (Jim) Chin, responsible for epidemiology and forecasting. CDC's David Heymann joined to guide research.

Indicative of his leadership qualities, Mann motivated extraordinary loyalty from these and other staff—to himself personally as well as to the program and vision. Rapid assessments of the impact of the epidemic in countries led to emergency, short-term (one year), and medium-term (three- to five-year) plans. Other important innovations were Mann's recognition of the importance of involving the civil sector and affected communities, including people living with HIV, in the AIDS response. All of this was outside the norm of WHO.

Mann's initial approach for GPA operations was to combine a vertical program, reflective of CDC's smallpox eradication experience, with the flexibility and horizontality of WHO's "Health for All" vision. He quickly recognized the skepticism and resentment about AIDS that existed among African leaders and public health officials, stemming from their offense at suggestions of an African origin for AIDS (Chapter 18) and political and cultural homophobia. Mann oversaw his first WHO meeting in Africa at WHO's regional headquarters in Brazzaville in November 1986, a meeting attended by senior health ministry staff from several dozen countries as well as invited researchers and guests.[14]

I had been in Kinshasa finishing some fieldwork (Chapter 13) and, in prelude to the meeting, was to help Ryder manage a high-level group of US visitors, including John LaMontaigne and Carl Western from NIH, Curran from CDC, and King Holmes, the world's leading expert on STIs, from the University of Washington. After visiting Projet SIDA, the group was to travel to Brazzaville, and I was to get them across the River Congo that separates the two capital cities. Distinguished as the group was, this logistical exercise was more difficult than expected, with lost passports, "wrong" passports reserved for travel to Israel, and other drama: In Brazzaville, the delegates' hotel was filled with sex workers who accosted clients in the bar and elevators and, without invitation, came knocking on the doors of hotel rooms.

In preparation for the meeting, Mann had asked Curran to impress on the attendees the severity of the impending health crisis, so that he could then speak about what needed to be done. Speaking without slides or other materials, Curran delivered as asked—quietly but convincingly predicting what the epidemic would bring in terms of disease and death and making it relevant at a personal level. He referred to the sex workers in the hotel the evening before, speculating on their rate of HIV infection, wondering if anyone in the audience had hired them. He reminded the almost exclusively male officials that women such as these were people's daughters, sisters, and wives, and that AIDS would become apparent in their own families. The disease was like no other—not only medically and demographically but also in social, political, and economic terms. But he reminded his audience that with crisis comes opportunity. Responding to AIDS could bring benefits such as strengthening international collaboration, establishing research, focusing on community empowerment, ensuring safe blood transfusion and needle and syringe hygiene, developing laboratories, and other needed actions. He ended on a note of uncertainty, reminding his stunned audience that, as the continent's health leaders, they had the responsibility to influence how this challenge played out. He handed the shaken group back to Mann, who now had their full attention to discuss technical and programmatic priorities.

Over time, from initially seeing AIDS prevention as a matter of individual choice, Mann began to focus on the importance of context that he had not dwelt upon as a researcher in Kinshasa. He spoke of three epidemics: the silent spread of HIV, the subsequent visible epidemic of disease and death, and the later socioeconomic and political impact. Discrimination against persons living with HIV was an obvious issue, but other challenges such as travel restrictions or calls for universal screening broadened his outlook beyond the infected individual. His burgeoning interest in women's health and role in society further sharpened his awareness of people's rights. Influencers included the likes of Lawrence (Larry) Gostin, a professor of public health law at Harvard University's school of public health, and the Australian judge Michael Kirby who provided Mann with advice on human rights and international law.[15] Along with others such as Curran, Mann recruited these individuals to a senior advisory body he set up—the Global Commission on AIDS.

Although GPA's expansion and visibility were remarkable and Mann's eloquence inspirational, they did not preclude increased demands for demonstration of impact. By the end of 1989 some 160 countries had AIDS control plans—an indication of widespread acceptance that AIDS was a problem—yet these were process indicators, not evidence of behavior change or declining HIV incidence. Mann had to walk the fine line between justifying GPA's work and budgets and simultaneously projecting what he thought could happen, up to 100 million HIV infections by the year 2000. Jealousy and resentment of his unorthodox methods in the sclerotic but powerful WHO bureaucracy also began to catch up, and other UN agencies vied for their own share of the AIDS response with its visibility and its money. "Fat AIDS" was a term increasingly heard.

All the while Mann was refining his focus on human rights and health. Major attention was initially focused on stigma and discrimination, but a broader insight was the realization of unequal vulnerability to HIV. Sex in a context of high HIV prevalence carried a different risk than in a low prevalence setting. Advice about condoms did not help a disempowered African woman living in poverty. Access to prevention was impeded for persons engaging in stigmatized behaviors such as male-to-male sex or criminalized activities such as drug injection.

Mann considered public health, ethics, human rights, and human well-being as complementary. He increasingly emphasized human dignity as core and solidarity a duty. Linking the individual with the many, he railed against silence, isolation, and exclusion.[16,17,18] His daughter Lydia described her father as more spiritual than religious but considered him strongly influenced by his sense of Jewish identity, committed to the intrinsic value of every individual.[3] She described how the whole family had been affected by their time in Kinshasa and the deprivation around them: "[you either ignore it] or you become a good person."[3] In a philosophic and conceptual evolution that was deeply personal and based on inner, fundamental beliefs, Mann attempted to bridge his nascent human rights awareness with traditional public health.

Not all understood, and some questioned, Mann's rights-based construct that he delivered with a passion that deflected practical questions about implementation. To some, especially colleagues educated in Europe, his thinking seemed slightly naïve, as if he were just discovering that social determinants influence people's lives, choices, and health. Social justice, defined by Gostin as a fair distribution of the benefits and burdens of society, seemed a more relevant paradigm to some than human rights, which, strictly speaking, are legal concepts.[19] More important than philosophic considerations, however, were the bureaucratic forces beginning to bear down on him, particularly his relations with his new boss Hiroshi Nakajima, appointed WHO Director General in 1989.

If the relationship between Mahler and Mann was an almost spiritual friendship, that between Mann and Nakajima was one of mutual disrespect, bordering on contempt. A traditionalist and WHO insider, Nakajima thought GPA should function as a regular WHO program. He was intensely jealous of Mann's power and influence, resented Mann's flouting of WHO systems, and considered him vain. He wanted AIDS dealt with as a biomedical issue and an STI, thought Mann should focus more on research, especially on therapeutics and vaccines, and was dismissive of the human rights emphasis. Mann's GPA successor, Michael (Mike) Merson, quoted Nakajima questioning the specificity of Mann's paradigm on human rights, "the... charter from the UN is not clear—it's vague."[8]

Mann was equally disdainful of Nakajima and his view on AIDS, and worried that GPA risked being undone. Relations only worsened over time, exemplified by restrictions on Mann's travel, other petty obstructions, and behind-the-scenes inducements for him to leave. On March 16, 1990, Mann abruptly resigned. He told Curran, his friend and still his supervisor, one hour later when he collected Curran, who had just flown in from Atlanta for a meeting of the Global Commission, from the airport. He then informed the other Global Commission members and his own staff, none of whom were aware or prepared. McCormick, also a friend and supporter from Kinshasa days, had been in discussions with Mann about work at GPA and was equally shocked.[9,20] Mann resigned after less than four years at WHO, but, just as in Zaire, he had accomplished a great amount in a short time.

Mann knew that his resignation would make international news. Although his position had become increasingly untenable, he overplayed his hand, thinking that CDC and the United States would not stand on the sidelines in the face of the crisis engendered. There he was mistaken; individuals never win against large bureaucracies, and organizations consider no one irreplaceable. Nakajima accepted Mann's resignation but insisted it be immediate. He appointed Merson, who had been serving as Director of WHO's Diarrheal Diseases Programme, as acting and later definitive Director of GPA. Relations between Merson and Mann, both CDC assignees, had long been tense. Although Merson went on to have a productive tenure, his initial selection by Nakajima was seen as cynical and was challenging for Mann's loyal staff. While still in Geneva, Curran arranged for Mann to serve out his CDC overseas tour of duty from his home in France, writing up prior work.

Although Mann was perceived as having the moral high ground after these events, he lost his global platform. And, while he retained stature and influence, he inevitably became less prominent. He turned to academia, accepting a position later in 1990 at Harvard, his alma mater, as professor of epidemiology and international health. In 1993 he became the founding Director of the François-Xavier Bagnoud (FXB) Center for Health and Human Rights at Harvard. Funding for this initiative had been given by an admirer of Mann, the Swiss Countess Albina du Boisrouvray, in honor of her son, a search-and-rescue pilot who died at age twenty-four in a mission over Mali in 1986.

Mann organized two conferences on health and human rights and, along with committed colleagues and friends, founded the *Journal of Health and Human Rights*. He also oversaw two editions of a major work, *AIDS in the World*, that updated the status of the epidemic in its multisectoral context.[21,22] At Harvard he was a revered teacher. Photographs of Jonathan Mann on the web most frequently show him as a bowtie-wearing professor (Figure 14.1). Supported by the School of Public Heath's Dean, Harvey Fineberg, with whom he developed a warm relationship, Mann introduced a tradition of giving graduating students a copy of the *Universal Declaration of Human Rights*[23] in addition to their academic diplomas.

To most, Mann's accomplishments after resigning from WHO would have seemed a productive record. Those who knew him, however, sensed dissatisfaction and restlessness, a yearning for more. Leaving Geneva, according to his daughter, had been difficult.[3] In late 1997 he resigned from Harvard

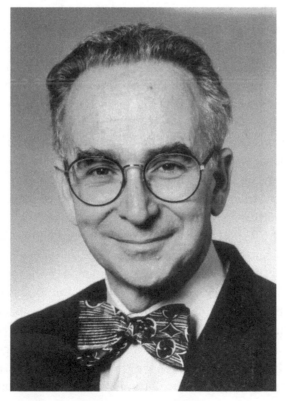

Figure 14.1. Jonathan Mann. (AP Photo/Keystone)

to take up the position of founding dean at the new school of public health at Allegheny University. He wanted to pursue the three-fold interaction between health and human rights he had defined—the impact of health policies on rights, the impact of rights policies on health, and the synergistic relation between rights and health. He also wanted to apply his conceptual framework to real life situations in an underprivileged urban setting. It was not to be, and Allegheny University did not come through on agreements or expectations.

The years subsequent to his resignation from WHO were not easy for a searcher like Mann. His marriage of 25 years foundered, and in 1996 he remarried. His second wife, Marie Lou Clements, was a distinguished vaccine researcher at Johns Hopkins School of Public Health who merits her own tribute. I recall seeing both together at a social gathering in Atlanta a while later, a middle-aged couple in a new relationship, Mann less stiff and formal than in earlier years, talking excitedly. It was the last time I saw him. On September 2, 1998, Mann and Clements boarded a Swissair flight from New York to Geneva, one taken frequently by global health and UN personnel. A new regime was in charge at WHO, headed by Norway's former Prime Minister, Gro Harlem Brundtland, and the couple was to have discussions in Geneva. The MD-11 crashed off the coast of Nova Scotia consequent to faulty wiring and an on-board fire. There were no survivors. I recall weeping when I heard the news on National Public Radio in my apartment in Atlanta. Mann was fifty-one when he died.

An outpouring of grief and adulation occurred when news of Mann's death spread around the world. Colleagues, some of them friends, penned earlier and later tributes and obituaries,[16,24,25,26] as did major international newspapers.[27] In 2008, when the tenth anniversary of the Swissair crash came around, I was Director of WHO's HIV/AIDS Department in Geneva. My suggestion to WHO leadership to host a memorial event was met with no enthusiasm amidst internal politics and prioritizations, but The Joint United Nations Programme on HIV/AIDS (UNAIDS) took up the suggestion.[28] Peter Piot, Justice Kirby, and others spoke fittingly to Mann's memory and influence. One absentee highlighted the issues in the world that Mann had cared about. We had arranged for Bila Kapita, Projet SIDA's senior medical patron and collaborator at Mama Yemo Hospital in Kinshasa (Chapter 13), to attend and speak. His flight was to take him through Brussels on the way to Geneva, but with his Congolese nationality it proved impossible to obtain a transit visa at short notice.

The FXB Center continues at Harvard and the *Journal of Health and Human Rights* continues to be published. Allegheny University declared bankruptcy, but some of its attributes were taken over by Drexel University whose Dornsife School of Public Health boasts a Jonathan Mann Global Health and Human Rights Initiative. The program aims to support research linking global health and human rights, expanding practical and educational networks, and advocating for the philosophy that Mann espoused.

Mann was human and therefore also had his faults. Having died young, he is frozen in time, protected from the challenges of the current century or his own later life. Whatever his strengths and weaknesses, those who knew him describe his personal warmth and concern for individuals. By any account, his influence defining the global AIDS response was unique, transformational, and lasting. He contributed to societal change in a world hungry for leadership in the face of a new and frightening health threat. His impact on CDC's work in AIDS, now seemingly distant, began at Projet SIDA and persisted on CDC's later international research and programmatic involvement under PEPFAR. As Curran commented, "It could be argued that his initial leadership and success set the stage for CDC's massive HIV efforts on the continent of Africa."[6]

Why past as prologue? Since Mann's death, a number of other pathogens have caused major epidemics. Outbreaks of SARS, H1N1 influenza, MERS, arbovirus infections, Ebola, and, most recently, COVID-19 have threatened global health security in escalating fashion. Concepts that motivated Mann—dignity, justice, vulnerability, marginalization, and the need for global solidarity—have continued to receive inadequate attention.[29] The response to the most serious of these challenges, the pandemic of COVID-19, has been fragmented and disjointed. When discussing Mann, colleagues and others continually remark on his leadership ability and the cohesion he forged in the early response to AIDS. His legacy makes us yearn for similar global health leadership today and in the future.

Notes

1. Bayer R. In Memoriam. Jonathan Mann, 1947–1948. Am J PH 1998;88:1608–1609.
2. BMJ. Obituaries. Jonathan Mann. 1988;317:754.
3. Author's interview with Lydia Kline, 2020.

4. Fee E, Parry M. Jonathan Mann, HIV/AIDS, and human rights. J Public Health Policy 2008;29:54–71.

5. Pepin J. The origins of AIDS. New York: Cambridge University Press; 2011:215–220.

6. "GREENBERG, ALAN," *The Global Health Chronicles*, accessed January 29, 2023, https://www.globalhealthchronicles.org/items/show/7907

7. "CURRAN, JAMES," *The Global Health Chronicles*, accessed January 24, 2023, https://www.globalhealthchronicles.org/items/show/7743

8. Merson M, Inrig S. The AIDS pandemic. Searching for a global response. Cham, Switzerland: Springer International Publishing; 2018.

9. McCormick JB, Fisher-Hoch S. Level 4: virus hunters of the CDC. New York: Barnes and Noble Books; 1999.

10. Author's conversation with Robin Ryder, 1987.

11. Declaration of Alma-Ata International Conference on Primary Health Care, Alma-Ata, USSR, September, 6–12, 1978. https://www.who.int/docs/default-source/documents/almaata-declaration-en.pdf?sfvrsn=7b3c2167_2

12. "PARRA, WILLIAM," *The Global Health Chronicles*, accessed November 19, 2022, https://www.globalhealthchronicles.org/items/show/7952

13. "RYDER, ROBIN," *The Global Health Chronicles*, accessed January 25, 2023, https://www.globalhealthchronicles.org/items/show/7730

14. Report of the first Regional Conference on AIDS in Africa, Brazzaville, November 11–13, 1986. World Health Organization; 1988. https://apps.who.int/iris/handle/10665/58406

15. Gostin LO, Lazzarini Z. Human rights and public health in the AIDS pandemic. New York: Oxford University Press; 1997.

16. Gostin L. A tribute to Jonathan Mann: health and human rights in the AIDS pandemic. J L Med & Ethics 1998;26:256–258.

17. Gostin LO. Public health, ethics, and human rights: a tribute to the late Jonathan Mann. J L Med & Ethics 2001;29:121–130. doi:10.1111/j.1748-720X.2001.tb00330.x

18. Cameron E. The deafening silence of AIDS. Health and Human Rights 2000;5:7–24.

19. De Cock KM, Mbori-Ngacha D, Marum E. Shadow on the continent: public health and HIV/AIDS in Africa in the 21st century. Lancet 2002;360:67–72. doi: 10.1016/S0140-6736(02)09337-6.

20. Author conversation with J. McCormick.

21. Mann J, Tarantola DJM, Netter TW, editors. AIDS in the World. Cambridge, MA: Harvard University Press; 1992.

22. Mann JM, Tarantola D, editors. AIDS in the World II. New York: Oxford University Press; 1996.

23. United Nations. Universal Declaration of Human Rights. https://www.un.org/en/about-us/universal-declaration-of-human-rights.

24. Piot P, Tarantola D. Obituary: Jonathan Mann. Bull WHO 1998;76:iii–iv.

25. Tarantola D. Obituary: Jonathan Mann and Mary Lou Clements-Mann. Independent, September 5, 1998.

26. Wojcik ME. On the sudden loss of a human rights activist: a tribute to Dr Jonathan Mann's use of international human rights law in the global battle against AIDS. J Marshall L Rev 1998;32:129–139.
27. Hilts PH. Jonathan Mann, AIDS pioneer, is dead at 51. The New York Times, September 4, 1998.
28. UNAIDS honors Jonathan Mann. The Epidemiology Monitor 2009;30:1–4. http://epi monitor.net/Epi-Docs/Archives/EM%20JAN%2009_Layout%201.pdf
29. De Cock KM, Jaffe HW, Curran JW. Reflections on 40 years of AIDS. Emerg Infect Dis 2021;27:1553–1560. doi:10.3201/eid2706.210284.

15

HIV-2 and Projet RETRO-CI
in Cote d'Ivoire

Kevin M. De Cock

By the mid-1980s a severe heterosexual AIDS epidemic was underway in Central and eastern Africa, but West Africa seemed relatively spared. In 1985, international researchers, including Max Essex's group from Harvard, published serologic evidence of infection in healthy Senegalese sex workers with a virus related to but distinct from the classic AIDS virus[1]—possibly a second strain of HIV. In what became an alphabet soup, Essex and colleagues reported isolation of human and monkey viruses: human T-lymphotropic virus type IV (HTLV-IV) from the sex workers,[2] and simian T-lymphotropic virus type III (STLV-III) from African green monkeys.[3] It later transpired that both these viruses were laboratory contaminants with another African green monkey virus, SIVagm.[4] In 1986 Montagnier's group in Paris isolated the true second HIV-like retrovirus from ill patients from Guinea Bissau and Cape Verde—the virus that would become known as HIV-2.[5]

Before joining Joe McCormick's Viral Special Pathogens Branch as an EIS officer in 1986, I had taught internal medicine at the University of Nairobi in Kenya. I was especially interested in AIDS in Africa, and McCormick strongly supported these interests.[6] I had just returned from investigating a yellow fever epidemic in Nigeria in mid-1987,[7,8] when I was invited to a restricted meeting on AIDS in Africa organized by NIH. The meeting was held prior to the third international AIDS conference, which was being hosted that year in Washington, DC. At the NIH-sponsored meeting, the Harvard group presented findings on their asymptomatic sex workers in Senegal, while a Swedish team from the Karolinska Institute described patients from Guinea Bissau with AIDS. French researchers reported on their recently described West African virus, HIV-2. It was all very confusing.

The implications of these divergent findings in 1987 were more than academic. If a novel human retrovirus was circulating in West Africa, then

Kevin M. De Cock, *HIV-2 and Projet RETRO-CI in Cote d'Ivoire* In: *Dispatches from the AIDS Pandemic*. Kevin M. De Cock, Harold W. Jaffe, and James W. Curran and Edited by: Robin Moseley, Oxford University Press.
© Oxford University Press 2023. DOI: 10.1093/oso/9780197626528.003.0015

its distribution, pathogenicity, and transmission would need investigation. Most importantly, we did not have specific diagnostics, and a new agent could threaten the global blood supply. I suggested to McCormick that we needed a Projet SIDA (Chapter 13) in West Africa. He agreed, and my second EIS year was devoted to that vision.

Negotiating Access to West Africa

At the AIDS conference in Washington, I strove to meet delegates from West Africa and explore collaboration. One new contact, Françoise Brun-Vézinet, the eminent French virologist who codiscovered HIV-2, would become unfailingly generous over ensuing years. At the conference, I recall her starting her presentation on HIV-2 in Cape Verde with the memorable comment that the islands of Cape Verde were green only by name, as she reported on serologic studies in this rocky archipelago.

McCormick and I conferred about which West African country could support a CDC research site. Along with Bill Heyward, then still in the AIDS division in Atlanta, we persuaded Jim Curran of the need for a mission to West Africa. A fourth member joined the team—John Krebs, a CDC zoologist with extensive field experience with Lassa fever in Sierra Leone. We prioritized three countries—Guinea, Burkina Faso, and Cote d'Ivoire—and aimed to conduct pilot studies in each. Three criteria for the proposed site were paramount: the prevalence of HIV-2 infection, the interest of local authorities in collaboration, and the quality of infrastructure to support research. We also had to consider what other international groups were already present to avoid conflicts.

Cote d'Ivoire's major city of Abidjan, referred to as "the Paris of West Africa," best met our criteria. We committed to collaboration with colleagues from Abidjan's University Hospital Medical Center at Treichville and its Infectious Diseases Department, and the Ministry of Health. Dennis Kux, the US ambassador, strongly supported our initiative from the start. Our pilot study entailed establishing a temporary laboratory at the hospital; collecting 200 blood specimens from five sentinel groups; performing preliminary testing for HIV-1 and HIV-2; and shipping specimens back to Atlanta for more refined testing. The study groups included hospitalized patients, pregnant women, blood donors, TB patients, and patients with STIs. We paid five medical students a small stipend to assist with the study, two of whom ended up working for us long-term and later obtained postgraduate degrees in public health.

Our results were presented in 1988 at the fourth international AIDS conference in Stockholm, but the study was more valuable than the poster displayed, as captured in a paper on the epidemiology published in the journal *AIDS*[9] and another in the *Journal of Infectious Diseases*[10] that documented for the first time infection with both HIV-1 and HIV-2 in a single patient. In addition, the study yielded isolates of HIV-2, and the specimens collected were invaluable for evaluation of diagnostic tests. Most significantly, we had clear evidence of the presence of both HIV-1 and HIV-2 and of high rates of HIV infection in Abidjan: 45 percent of all patients on the infectious diseases ward at Treichville's university hospital were positive for one or both viruses.[9]

Amid the technical discussions, there was also need for political negotiations. Moving forward would require support from the US Embassy and State Department and informal approval from other US agencies. Approval from the government of Cote d'Ivoire would involve not only the Minister of Health—who undoubtedly would have to obtain agreement from the longstanding President, Félix Houphouët-Boigny, about a topic as sensitive as collaboration with the US government on AIDS—but also the country's technical counterparts. Cote d'Ivoire was a bastion of French influence, and the establishment of an American scientific outpost would surely cause unease. During a WHO-sponsored evaluation of Cote d'Ivoire's AIDS situation in the fall of 1987, I was quizzed in public by Professor Marc Gentilini, France's most eminent tropical medicine specialist who was leading the WHO team, about CDC intentions. And CDC leadership needed to agree that this proposal merited support and funding, at a cost of one million dollars for the first year.

Our principal interlocutors were Koudou Odehouri, head of the National AIDS Control Programme, and Auguste Kadio, the taciturn head of infectious diseases at the University. Odehouri introduced me to the Minister of Health, Alphonse Djédjé Mady, and, despite my being in a somewhat junior position at CDC, I negotiated our aspirations. Djédjé Mady expressed support for collaboration and requested an emphasis on training. It was the first of several meetings I had with him that were memorable for his graciousness and eloquent explanation of Ivorian expectations. I understood we would have to invest in local capacity building and that the clinical needs of patients with HIV/AIDS would have to be addressed.

Becoming Projet RETRO-CI

Anne Porter, our English laboratory technologist, and I began full time work in Abidjan in June 1988. The first priority was dealing with containers of equipment shipped from Atlanta and setting up the laboratory. We then hired our first research physicians (Georgette Adjorlolo from Cote d'Ivoire and Malian dermatologist Mamadou Diallo), invested in administration, and recruited a data manager and statistician from Belgium, Marie-France Lafontaine. This exercise of building an international team and equipping a project took time and effort (Figure 15.1). Communication with Atlanta made heavy use of the new technology of fax, the machine installed in the kitchen of my house. Our French infectious disease colleague, Jacques Moreau, proposed the name RETRO-CI, derived from "retrovirus" and "Cote d'Ivoire." Lafontaine and Porter were replaced after two years by, re-spectively, Ronan Doorly and Kari Brattegaard, increasing our internation-alism to include Ireland and Norway. "You are who you hire" is a phrase that has resonated with me since these early experiences.

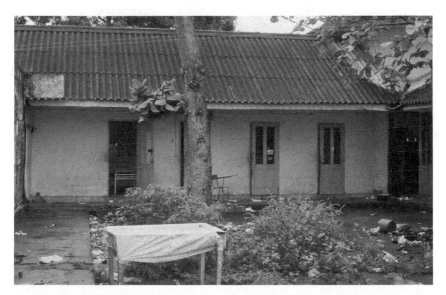

Figure 15.1. Abandoned building, Infectious Diseases Service, Treichville University Hospital, Abidjan, Cote d'Ivoire, 1988. CDC funded renovations to house the Projet RETRO-CI laboratory and epidemiology infrastructure. (Kevin De Cock, personal collection)

How Much AIDS, How Much Death from AIDS?

The clean entrance to the infectious disease ward at Treichville's university hospital belied the sorry state of its remotest rooms. *"Salle 24"* was where the most skeletal patients were relegated. The ward used old cholera beds whose plastic mattresses had a hole in the middle for collecting fecal material in a bucket underneath. The beds were now filled with patients with AIDS and its associated chronic diarrhea. A characteristic smell, which I came to associate with death, pervaded the ward. The emaciated patients lay listless, the scene one of utter misery. We regularly showed visitors this tableau to impress on them the then dire nature of AIDS in Africa. When US Vice President Dan Quayle visited Cote d'Ivoire in early 1991, he blanched when I took him around, gritting his teeth and remarking when he left that he would never forget this scene (Figure 15.2).

Questions of public health importance in 1988 focused on the level of HIV disease and death in Cote d'Ivoire and the relative contributions of HIV-1 and HIV-2. Influenced by Jonathan Mann's earlier work in Kinshasa

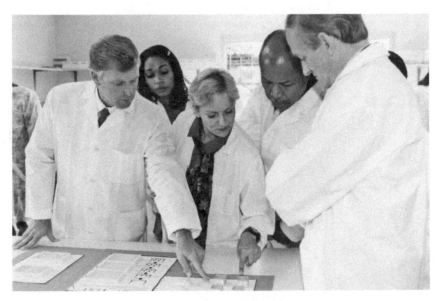

Figure 15.2. US Vice-President Dan Quayle visiting Projet RETRO-CI, 1991. Pictured (l-r): Vice President Quayle, Helene Gayle, Kari Brattegaard, Department of Health and Human Services Secretary Louis Sullivan, Kevin De Cock. (Kevin De Cock, personal collection)

(Chapter 13), we implemented a rudimentary surveillance study (Figure 15.3). By capturing all new AIDS cases admitted to Abidjan's largest hospitals over a specific time and applying this numerator to the denominator of the city's population, we could estimate a minimum AIDS incidence. Also, we could show the relative proportions of cases due to both viruses. We interviewed and took blood samples from more than 1,500 patients and calculated rates using a report on the estimated population of the city specially provided by a French demographer, Bernard Barrere.

The study showed that in 1988, the minimum incidence of AIDS in Abidjan—where AIDS was not known to be a problem—exceeded the incidence in Kinshasa and that in New York City and approached the AIDS incidence in San Francisco.[11] Four percent of the AIDS cases were considered attributable to HIV-2. For every woman with AIDS, four men were affected. Elsewhere this would be indicative of a severe epidemic among MSM or IDUs, but here it was an epidemic initiated by commercial sex. A restricted

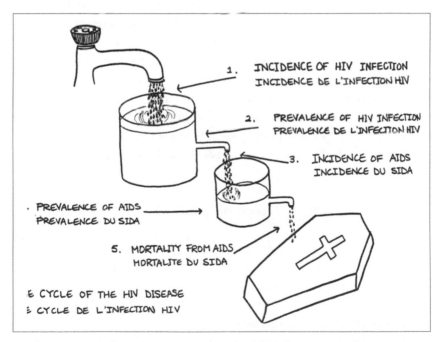

Figure 15.3. Drawing representing "the cycle of HIV disease," Abidjan, Cote d'Ivoire, 1988. This figure illustrated the epidemiologic concepts of HIV incidence and prevalence, AIDS incidence and prevalence, and AIDS mortality. (Kevin De Cock, personal collection)

group of sex workers serviced the large community of male immigrants working in Abidjan. Over twenty countries of origin were represented in our study population, and regional migration, primarily by single men without their families, supported a sex industry and high rates of STIs. With time, this AIDS ratio of men to women equaled out as infection entered the general population.[12]

In Abidjan, the body of each person who dies must pass through one of a limited number of mortuaries for certification. I reasoned that we could test cadavers for HIV, apply an AIDS case definition from inspection or hospital records, and, again, using our demographic report for population denominators, estimate the mortality rate from AIDS in Abidjan. We studied almost seven hundred cadavers, approximately 7 percent of estimated annual deaths in the city.[13] The rates of HIV infection in males and females who had died were 41 percent and 32 percent, respectively. AIDS was the leading cause of death in men, with 15 percent of male cadavers meeting a strict case definition, and the second cause (13%) in women. The leading cause of death in women was maternal mortality, including deaths from abortion.

Results of these initial studies were presented at the international AIDS conferences in 1989 and 1990 and published, respectively, in *The Lancet*[11] and *Science*,[13] putting RETRO-CI on the world map. Subsequent analysis of hospital registers showed a substantial increase in in-patient death rates on the medical but not surgical wards of Abidjan's hospitals over the previous five years, evidence of the evolution of the hitherto undetected AIDS epidemic.[14] These early experiences emphasized to us how much there is to learn from the dead, something surprisingly neglected.[15]

Diagnosing HIV-2

Although we took advantage of research opportunities as they presented themselves, we emphasized the fundamental raison d'être for RETRO-CI's establishment: to understand HIV-2. For this, we urgently needed advice on distinguishing HIV-1 from HIV-2 infection, given that our enzyme immunoassays frequently reacted to both viruses. Specimens positive on the screening enzyme immunoassays had to be confirmed with a supplemental test, initially Western blots. These were expensive and laborious, and their interpretation was subjective. HIV-2-specific reagents were in short supply, and few international diagnostic companies focused on this specialized area.

In early 1989, about eight months after our arrival in Abidjan, we hosted some of CDC's most senior officials for our first site visit; the visitors outnumbered our full-time staff. Such visits assessed our science and guided research priorities, but also served to assure the Cote d'Ivoire government and the US Embassy of CDC's high-level commitment. During discussions of our diagnostic challenges, I recall Harold Jaffe, then a senior AIDS epidemiologist in Atlanta, saying with world-weary directness that if we could not diagnose HIV-2 then there was really no reason for us to be there. This comment engendered both motivation and sleeplessness in all our staff.

Type-specific diagnosis of HIV infection was facilitated by introduction of commercially available, HIV-2-specific Western blots as well as tests based on synthetic peptides presented on strips. We spent hundreds of thousands of dollars procuring and evaluating diagnostics and introducing simpler and cheaper testing algorithms.[16,17,18,19,20,21,22,23,24,25] As laboratory director, Brattegaard expanded capacity to include immunologic testing for CD4+ lymphocyte counts, and later microbiology for STIs. In due course, we developed confidence in our ability to diagnose HIV-2 in adequate numbers for epidemiologic research, assess infected persons' immunologic status, and diagnose diverse bacterial infections.

We aimed to conduct simple studies before more complex ones and designed them in collaboration with Ivorian colleagues. As CDC had done at Projet SIDA, we pushed for establishment of a local ethics committee. Odehouri and other colleagues argued for interest and assistance in the clinical realm. Although we could not respond directly at that time, a solid body of clinically relevant work was conducted over subsequent years.

Another recollection from the site visit was Curran's exhortation to initiate cohort studies to compare the natural history of HIV-1 and HIV-2 infections. He gave advice on administration, emphasizing its importance but reminding me that we would be judged on science. Nonetheless, managerial links with CDC headquarters needed strengthening and the time-honored practice of linking a PHA with an epidemiologist proved fruitful.

Harold Van Patten,[26] a CDC PHA with experience in STIs and AIDS, was to join our group (he was later succeeded by Leo Weakland), but adding staff required agreement from the US Embassy. Regarding his own appointment, Van Patten recalled that an embassy official told CDC, "I'm going to recommend to the Ambassador that we not approve Harold coming," and when asked what CDC could do to help, reportedly responded, "Could CDC buy us a truck, and maybe we could find a way to have Harold come."[26] As Van Patten added, "Basically, they traded a truck for my assignment there."[26]

Van Patten showed his mettle when he called me one afternoon, early in his tenure, to say with remarkable sangfroid that he had been held up at gunpoint with his visiting son, had his car shot up, but was otherwise all right. We had several other security incidents over the years but, fortunately, no serious outcomes other than fright.

The *Clinique de Confiance*

Sometime in mid-1989, Odehouri asked me to act as translator for a meeting with the Ghanaian Ambassador. The Ambassador asked for assistance with HIV/AIDS prevention for his community and stated that he was especially worried about HIV risks for his countrywomen, thousands of whom were sex workers in Cote d'Ivoire.

We met leaders of the Ghanaian community, including the Chief, his associates, and the senior women's representative, the "Queen Mother." The discussions about prostitution were open, the Chief referring to "our sisters in Treichville," the quartier of Abidjan known for its sex work. Marie Laga was visiting from Antwerp's ITM, and we were invited to the Chief's home, where we discussed collaboration with the sex worker community. I wondered about perceptions of risk. The Chief had nine wives, some of them very young, and twenty-eight children. Marie and I were quizzed about HIV transmission risks, whether razors played a role, and prevention. Typical of the time and attitudes in many countries, there was joking and skepticism about condom use. Amid much laughter, a condom was filled with water to show how much it could stretch.

Commercial sex played a critical role in initiating the AIDS epidemic in both Cote d'Ivoire and Ghana. At the WHO regional meeting on AIDS in Brazzaville in 1986 (Chapter 14), I had heard that the first AIDS cases in Ghana were in sex workers returning from Abidjan. As mentioned above, our early data in Abidjan showed a 4:1 male-to-female sex ratio.[11,12] In Ghana, early on, the opposite was true, with more cases of AIDS in women than men, many of the women having returned from sex work outside of their own country. There is a rich social science literature on prostitution in West Africa, given that it is a thriving regional business. Ghanian women of the Krobo and Ashanti ethnic groups were disproportionately involved and affected by HIV. The historical roots for this phenomenon among the Krobo date back to the 1960s with the construction of the Akosombo dam and associated population displacement.

RETRO-CI replicated East and Central African studies showing HIV associations with other STIs, especially genital ulcers, as well as with lack of male circumcision[27] Although HIV-2 was relatively uncommon, the same risk factors applied as for HIV-1. Following the demise of research at Projet SIDA in Kinshasa in 1991, we collaborated with Laga and Peter Piot to transfer that STI expertise to Abidjan.[28] We rented a house to serve as a clinic for sex workers, at that time all female. Laga recruited a quiet Belgian epidemiologist, Peter Ghys, recognizable for his walrus mustache, to lead this body of work.

It was Ghys who gave our sex worker clinic its name, *La Clinique de Confiance*, a play on words. *Confiance d'accord, mais prudence d'abord* ("Trust OK, but caution first") was the health message displayed throughout the town on billboards advertising Prudence™ condoms. The major funder of these condom promotion efforts was the US Agency for International Development—its overseas advocacy in marked contrast to reticent condom advice from the US government domestically. *Clinique de Confiance* was a term instantly recognized in relation to this message. More subtly, the initials were CDC.

News of free services and condoms spread, important studies were conducted, and HIV prevention and STI treatment services provided. Over eight thousand women were seen in the clinic during 1992 2002.[28,29,30,31,32] The initial overall HIV prevalence was 89 percent, reminiscent of that in Nairobi in East Africa. One third of the women had gonorrhea, one fifth suffered from syphilis and genital ulcers, and only one fifth reported using condoms. The serologic profile of dual reactivity to HIV-1 and HIV-2 among them was exceptionally common, 30 percent overall. This proportion of dual reactivity among HIV-infected persons was much greater than in other groups, reflecting the very high level of exposure to both AIDS viruses in these women.[30]

We were dismayed by these findings and strove to keep the women coming back to the clinic. Although loss-to-follow up was high, reported condom use increased substantially and rates of STIs and new HIV infections decreased.[31] Before our intervention 16 percent of women became infected with HIV annually, and this rate more than halved over time. Ample evidence from these and other studies emphasized the substantial role sex work played in the overall epidemic,[33] the size of the sex worker population, the women's unstable and migratory lifestyle, and their extremely high rates of HIV and other STIs. Much, much more attention is still required to this driver of epidemic AIDS in West Africa, and simple interventions as Projet Retro-CI delivered have substantial impact. Underinvestment in HIV prevention among sex workers in Africa remains one of the deficiencies of the global AIDS response.

No effective treatment for AIDS was available at that time, and donor programs did not support HIV/AIDS care. Most of the HIV-infected women in our studies returned home to die when they inevitably became ill. If they had no money, they would end up at the University Hospital in Treichville, to die neglected and alone. AIDS was discussed yet less visible in the expatriate community that generally used the private medical sector. A Belgian woman was admitted to the Infectious Diseases Service with terminal HIV-2 disease. She had worked as a barmaid and occasional sex worker in an upscale Abidjan restaurant. Another infected Belgian woman was *Soeur* Katherine, a missionary nun who contracted HIV through a postoperative blood transfusion and rapidly progressed to AIDS. She then played an important leadership role in AIDS advocacy. Both were repatriated to die in the home country they had not seen for many years.

Blood safety was beyond our remit but, mindful of its public health importance and our experience at Projet SIDA,[34] we conducted epidemiologic studies assessing the risks from transfusion and showing the importance of recruiting low-risk donors.[35,36] RETRO-CI's work helped stimulate international funders to eventually invest in a safe national blood transfusion service, an achievement that always made me think of Soeur Katherine.

Pathology

Clinical understanding of African AIDS continued to be lacking. A common feature was wasting, referred to in East Africa as "slim disease" (Chapter 13). There was much speculation about "slim" and putative gastrointestinal causes associated with malabsorption of food and nutrients. We knew that TB frequently complicated HIV and that bacterial infections were common. Nonetheless, our grasp of the spectrum of HIV disease was poor. Facilities for investigating patients were lacking. Diagnostic imaging of the brain was out of reach, bacteriology was limited, and TB culture unavailable.

Together with my friend Sebastian Lucas, a leading pathologist in the United Kingdom with whom I had collaborated in Nairobi years earlier, we speculated on the utility of autopsies in African patients with AIDS. Under Cote d'Ivoire's "Napoleonic" legal code, infectious disease deaths could be investigated by autopsy. Lucien Abouya, a collaborating medical student, had compared autopsy lung findings in HIV-positive and HIV-negative patients dying on the University Hospital's respiratory diseases ward, so I asked Lucas to complete the pathology reading of lung material. Striking findings were that TB caused 40 percent of these HIV-positive pulmonary and that PCP was rare ([37]). The published paper included an early plea for research on pre-ventive therapy for TB in persons living with HIV.

With support from multiple groups including his home institution, University College, London (UCL), Lucas established histopathology work at an industrial scale in Projet RETRO-CI. We screened consecutive adult hospital admissions, testing over five thousand patients. A remark-able 50 percent were HIV-infected, and 38 percent of those died within a week of admission. Almost three hundred adult autopsies were conducted, representing about a quarter of all HIV-positive deaths and close to one half those with HIV-2.[38] Lucas and RETRO-CI technical staff, led by UCL tech-nologist Chris Peacock, produced 8,500 microscopy slides for reading per month—five times the rate in the university department in London. The hospital mortuary was not air conditioned, and the work was physically ex-hausting. Close working relationships were established with the existing pa-thology department whose staff were eager collaborators, and infrastructure was strengthened.

An immediate reward for our efforts was appreciation from clinicians who were now getting world class pathology services in real time. Fully one third of HIV deaths were attributable to TB, and another fifth to bacterial infections or toxoplasmosis.[38] Among patients with HIV wasting syndrome or slim disease, the extent of wasting was directly correlated to the degree of immunosuppression and the prevalence of disseminated TB, with one half of skeletally thin decedents having this pathology.[39] The team also conducted autopsies in children who had been screened with rapid HIV tests in the mortuary. To our surprise, in view of findings in adults, PCP was common in infants and TB rare.[40]

The results from this work also had practical implications. Most impor-tantly, the clinical index of suspicion for TB had to be much higher. Over half of adult AIDS patients in Abidjan were dying of infections that were either preventable or treatable. Children of HIV-infected mothers might benefit from *Pneumocystis* prophylaxis. Lucas and I became convinced that the clinical care of patients with AIDS had to be addressed. The world would be judged to have shown great interest in AIDS in Africa, but little interest in Africans who had AIDS.[41]

The principal paper from the autopsy study appeared in the journal *AIDS* in December 1993,[38] while other, more specialized reports, were published later.[42,43,44,45] Most rewardingly, Joep Lange,* a leading Dutch researcher and advisor to WHO on clinical care, wrote an accompanying editorial. He reiterated our conclusions on the implications for preventive treatment and care (38,41) and called the work a landmark study ([46]).

We conducted further hospital studies to document the bacterial infections associated with HIV[47] and to describe the clinical picture in HIV-infected children.[48] An English clinician and PhD candidate, Alison Grant, later joined RETRO-CI to better define the spectrum of disease in living adult patients[49,50,51,52] The pathology and clinical epidemiologic findings later led Alan Greenberg, who would succeed me as Projet Retro-CI director, to propose a clinical trial of cotrimoxazole to prevent OIs, an example of studies building on conclusions from earlier work.

Understanding HIV-2

The scientific and public health uncertainty surrounding HIV-2 concerned its pathogenicity, transmission, and natural history. HIV-1 was spreading throughout West Africa, but HIV-2 apparently remained stable and most concentrated in Guinea Bissau.[12,53,54,55,56] Individual cases of HIV-2 had been described in various countries outside of West Africa, but epidemic spread had not occurred. Our studies of various patient populations showed similar clinical patterns in those reactive to HIV-1, HIV-2, or both viruses[57,58] HIV-2 infection was shown to be a risk factor for TB,[59] and Lucas's autopsy study demonstrated pathology indicative of AIDS in persons dying with HIV-2.[38] Any lingering doubt about HIV-2 being an AIDS-causing virus was erased, yet lack of pandemic spread was striking.

---

* Joep Lange and his partner, Jacqueline van Tongeren, died in the crash of Malaysia Airlines Flight MH 17 over Ukraine in 2014. (Yasmin S. The impatient Dr. Lange: one man's fight to end the global HIV epidemic. Baltimore: Johns Hopkins University Press; 2018).

A subtle question concerned the relative aggressiveness of the two viruses. Cohort studies in Senegal showed that persons with HIV-2 progressed more slowly and had more favorable survival, observations that had also been reported from Guinea Bissau and The Gambia. Laboratory studies in our cohort of pregnant women showed similar but lesser evidence of immune deficiency in those with HIV-2 compared to HIV-1 infection.[60] We compared two-year outcomes in patients with TB according to their HIV serostatus.[61] Persons with HIV-1 had a two-and-a-half-fold higher annual mortality than those with HIV-2, but the latter were still four times more likely to die than HIV-negative patients. The scientific consensus was that HIV-2 progressed to immune deficiency more slowly than HIV-1. A later claim from the team in Senegal that HIV-2 protected their long-studied women from acquiring HIV-1 was refuted by epidemiologic and laboratory evidence from RETRO-CI and other groups.[62,63,64]

The most direct route of HIV transmission to study was that from mother to child. From 1990 through 1992, we tested over 18,000 women and followed 613 of them with their infants for a two-year period. Rates of other STIs in this population were high.[65] Although, as expected, a quarter of women with HIV-1 transmitted the infection to their infants, the rate of transmission of HIV-2 was only 1 percent and corresponding child survival was substantially better.[66] In another study, responses to questions posed to women with HIV-2 about their prior reproductive history showed child survival rates similar to those for HIV-negative women.[67] Although indirect, this was an efficient demonstration of lack of vertical transmission and was consistent with our finding of low rates of HIV-2 in living children.[68]

To compare sexual transmission of the two viruses, we examined female partners of hospitalized men who had HIV-1 or HIV-2. The proportions of spouses of HIV-1-infected and HIV-2-infected men who were concordantly seropositive were similar, 49 percent and 44 percent, respectively. We concluded that HIV-1 and HIV-2 appeared equally transmitted within couples when the men had progressed to severe immune deficiency.[69]

The paradox of reduced efficiency of mother-to child transmission of HIV-2 compared to HIV-1 but similar sexual transmission of the viruses was likely related to stage of disease of the infected index. Evolving molecular science showed that viral load was lower for HIV-2 than for HIV-1 early in the course of infection, and this likely caused lower transmission. With time and progression of immune deficiency, however, isolation of HIV-2 became easier—indicating more virus and greater transmissibility. These differences in viral load throughout most of the natural history of the two viral infections resulted in lower transmissibility for HIV-2, less population spread, and, ultimately, lack of an HIV-2 pandemic.[70] With these conclusions about HIV-2 transmission and disease, I felt that Projet Retro-CI had accomplished CDC's initial charge from 1987.

Interventional Epidemiology

Greenberg served as RETRO-CI Director from 1993 to 1997. He reorganized, expanded, and strengthened the project. In an emotional interview, he remembered, "It was this United Nations. . . by the time I left there were about a hundred staff from 14 countries. . . something like 50 to 60 languages that were spoken. There were people from all over West Africa. . . It was an incredibly vibrant and interesting place."[71] Based on the country's expanding HIV-1 epidemic and a better understanding of HIV transmission and disease, Greenberg prioritized "interventional epidemiology" and developing virology capacity.

The landmark ACTG 076 trial, conducted mostly in the United States, had evaluated zidovudine (also called azidothymidine, or AZT) delivered antenatally and during labor to women with HIV, and after birth to their infants, to reduce transmission from mother to child. The results were published in 1994 and showed a two thirds reduction in transmission.[72] Aware that the great majority of infected women and children in the world were African, researchers determined to adapt this advance to lower-income settings. CDC initiated trials in Abidjan and Bangkok, Thailand, of a shorter and simpler course of zidovudine, all this before the advent of ART or programmatic funding for treatment.

A firestorm ensued concerning comparison groups and the use of placebos.[73] Marcia Angell, editor of the New England Journal of Medicine, condemned the trials as unethical.[74] Others were equally strong defending use of placebos as both ethical and necessary where the ACTG 076 regimen was unfeasible.[75] NIH Director Harold Varmus and CDC Director David Satcher defended the studies before Congress and wrote strongly supportive commentaries.[76,77] Bitterness on both sides of the argument persisted long into the future.

Editors of The Lancet appeared conflicted. The journal published a critical editorial,[78] but later published the trial results from Abidjan and Bangkok, along with those of a third, French-sponsored study in West Africa.[79,80,81] Short-course zidovudine reduced transmission from HIV-infected breastfeeding women by over one third, a stunning advance and the basis for subsequent research that ultimately showed transmission to infants could be reduced to less than 5 percent in African populations.

The other impactful trial was a placebo-controlled study of cotrimoxazole.[82] As described earlier, clinical and autopsy studies suggested that many causes of illness and death in persons with HIV in Abidjan were preventable. Prophylaxis of OIs, the mainstay of care in the era preceding effective ART, had essentially been ignored in Africa.[41] For their cotrimoxazole trial, Greenberg and colleagues selected HIV-infected TB patients as their study population; because such patients were already ill but under treatment for TB, they were highly at risk of other opportunistic events potentially amenable to cotrimoxazole prophylaxis.[38,41,46,83] The study showed that hospitalizations and mortality were almost halved in the group receiving the active drug.[82]

Both clinical trials influenced global health policy and practice. Stefan Wiktor was first author on both papers, both in *The Lancet*[79,82], and followed Greenberg as Director in 1997. During this time, John Nkengasong,[84] the Cameroonian-born, Belgian-trained virologist, developed RETRO-CI's virology laboratory into a continental center of excellence for research and program implementation. Giving up tenure at ITM, to his wife Susan's initial dismay, he took a new RETRO-CI position at personal risk, describing his first meeting with Greenberg in Abidjan:

> He pointed. . . and said, "John, I see a dilapidated building, but I see a virology lab there . . . what do you see here?" And I said, "Yes, I see a virology lab." But. . . I was completely discouraged. . . But I saw in him, the seriousness and the commitment. . . So, I went back to Belgium, convinced my wife and I took a one-year contract (84).

Nkengasong described his own journey from basic virology to participation in early efforts to increase access to therapy in West Africa and beyond. "My office was overseeing the infectious disease clinic. . . and people are dying and shouting and crying. . . It was very stressful to see that it was real."[84] Nkengasong was central to establishment of WHO's drug resistance network, HIV ResNet, and in laboratory evaluation of initial ART provision in Cote d'Ivoire.[85,86,87,88] In later years from CDC in Atlanta, he was central to laboratory expansion under PEPFAR (Chapter 22). Looking back to when he left Abidjan in 2002, he remarked, "we had about 8,000 patients on treatment as part of the UN drug access initiative. . . it was really helpful in informing. . . how you could expand ART treatment without all the complexities of the viral load testing."[84]

Concluding Projet RETRO-CI

For everyone, leaving Abdjan was emotionally wrenching. For those who had passed through, RETRO-CI profoundly influenced their subsequent careers. Several of us received decorations from the Ivorian government. Greenberg and I reminisce about Gouba, the gentle and dignified Burkinabe cook we employed who later died of AIDS, along with his wife and child. Every time someone left, resident philosopher Ehounou Ekpini, one of the medical students I had first hired, gave a speech. *"Partir, ce n'est qu'un aurevoir; tout de même partir c'est mourir un peu,"* he would say ("leaving is only a goodbye; all the same, leaving is to die a little").

Stefan Wiktor was followed by Terry Chorba as RETRO-CI Director, but a coup d'état in late 1999 predicted a difficult future. The project had evolved from a research site into a support structure for rapidly expanding AIDS programs that began to include delivery of antiretroviral medications. Another public health leader who subsequently stepped in as Director was Marie Laga from ITM. RETRO-CI slowly evolved into an implementation site for PEPFAR, and, although the research mission faded, it had fulfilled its original mission and continued to contribute to national and regional public health efforts.

Although HIV-2 is slowly receding in West Africa, hundreds of thousands or more remain infected. Overall attention to it is so scarce that some researchers have proposed it be recognized as a neglected tropical disease.[89] HIV-2 is naturally resistant to a group of drugs called non-nucleoside reverse transcriptase inhibitors and to several other antiretrovirals, and its treatment is understudied. A retrospective analysis of RETRO-CI data published in 2020, but based on much earlier data and specimens, showed a less favorable immunologic response to ART in patients with HIV-2 compared to those with HIV-1.[90] RETRO-CI answered the important public health questions concerning HIV-2 that were posed in the 1980s, but unaddressed issues remain in this era of therapy.

We had invested heavily in capacity building, and nearly all our colleagues, wherever they went, continued to work on African health issues. The RETRO-CI diaspora is too numerous to name, but it has had global impact. Greenberg led HIV epidemiology at CDC before transitioning to academia in 2005. Wiktor headed hepatitis work at WHO in Geneva. Ekpini has worked on HIV at WHO and continues in senior health positions at the United Nations Children's Fund (UNICEF), Adjorlolo went to the Elizabeth Glazer Pediatric AIDS Foundation, and Diallo, along with Sidibe Kassim, Gaston Djomand, and, from the laboratory, Karidia Diallo, remain at CDC working on African health issues. Brattegaard has consulted on laboratory and other aspects of global health. Ghys is responsible for global HIV estimates at UNAIDS, and Laga has been a leading figure at ITM. From 2016 to 2022, Nkengasong served as the first director of the Africa CDC after which he was appointed as Global AIDS Coordinator in the Biden Administration, and so the work goes on. Through them all, RETRO-CI lives.

Notes

1. Barin F, Denis F, Allan JS, et al. Serological evidence for virus related to simian T-lymphotropic retrovirus III in residents of West Africa. Lancet 1985;326:1387–1389.
2. Kanki PJ, Barin F, M'Boup, et al. New human T-lymphotropic retrovirus related to simian T-lymphotropic virus type III (STLV-IIIAGM). Science 1986;232:238–243.
3. Kanki PJ, Alroy J, Essex M. Isolation of T-lymphotropic retrovirus related to HTLV-III/LAV from wild-caught African green monkeys. Science 1985;230:951–954.
4. Connor S. Laboratory mix-up solves AIDS mystery. New Scientist 1988;117:32.
5. Clavel F, Brun-Vezinet F, Chamaret S, et al. Isolation of a new human retrovirus from West African patients with AIDS. Science 1986;233:343–346.
6. McCormick JB, Fisher-Hoch S. Level 4: virus hunters of the CDC. Atlanta, GA: Turner Publishing; 1996.
7. Nasidi A, Monath TP, De Cock K, et al. Urban yellow fever in western Nigeria, 1987. Trans Roy Soc Trop Med Hyg 1989;83:401–406.
8. De Cock KM, Monath TP, Nasidi A, et al. Epidemic yellow fever in eastern Nigeria, 1986. Lancet 1988;1:630–632.
9. Odehouri K, De Cock KM, Krebs JW, et al. HIV-1 and HIV-2 infections associated with AIDS in Abidjan, Cote d'Ivoire. AIDS 1989;3:509–512.
10. Rayfield M, De Cock K, Heyward W, et al. Mixed human immunodeficiency virus (HIV) infection in an individual: demonstration of both HIV type 1 and type 2 proviral sequences by using polymerase chain reaction. J Infect Dis 1988;158:1170–1176.
11. De Cock KM, Porter A, Odehouri K, et al. Rapid emergence of AIDS in Abidjan, Ivory Coast. Lancet 1989;2:408–411.

12. Djomand G, Greenberg AE, Sassan-Morokro M, et al. The epidemic of HIV/AIDS in Abidjan, Cote d'Ivoire: a review of data collected by Projet RETRO-CI from 1987 to 1993. J Acquir Immune Defic Syndr 1995;10:358–365.
13. De Cock KM, Barrere B, Diaby L, et al. AIDS: the leading cause of adult death in the West African city of Abidjan, Cote d'Ivoire. Science 1990;249:793–796.
14. De Cock KM, Barrere B, Lafontaine MF, et al. Mortality trends in Abidjan, Cote d'Ivoire, 1983–1988. AIDS 1991;4:393–398.
15. De Cock KM, Zielinski-Gutiérrez E, Lucas SB. Learning from the dead. N Engl J Med 2019;381:1889–1891.
16. De Cock KM, Porter A, Kouadio J, et al. Rapid and specific diagnosis of HIV-1 and HIV-2 infections: an evaluation of testing strategies. AIDS 1990;4:875–878.
17. De Cock KM, Maran M, Kouadio JC. Rapid test for distinguishing HIV-1 and HIV-2. Lancet 1990;336:757.
18. De Cock KM, Porter A, Kouadio J, et al. Cross-reactivity on Western blots in HIV-1 and HIV-2 infections. AIDS 1991;5:859–863.
19. George JR, Rayfield MA, Phillips S, et al. Efficacy of US Food and Drug Administration-licensed HIV-1 screening enzyme immunoassays for detecting antibodies to HIV-2. AIDS 1990;4:321–326.
20. Pau C-P, Granade TC, Parekh B, et al. Misidentification of HIV-2 proteins by Western blots. Lancet 1991;337:616–617. doi: 10.1016/0140-6736(91)91683-l.
21. Parekh B, Pau C-P, Granade TC, et al. Oligomeric nature of transmembrane glycoproteins of HIV-2: procedures for their efficient dislocation and preparation of Western blots for diagnosis. AIDS 1991;5:1009–1013.
22. George R, Ou C-Y, Parekh B, et al. Prevalence of HIV-1 and HIV-2 mixed infections in Cote d'Ivoire. Lancet 1992;340:337–339.
23. Gershy-Damet GM, Koffi K, Abouya L, et al. Salivary and urinary diagnosis of human immunodeficiency viruses 1 and 2 infection in Côte d'Ivoire. Trans Roy Soc Trop Med Hyg 1992;86:670–671.
24. Brattegaard K, Kouadio J, Adom M-L, Doorly R, George JR, De Cock KM. Rapid and simple screening and supplemental testing for HIV-1 and HIV-2 infections in West Africa. AIDS 1993;7:883–886.
25. Brattegaard K, Soroh D, Zadi F, Digbeu H, Vetter KM, De Cock KM. Insensitivity of a synthetic peptide-based test (Pepti-LAV 1-2) for the diagnosis of HIV infection in African children. AIDS 1995;9:656–657.
26. "VAN PATTEN, HAROLD," The Global Health Chronicles, accessed January 29, 2023. https://www.globalhealthchronicles.org/items/show/7976.
27. Diallo MO, Ackah AN, Lafontaine M-F, et al. HIV-1 and HIV-2 infections in men attending sexually transmitted diseases clinics in Abidjan, Cote d'Ivoire. AIDS 1992;6:581–585.
28. Diallo M, Ghys PD, Vuylsteke B, et al. Evaluation of simple diagnostic algorithms for Neisseria gonorrhoeae and Chlamydia trachomatis cervical infections in female sex workers in Abidjan, Cote d'Ivoire. Sex Transm Infect 1998;74(Suppl 1):S106–S111.
29. Ghys PD, Diallo MO, Ettiegne-Traore V, et al. High prevalence of genital ulcers due to HIV-related immunosuppression in female sex workers in Abidjan, Cote d'Ivoire. J Infect Dis 1995;172:1371–1374.

30. Ghys PD, Diallo MO, Ettiegne-Traore V, et al. Dual seroreactivity to HIV-1 and HIV-2 in female sex workers in Abidjan, Cote d'Ivoire. AIDS 1995;9:955–958.

31. Ghys PD, Diallo MO, Ettiegne-Traore V, et al. Increase in condom use and decline in HIV and sexually transmitted diseases among female sex workers in Abidjan, Cote d'Ivoire, 1991–1998. AIDS 2002;16:1–8.

32. Kamenga M, De Cock KM, St Louis M, et al. The impact of human immunodeficiency virus infection on pelvic inflammatory disease: a case-control study in Abidjan, Ivory Coast. Am J Obstet Gynecol 1995;172:919–925.

33. Sassan-Morokro M, Greenberg AE, Coulibaly I-M, et al. High rates of sexual contact with female sex workers, sexually transmitted diseases, and condom neglect among HIV-infected and uninfected men with tuberculosis in Abidjan, Cote d'Ivoire. J Acquir Immune Defic Syndr 1996;11:183–187.

34. Greenberg AE, Nguyen-Dinh P, Mann JM, et al. The association between malaria, blood transfusions, and HIV seropositivity in a pediatric population in Kinshasa, Zaire. JAMA 1988;259:545–549.

35. Savarit S, De Cock KM, Schutz R, Konate S, Lackritz E, Bondurand A. Risk of HIV infection from HIV antibody-negative blood transfusion in a West African city. BMJ 1992;305:498–501.

36. Schutz R, Savarit D, Kadjo JC, et al. Excluding blood donors at high risk donors of HIV infection in a west African city. BMJ 1993; 307:1517–1519. doi: 10.1136/bmj.307.6918.1517.

37. Abouya L, Beaumel A, Lucas SB, et al. *Pneumocystis carinii* pneumonia: an uncommon cause of death in African patients with AIDS. Am Rev Respir Dis 1992;145:617–620.

38. Lucas SB, Hounnou A, Peacock C, et al. The mortality and pathology of HIV infection in a west African city. AIDS 1993;7:1569–1579.

39. Lucas SB, De Cock KM, Hounnou A, et al. Contribution of tuberculosis to slim disease in Africa. BMJ 1994;308:1531–1533.

40. Lucas SB, Peacock CS, Hounnou A, et al. Disease in children infected with HIV in Abidjan. BMJ 1996;312:335–338.

41. De Cock KM, Lucas SB, Lucas S, Agnes J, Kadio A, Gayle H. Clinical research, prophylaxis, therapy and care for HIV disease in Africa. Am J Public Health 1993;83:1385–1389.

42. Lucas SB, Hounnou A, Peacock C, Beaumel A, Kadio A, De Cock KM. Nocardiosis mimicking tuberculosis in HIV-positive patients: an autopsy study in West Africa. Tuberc Lung Dis 1994;75:301–307.

43. Lucas SB, Diomande MI, Hounnou A, et al. HIV-associated lymphoma in Africa: an autopsy study in Cote d'Ivoire. Int J Cancer 1994;59:20–24.

44. Lucas SB, Hounou A, Bell J, et al. Severe cerebral swelling is not observed in children dying with malaria. QJM 1996;89:351–353.

45. Bell JE, Lowrie S, Koffi K, et al. The neuropathology of HIV-infected African children in Abidjan, Cote d'Ivoire. J Neuropathol Exp Neurol 1997;56:686–692.

46. Lange JMA. HIV-related morbidity and mortality in sub-Saharan Africa: opportunities for prevention. AIDS 1993;7:1675–1676.

47. Vugia DJ, Kiehlbauch JA, Yeboue K, et al. Pathogens and predictors of fatal septi-
    cemia associated with human immunodeficiency virus infection in Ivory Coast, West
    Africa. J Infect Dis 1993;168:564–570.
48. Vetter KM, Djomand G, Zadi F, et al. Clinical spectrum of HIV disease in children in
    a West African city. Pediatr Infect Dis J 1996;15:438–442.
49. Grant AD, Djomand G, Smets P, et al. Profound immunosuppression across the spec-
    trum of opportunistic disease among hospitalized HIV-infected adults in Abidjan,
    Cote d'Ivoire. AIDS 1997;11:1357–1364.
50. Grant AD, Djomand G, De Cock KM. Natural history and spectrum of disease in
    adults with HIV/AIDS in Africa. AIDS 1997;11(Suppl B):S43–S54.
51. Grant AD, Kassim S, Domoua K, et al. Spectrum of disease among HIV-infected
    adults hospitalised in a respiratory medicine unit in Abidjan, Cote d'Ivoire. Int J
    Tuberc Lung Dis 1998;2:926–934.
52. Grant AD. Spectrum and natural history of HIV disease in Abidjan, Cote d'Ivoire.
    PhD Thesis, London School of Hygiene and Tropical Medicine; 1998.
53. De Cock KM, Brun-Vezinet F. Epidemiology of HIV-2. AIDS 1989;3(Suppl
    1):S89–S95.
54. De Cock KM, Brun-Vezinet F, Soro B. HIV-1 and HIV-2 infections and AIDS in West
    Africa. AIDS 1991;5(Suppl 1):S21–S28.
55. De Cock KM, Brun-Vezinet F. The epidemiology of HIV-2 infection. In: Mann J,
    Tarantola D, Netter TW, eds. AIDS in the world. Cambridge, MA: Harvard University
    Press; 1993:275–277.
56. Kanki PJ, De Cock KM. Epidemiology and transmission of HIV-2. AIDS 1994;8(Suppl
    1):S85–S93.
57. De Cock KM, Odehouri K, Colebunders RL, et al. A comparison of HIV-1 and HIV-
    2 infections in hospitalized patients in Abidjan, Cote d'Ivoire (West Africa). AIDS
    1990;4:443–448. doi: 10.1097/00002030-199005000-00010.
58. Gnaore E, Sassan-Morokro M, Kassim S, et al. A comparison of clinical features
    in HIV-1 and HIV-2 associated tuberculosis. Trans Roy Soc Trop Med Hyg
    1993;87:57–59.
59. De Cock KM, Gnaore E, Adjorlolo G, et al. Increased risk for tuberculosis in persons
    with HIV-1 and HIV-2 infections in Abidjan, Cote d'Ivoire. BMJ 1991;302:496–499.
60. Kestens L, Brattegaard K, Adjorlolo G, et al. Immunological comparison of HIV-
    1-, HIV-2- and dually-reactive women delivering in Abidjan, Côte d'Ivoire. AIDS
    1992;6:803–807.
61. Kassim S, Sassan-Morokro M, Ackah A, et al. Two-year follow-up of persons
    with HIV-1- and HIV-2-associated pulmonary tuberculosis treated with short-
    course chemotherapy in West Africa. AIDS 1995;9:1185–1191. doi: 10.1097/
    00002030-199510000-00011.
62. Travers K, Mboup S, Marlink S, et al. Natural protection against HIV-1 infection pro-
    vided by HIV-2. Science 1995;268:1612–1615.
63. Greenberg AE, Wiktor SZ, DeCock KM, Smith P, Jaffe HW, Dondero TJ. HIV-2 and
    natural protection against HIV-1 infection. Science 1996;272:1959–1960.

64. Wiktor SZ, Nkengasong JN, Ekpini ER. Lack of protection against HIV-1 infection among women with HIV-2 infection. AIDS 1999;13:695–699.

65. Diallo MO, Ettiegne-Traore V, Maran M, et al. Sexually transmitted diseases and human immunodeficiency virus infections in women attending an antenatal clinic in Abidjan, Cote d'Ivoire. Int J STD AIDS 1997;8:636–638.

66. Adjorlolo G, De Cock KM, Ekpini E, et al. Prospective comparison of mother-to-child transmission of HIV-1 and HIV-2 in Abidjan, Ivory Coast. JAMA 1994;272:462–466.

67. De Cock KM, Zadi F, Adjorlolo G, et al. Retrospective study of maternal HIV-1 and HIV-2 infections and child survival in Abidjan, Cote d'Ivoire. BMJ 1994;308:441–443.

68. Gayle HD, Gnaore E, Adjorlolo G, et al. HIV-1 and HIV-2 infections in children in Abidjan, Cote d'Ivoire. J Acquir Immune Defic Syndr 1992;5:513–517.

69. N'Gbichi J-M, De Cock KM, Batter V, et al. HIV status of female sex partners of men reactive to HIV-1, HIV-2, and both viruses in West Africa. AIDS 1995;9:951–954.

70. De Cock KM, Adjorlolo G, Ekpini E, et al. Epidemiology and transmission of HIV-2. Why there is no HIV-2 pandemic. JAMA 1993;270:2083–2086.doi: 10.1001/jama.270.17.2083.

71. "GREENBERG, ALAN," The Global Health Chronicles, accessed January 29, 2023. https://www.globalhealthchronicles.org/items/show/7907

72. Connor EM, Sperling RS, Gelber R, et al. Reduction of maternal-infant transmission of human immunodeficiency virus type 1 with zidovudine treatment. N Engl J Med 1994;331:1173–1180.

73. Lurie P, Wolfe SM. Unethical trials of interventions to reduce perinatal transmission of the human immunodeficiency virus in developing countries. N Engl J Med 1997;337:853–856.

74. Angell M. The ethics of clinical research in the Third World. N Engl J Med 1997;337:847–849.

75. De Cock KM. Publicity, politics, and public health: the case of placebo-controlled trials for the prevention of mother-to-child transmission of HIV in resource-poor countries. International AIDS Society Newsletter 1997;8:9–10.

76. Varmus H, Satcher D. Ethical complexities of conducting research in developing countries. N Engl J Med 1997;337:1003–1005.

77. The conduct of clinical trials of maternal–infant transmission of HIV supported by the United States Department of Health and Human Services in developing countries. Washington, DC: US Department of Health and Human Services, July 1997.

78. Editorial. The ethics industry. Lancet 1997;350:897.

79. Wiktor SZ, Ekpini E, Karon JM, et al. Short-course oral zidovudine for prevention of mother-to-child transmission of HIV-1 in Abidjan, Côte d'Ivoire: a randomised trial. Lancet 1999;353:781–785.

80. Dabis F, Msellati P, Meda N, et al. 6-month efficacy, tolerance, and acceptability of a short regimen of oral zidovudine to reduce vertical transmission of HIV in breastfed children in Côte d'Ivoire and Burkina Faso: a double-blind placebo-controlled multicentre trial. DITRAME Study Group. DIminution De La Transmission Mère-Enfant. Lancet 1999;353:786–792. doi: 10.1016/s0140-6736(98)11046-2.

81. Shaffer N, Chuachuuwong R, Mock PA, et al. Short course zidovudine for perinatal HIV-1 transmission in Bangkok, Thailand: a randomized controlled trial. Lancet 1999;353:773–780.

82. Wiktor SZ, Sassan-Morokro M, Grant AD, et al. Efficacy of trimethoprim-sulphamethoxazole prophylaxis to decrease morbidity and mortality in HIV-1-infected patients with tuberculosis in Abidjan, Cote d'Ivoire: a randomized controlled trial. Lancet 1999;353:1469–1475.

83. Greenberg AE, Lucas SB, Tossou O, et al. Autopsy-proven causes of death in HIV-infected patients treated for tuberculosis in Abidjan, Cote d'Ivoire. AIDS 1995;9:1251–1254.

84. "NKENGASONG, JOHN," *The Global Health Chronicles*, accessed January 29, 2023. https://www.globalhealthchronicles.org/items/show/8138.

85. Adjé C, Cheingsong R, Roels TH, et al. High prevalence of genotypic and phenotypic HIV-1 drug-resistant strains among patients receiving antiretroviral therapy in Abidjan, Côte d'Ivoire. J Acquir Immune Defic Syndr 2001;26:501–506. doi: 10.1097/00126334-200104150-00018.

86. Adjé-Touré C, Celestin B, Hanson D, et al. Prevalence of genotypic and phenotypic HIV-1 drug-resistant strains among patients who have rebound in viral load while receiving antiretroviral therapy in the UNAIDS-Drug Access Initiative in Abidjan, Côte d'Ivoire. AIDS 2003;17(Suppl 3):S23–S29. doi: 10.1097/00002030-200317003-00004.

87. Bilé EC, Adjé-Touré C, Borget MY, Kalou M, Diomande F, Chorba T, Nkengasong JN. Performance of drug-resistance genotypic assays among HIV-1 infected patients with predominantly CRF02_AG strains of HIV-1 in Abidjan, Cote d'Ivoire. J Clin Virol 2005;32:60–66. doi: 10.1016/j.jcv.2004.07.008.

88. Adjé-Touré CA, Cheingsong R, Garcìa-Lerma JG, et al. Antiretroviral therapy in HIV-2-infected patients: changes in plasma viral load, CD4+ cell counts, and drug resistance profiles of patients treated in Abidjan, Côte d'Ivoire. AIDS 2003;17(Suppl 3):S49–S54.

89. Gottlieb GS, Raugi DN, Smith RA. 90-90-90 for HIV-2? Ending the HIV-2 epidemic by enhancing care and clinical management of patients infected with HIV-2. Lancet HIV 2018;5:e390–e399. doi: 10.1016/S2352-3018(18)30094-8.

90. Minchella PA, Adjé-Touré C, Zhang G, et al. Long-term immunological responses to treatment among HIV-2 patients in Côte d'Ivoire. BMC Infect Dis 2020;20:213. doi: 10.1186/s12879-020-4927-x.

16

The HIV/AIDS Collaboration in Thailand

Kevin M. De Cock

As CDC's global presence increased, the EIS program slowly expanded its international influence.[1,2,3] Other programs based on EIS were developed outside of the United States, but the misunderstood name "Epidemic Intelligence Service" was replaced by the more descriptive "Field Epidemiology Training Program" (FETP). Over the years several dozen FETPs have been established across the world, always in association with the host country's ministry of health. Some have been short lived, others successfully maintained—with funding and national commitment usually the deciding factors. Former CDC Director Tom Frieden often said that CDC's most important contribution to global health may well be its support for the FETPs worldwide.[4]

The first and possibly most successful FETP was established in Thailand in 1980. The CDC advisor for the program was David Brandling-Bennett who later took up positions at WHO and the Bill and Melinda Gates Foundation. AIDS became a concern in Thailand in the 1980s as the country had an extensive sex industry as well as a large population of IDUs. In 1983, Bruce Weniger,[5] fresh from EIS in CDC's Division of Parasitic Diseases, where he had witnessed the increasing requests for the drug pentamidine for cases of PCP, went to Thailand as CDC's second assignee for the still young FETP.

Weniger's CDC connections enabled him to access HIV tests and to assist with the first systematic examination in Thailand of specific groups at risk. A 1985 study of 600 subjects that included male and female sex workers, IDUs, blood donors, and patients with thalassemia (a blood disorder that can require frequent transfusions), found only one positive specimen— taken from a twenty-year-old male sex worker who had worked in a gay bar in Bangkok.[5,6] Notably, all specimens from drug injectors were negative. Weniger recounted that the United States Army's Armed Forces Research Institute of Medical Sciences (AFRIMS) in Bangkok identified another four infected male sex workers later that year.[7]

Kevin M. De Cock, *The HIV/AIDS Collaboration in Thailand* In: *Dispatches from the AIDS Pandemic*. Kevin M. De Cock, Harold W. Jaffe, and James W. Curran and Edited by: Robin Moseley, Oxford University Press.

In the late 1980s, Projet SIDA (Chapter 13) was thriving, and work was on-going to establish a research site in West Africa—what would become Projet RETRO-CI (Chapter 15). Both were part of the International Activity, under Bill Heyward, in Jim Curran's AIDS division in Atlanta. Heyward wanted to expand the reach of his group and began to look toward Asia. In 1990, he assigned Weniger, now back from his FETP service, to initiate AIDS work in Thailand. Helene Gayle (Figure 16.1), who later headed the International Activity, expanded on the reasons for this international research:

> We then had the three different activities [Kinshasa, Abidjan, and Bangkok], and each one was formed for a slightly different reason. . . Thailand was [started] because they had the huge injection drug use population, to understand that better. . . .and the research evolved as it went on. They became sites for vaccine research and other kinds of research, as well as prevention research.[8]

In addition to the large IDU population, Thailand's large sex industry was a potential risk for widespread heterosexual transmission, another reason for CDC focusing on this area of the world. Nancy Young joined the collaboration as laboratory director and Khanchit Limpakarnjanarat, a Thai former CDC EIS officer, as epidemiologist, later becoming the de facto deputy director of the whole operation.

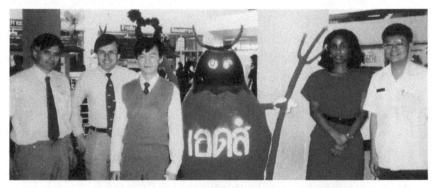

Figure 16.1. Thailand site visit, circa 1991. Pictured (l–r): Bruce Weniger, Jim Curran, Wat Utaivoravit, "AIDS Devil," Helene Gayle, Khanchit Limpakarnjanarat. (Kevin De Cock, personal collection)

Descriptive Epidemiology

Injection Drug Users

At WHO, the HIV/AIDS epidemiology group, under the leadership of Jim Chin in Jonathan Mann's GPA (Chapter 14), had categorized the world's HIV epidemic into three patterns.[9] Pattern I and II countries were characterized, respectively, by established epidemics in high-risk groups (such as in the United States) or in the general population (as in countries in East and Central Africa). In comparison, Pattern III countries had few cases or had experienced HIV introduction only recently. Despite ominous signs, Thailand was still considered a Pattern III country when Weniger returned there in 1990, but he rapidly and usefully showed that this classification no longer held.[6] The first few years of CDC's collaborative work on AIDS in Thailand provided important descriptive data on the epidemic. Collaboration between CDC's epidemiology and laboratory experts was especially productive.

For CDC staff, working in Thailand in 1990 was quite different from the experience in sub-Saharan Africa. Thailand was already what today would be called a middle-income country, a stark comparison to the poverty of Africa. CDC staff complained of traffic jams and smog. The HIV epidemic was new, so even if HIV prevalence was expanding, its impact—people ill and dying from AIDS—was not yet visible. Technical capacity—clinical, laboratory, and epidemiologic—was much greater than it had been early on in CDC's other international collaborations. Disease surveillance was prioritized, a long-term benefit from the FETP. There was also strong research capacity, preexisting international collaboration, and active local and regional dissemination of data and academic publishing. Combined with political will, the Thai open mindedness and strong science laid foundations for international leadership in the prevention of heterosexual and mother-to-child transmission—all before hospitals were crowded with sick and dying AIDS patients.

Weniger and colleagues insightfully described sequential "waves" of HIV infection "washing over" various sectors of Thai society, a likely harbinger of the epidemiologic future for the region. Their review of the epidemiology of HIV in Thailand published in the journal *AIDS* in 1991[6] became widely cited. The waves involved IDUs, female sex workers, sexually active heterosexual men, and the general (adult and child) population. MSM also became increasingly infected but, apart from sex workers, were not included in early studies. What was unanticipated was that some of these waves, apparently both sequential and linked, were independent of one another according to the new discipline of molecular epidemiology.[10,11,12,13,14] These early studies and the subsequent mounting of prevention efforts would not have been possible without the pragmatic approach to HIV/AIDS by the Thai authorities at the highest level, quite different from that in many other countries.

Although the first few documented HIV infections were in MSM, the initial avalanche was in IDUs. Weniger speculated that incarcerated drug users from the West may have introduced infection into Thai prisons, spreading to the community upon intermittent release of prisoners[5,6,7] Studies from the Thanyarak Hospital and the Bangkok Metropolitan Administration Health Department involved predominantly heroin users attending methadone treatment. Rates of HIV infection increased from around 1 percent to between one third and one half of all treatment attendees over the course of 1988. These proportions concerned prevalence; measurements of the incidence during this period, the rate of new infections over time in 1988 to 1989, showed 3 percent to 5 percent of injectors becoming infected *per month*. Sentinel surveys conducted in 1989 among IDUs throughout the country showed high rates of infection everywhere, even among persons from the remote hill tribe populations.

The dominant risk factor for HIV infection in people who inject drugs is the sharing of injection paraphernalia. As many as one fifth of Thai drug users attending detoxification programs reported prior incarceration, and previous imprisonment was shown to be a risk factor for HIV infection consistent with ubiquitous needle sharing in local jails and prisons.[6,15,16] Drug injectors formed an obvious bridge for sexual transmission to the general heterosexual population.

In close collaboration with the Thai authorities, including the Office of the Narcotics Control Board, CDC researchers used a form of the "capture–recapture" methodology widely applied in animal ecology to estimate the size of the drug-using population in Bangkok. By cross-matching the list of all persons receiving methadone treatment in Bangkok (the first capture) with the list of individuals who had been detained at police stations and had urine tests positive for opioid metabolites (the second capture), it was possible to estimate the total number of opioid users. Applying assumptions about the proportion who injected (89%) and the proportion who were HIV-infected (one third), the researchers concluded that there were about 12,000 HIV-positive IDUs in Bangkok in 1991.[17]

Unsurprisingly, HIV spread widely throughout drug-injecting communities in the region—including in Burma (Myanmar), Laos, Vietnam, Malaysia, India, and China.[6] Weniger commented on the unintended consequences of some drug-use interventions:

> In the early days opium was the drug of choice. . . grown and cultivated in that famous Golden Triangle where Myanmar and Laos and Thailand meet. Then it's transported along smuggling routes to go to other parts of the world. But smoking opium doesn't transmit HIV. . . as drug suppression efforts became more successful, opium smuggling was replaced with heroin production . . . there were refineries located closer to the sources of the opium poppies, so that there would be less volume of drug to smuggle and transport. So, what was being transported was then heroin, which is injected . . . So ironically the success of drug suppression helped increase the risk of blood-borne diseases like HIV.[5]

Female Sex Workers and Heterosexual Men

Public health authorities in Thailand estimated that in 1990 there were close to 100,000 female sex workers nationally, with almost 30,000 in Bangkok.[6] Based on 1988 data, there may have been one sex worker for every 146 men aged fifteen to forty-four; higher estimates were that 2.4 percent of women aged fifteen to twenty-nine were engaged in the sex trade. Weniger described the "traditional double standard in sexual behavior" responsible for the brisk heterosexual epidemic that emerged, initially affecting lower socioeconomic, brothel-based women in northern Thailand.[18] Although traditionally most women abstained from premarital or extramarital sex, almost one third of men in 1989–1990 reported sex outside of their marriage or steady relationship. Around three quarters of men reported having paid for sex at some time. In 1989, HIV prevalence in brothel-based sex workers reached 37 percent to 44 percent, with initial monthly incidence as high as 10 percent. As Weniger recalled,

> [T]here were really two types of female sex workers. The brothel-based ones were the ones that were very low cost, $3, $5, $8, and working in establishments. They would call them tea houses or brothels. Then there were more freelance workers who might work in bars, meet customers, go

to a short-stay motel around the corner or high-class places even. The rates of HIV were different in those places.[5]

Infection rates in these "indirect" sex workers who charged higher rates increased to a median prevalence of around 5 percent.

If Weniger's "second wave" of HIV was in female sex workers, the third was in heterosexual men for whom the strongest risk factors were frequenting sex workers and having had prior STIs.[6] For this third wave, a particularly useful line of investigation was linked to the Thai practice of military conscription by lottery, which, despite its biases through nonsystematic exclusions, offered close to a national random sample of young men. In the early 1990s the prevalence of HIV in conscripts in northern Thailand was more than 10 percent,[19] but in subsequent years it fell sharply because of reduced sex worker contact, reduced STI incidence, and greatly increased condom use.[20] This exemplified the impact of Thailand's famous "100% Condom Only" campaign for which Weniger credits an FETP graduate, Wiwat Rojanapithayakorn:

> He [Rojanapithayakorn] came up with this, where although prostitution was technically illegal, the police knew where these places were... Working with the police, he went to these places and set up a program where... the owners of these establishments were mandated to require their employees to always use condoms, and if their customer refused, to explain to the employee "don't have sex with this person."[5]

Rojanapithayakorn went on to win the Prince Mahidol of Thailand prize for this work, one of Asia's most prestigious awards. Great credit is also due to Mechai Viravaidya, a champion of family planning and condom promotion. Condoms were often called "Mechais" in Thailand, and Viravaidya later became a cabinet member overseeing the country's AIDS portfolio. He also was a close adviser to Mann at WHO and to many others in the public health world.

Inevitably, spread of HIV to low-risk women and their infants did occur, but only to a limited degree. The Thai outbreak had threatened to ignite into a generalized population epidemic analogous to the experience in Africa, but HIV ultimately settled in concentrated fashion in key populations at highest risk—sex workers, MSM, transgender women, and IDUs. Thailand's pragmatic and nonjudgmental approach to control of HIV and STIs within the sex work industry and among sexual minorities, along with its robust disease surveillance and openness about sharing data, helped limit expansion of the epidemic.

Laboratory Insights

CDC is at its best when its strong laboratory capacity integrates with epidemiology and public health efforts. This was exemplified by the work of CDC research scientist Chin-Yih Ou[21] and his collaborators in Thailand. After graduating in laboratory sciences in Taiwan, Ou arrived in the United States in 1977 for doctoral studies in molecular biology at the Oak Ridge National Laboratory in Tennessee. His training there in cloning, sequencing, and other molecular techniques focused on murine leukemia virus, a retrovirus. This was to prove useful when he accepted a position in the AIDS division at CDC in 1986 under Gerald ("Gerry") Schochetman[22] and set up systems for the molecular diagnosis of HIV.

Antibody testing for HIV had just become available but the gold standard for diagnosis remained viral culture, which at CDC was performed in the laboratory directed by Paul Feorino (Chapter 9). Ou described how he read about the concept of polymerase chain reaction (PCR) for detecting genomic material, how he thought this could be applied to the diagnosis of HIV, and what it took to put this into practice.[21,23,24] There is irony in the fact that developing the concept of PCR led Kary Mullis to receive the Nobel Prize for Chemistry in 1993 but did not prevent him from later becoming a denialist who refuted HIV as the cause of AIDS. Ou taught himself the new technology and was the first at CDC to use it. As he recounted, "There was nobody to learn from. You just looked into the publications and started from there. You just needed to try it a few times."[21] His tenacity, exemplified by his cleaning of his own laboratory to exclude any cross contamination, paid off. He later played a critically important role in the investigation of a cluster of HIV infections among patients of an HIV-infected dentist in Florida that attracted international attention.[25]

Ou's initial application of PCR for HIV—for the diagnosis of infection in infants in whom maternal antibodies could persist beyond one year—resulted in publications in *Science* and the *New England Journal of Medicine*.[23,26] His laboratory also began to study HIV genetic diversity, looking at specimens from different parts of the world. He first visited Thailand and met Weniger in 1990, and they agreed to collaborate with Thai colleagues to examine the genetic characteristics of the country's circulating virus.

To their surprise, two different subtypes or "clades" of HIV (Chapter 18) were circulating and could be tracked epidemiologically.[10] Drug injectors mostly had subtype B infections, closely related to the predominant virus in North America. By contrast, persons infected sexually had a subtype more closely related to isolates of African origin, initially referred to as A but later reclassified as subtype E.* These observations upset the earlier hypothesis that transmission across various groups was responsible for the apparent succession of epidemic waves across Thai society. Rather, it seems that different viral introductions through drug injection and unprotected sex had instigated independent epidemics, with subtype B likely introduced from westerners with HIV, and E from Africa.

This work was an early example of the burgeoning discipline of HIV molecular epidemiology, which was to become increasingly important over time for epidemiologic investigations as well as prevention studies, including those for HIV vaccines.[10,11,12,13,14] Whether different subtypes of HIV influence transmissibility of infection or disease progression remains controversial.[27] The spectrum of disease associated with subtype B and E infections in Thailand was similar.[28]

From Weniger to Mastro

As with CDC's African field work, the early descriptive research in Thailand was foundational for deeper analytic work that in turn led to intervention studies of HIV prevention methodologies (Figure 16.2). Weniger was succeeded as the collaboration's director in 1993 by CDC epidemiologist Tim Mastro, who had been working with the Thai collaboration since 1990. Like Weniger, Mastro had prior experience in Thailand. Before joining CDC he had worked on the Thai–Cambodia border for the American Refugee Committee and then the United Nations. Mastro's earlier work serendipitously led to EIS and then further international involvement. That both he and Weniger were married to Thai citizens unquestionably gave them insight and facilitated their integration into the local environment.

---

* The full name of subtype E is now CRF01_AE, indicating it is a circulating recombinant form including components of subtype A.

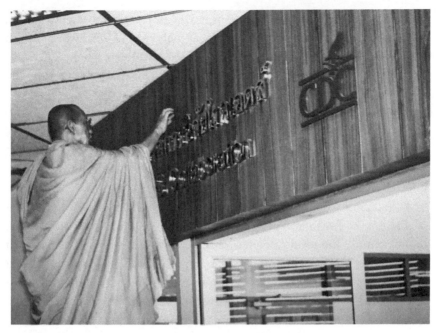

Figure 16.2. Thai monk blessing CDC office in Thailand, 1995. (Courtesy of Tim Mastro)

Preventing Sexual Transmission

Mastro sharpened the group's epidemiologic focus and, innovatively, involved mathematical modelers to estimate the risk of HIV transmission from different exposures. Military recruits were known to have high rates of new HIV infections from contact with female sex workers. Mastro and colleagues published estimates of the risk of female-to-male transmission that ranged from 3.1 percent to 5.6 percent per episode of vaginal intercourse with an HIV-infected woman[29,30] Such rates were approximately tenfold higher than estimates in Europe and North America, where this topic was more difficult to study because heterosexually acquired HIV was less common. Relevant factors explaining these higher-than-expected rates of transmission included the likelihood that many of the women with HIV had been recently infected and therefore probably had high viral loads, increasing infectiousness. High rates of other STIs and almost universal lack of male circumcision were also surely relevant.

Despite Thailand's innovative efforts in HIV prevention, women—not just those who were sex workers—remained at high risk, especially in northern Thailand.[31] In Bangkok, the prevalence of HIV infection in women attending antenatal clinics increased from 1.0 percent to 2.3 percent between 1991 and 1996, with 23 percent and 50 percent of uninfected and infected women, respectively, reporting more than one lifetime sex partner.[32] Having had two lifetime partners increased the likelihood of HIV infection threefold, while having more than two partners increased the risk almost six times. Having a partner with known HIV risk factors increased women's chances of being infected, as did having a history of STIs.

Although the proportion of women reporting more than one lifetime sex partner was higher than expected from prior surveys, the great majority were monogamous. The results emphasized that, for most women at least, their own behavior was neither protective nor a risk factor for acquiring HIV; their likelihood of becoming infected and later transmitting HIV to their infants or dying of AIDS was determined by the risk profile of their partner.[33]

"The Chiang Rai Health Club" was the name for a prospective, ten-year cohort study of female sex workers in northern Thailand that was initiated in 1991 and provided preventive interventions and follow-up.[34,35] Although the 100 percent condom program described earlier certainly reduced HIV transmission, the risk for sex workers remained high. From 1991 to 1994, despite STI management and preventive efforts, 20.3 percent of brothel-based female sex workers became infected with HIV annually (for those working in other venues the proportion was 0.7%). In Bangkok, the prevalence of HIV infection was actually higher in the most recent entrants into the sex trade (12.5% in women who had begun sex work since 1994) compared with those who had started in earlier years (5.5% in women who had started before 1989).[36]

Peter Kilmarx (Figure 16.3), a former EIS officer and Peace Corps volunteer in the Democratic Republic of Congo (DRC) ([37]), joined the collaboration in 1996 and was posted to the CDC field site in Chiang Rai in the far northern (Golden Triangle) region of Thailand. The difficulty that women faced ensuring male condom use led to interest early on in female-controlled interventions. Greatest attention was given to vaginal microbicides, products that women could apply vaginally prior to sexual intercourse, with the aim of blocking HIV transmission. Kilmarx and collaborators conducted a safety and acceptability study of Carraguard,* a carrageenan-derived gel, in a cohort of women in Chiang Rai.[38] The work was supported in part by the newly established Bill and

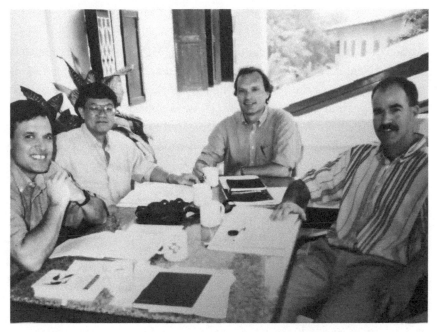

Figure 16.3. Chiang Rai study team, 1996. Pictured (l–r): Mike St Louis,
Khanchit Limpakarnjanarat, Tim Mastro, Peter Kilmarx. (Courtesy of Tim
Mastro)

Melinda Gates Foundation, and both Bill Gates Senior and Melinda
Gates visited the study site. Although this important work showed
the product to be safe and acceptable, later efficacy trials in southern
Africa showed that it did not prevent HIV infection. As discussed in
Chapter 19, the research agenda was subsequently taken over by ART-
based prevention.

In parallel to the country's public health focus, the collaboration did
not begin research on HIV in MSM until the late 1990s. The instigator of
this work was Frits van Griensven, an energetic Dutch behavioral scientist
recruited by Mastro in 1998. Himself gay and with deep understanding of
local mores, van Griensven was an effective researcher who played an important role in building Thailand's capacity and infrastructure for later studies
on interventions among MSM.[39] His contributions for work with MSM and
transgender populations were later recognized by a knighthood conferred by
the Netherlands government. MSM now account for almost half of new HIV
infections in Thailand.

Preventing Mother-to-Child Transmission

Although CDC's early international work on HIV might sometimes have seemed disparate, a strong linkage across all sites concerned mother-to-child transmission. After the results of the landmark ACTG 076 study of zidovudine to prevent vertical transmission were published in 1994,[40] the race was on to see how this could be implemented in lower-resourced settings. The CDC sites in Abidjan and Bangkok, primed after years of preparatory work for longer-term intervention studies,[41] provided appropriate as well as contrasting settings. Avoidance of breastfeeding was nearly impossible in the African setting because of uncertainty about access to clean water for the safe preparation of infant formula. This was not the case in Bangkok. Two CDC-supported trials of the same intervention—short-course, oral zidovudine—were therefore complementary, shedding light on the relative importance of breastfeeding and the impact of this simplified intervention on perinatal HIV transmission.[42,43]

Nathan Shaffer[44] joined CDC in 1986 as an EIS officer in the Enteric Diseases Branch, an elite assignment because of the technical strength of the group and its frequent investigations into outbreaks of foodborne and waterborne diseases. After EIS, he joined CDC's Malaria Branch and took the well-traveled route to Kinshasa, becoming involved in the project's family studies and developing an interest in vertical transmission of HIV. Margaret Oxtoby, a pediatrician and lead of the perinatal HIV group in CDC's AIDS division in Atlanta, soon invited him to join her HIV studies on women and children being conducted in New York, New Jersey, and Atlanta. When a full-time position opened in Thailand in 1995, Shaffer seized the opportunity.

Technology for measuring CD4+ T-lymphocyte counts, the key indicator of immune deficiency, had become available for field use, and PCR had been introduced. The concept of viral load, the amount of virus detectable in plasma, had emerged in the mid-1990s as a driver of HIV disease progression but was also critically relevant to transmission. Shaffer's study in the *Journal of Infectious Diseases*, described in Chapter 19, clearly demonstrated viral load as the most important determinant of transmission from mothers to their infants.[45]

Also actively involved in this area of work was RJ Simonds,[46] who joined Oxtoby's group in the AIDS division as an EIS officer in 1990. When looking at EIS positions, Simonds told Curran that he knew nothing about AIDS. (Shaffer had similarly told his malaria supervisors he knew nothing about malaria when they took him on.) As described by Simonds, Curran's reply was indicative of the CDC belief that any EIS officer could rapidly learn what needed to be done. "Oh, RJ, don't worry about that," Simonds quoted Curran as saying. "A few years ago, nobody knew anything (about AIDS). You'll catch on."[46] Simonds's initial career closely tracked Shaffer's pathway, and later interviews with both showed they brought strong characteristics of curiosity and commitment to social justice with them when they came to CDC.

The placebo-controlled trial of short-course zidovudine in Bangkok showed that the active intervention halved transmission, to just under 10 percent,[42] with reduction of maternal viral load the predominant mechanism of action.[42,47] This successful trial was unquestionably one of the collaboration's most important achievements, but what was particularly impressive was how Thailand health officials rapidly took the research to nationwide program scale-up. Both Shaffer and Simonds continued with important global health work, especially relating to the prevention of mother-to-child transmission. Along with Mastro, they expressed pride that Thailand became the first country in Asia to reduce vertical transmission to less than 2 percent, arbitrarily defined as elimination of transmission in nonbreastfeeding HIV-infected women.

Despite the success of the short-course zidovudine trial, the same controversy around the use of placebos that engulfed the African studies played out in reference to the Thai work.[48,49,50,51,52] The debates continued over years, yet this work led directly to endorsement of the short-course regimen by WHO, to early and wide-scale program implementation in Thailand, and the saving of countless children's lives.

Preventing HIV in Injecting Drug Users

In the move from descriptive studies to more complex analytic work, Mastro prioritized prospective cohort studies—the long-term follow-up of individuals from specific groups for documentation of their HIV exposures and associated risk factors and for determining incidence of HIV infection. Subsequent work would allow rigorous evaluation of preventive interventions, including vaccines. While northern Thailand was most suited for cohort studies of female sex workers, exemplified by the Chiang Rai Health Club, Bangkok offered ample opportunity for addressing HIV in IDUs through the Bangkok Metropolitan Administration, which was responsible for provision of drug treatment services through its large network of clinics.

Mastro and his modeling colleagues extended their work estimating the efficiency of HIV transmission to the IDU population.[53,54] The models took account of each person's reported frequency of needle sharing and number of injections. The investigators estimated a risk of HIV infection of 8 per 1,000 episodes of needle sharing with an infected person, almost three times the estimated risk of infection in US healthcare workers from needlestick exposure to blood of infected individuals.[53,54]

These cohort studies were important to increase understanding of the basic epidemiology and social context of HIV, determining the rate of infection, the circumstances in which people acquired HIV, and the social, economic, and cultural characteristics of the people at risk. Cohort studies were also necessary to demonstrate that it was possible to follow the same individuals over time so that interventions to reduce new HIV infections could be evaluated.[55,56] In that regard, no intervention was considered more important than an HIV vaccine, an aspiration that began when HIV was discovered as the cause of AIDS.

The first vaccine to go into human efficacy trials (so-called "Phase III trials," implemented after the earlier two phases have established safety and basic immunogenicity) was a product called AIDSVAX.[57] This vaccine was produced by the company VaxGen, a spinoff from Genentech in California. One of the VaxGen founders was Don Francis, who had retired from CDC in 1993. The vaccine was based on the envelope gp120 glycoprotein of HIV and eventually was formulated with both the B and E subtype antigens for Thailand (AIDSVAX B/E) and with two B antigens for the United States (AIDSVAX B/B). Phase III trials were conducted in IDUs in Thailand and gay men in the United States and a few other sites.

Whether or not to proceed with these trials pitted theoretical and empirical views against each other.[58] The theoretically minded camp argued that a vaccine required better understanding of the essentials of immunity against HIV and measurable correlates of protection. The empiricists argued that this was all theoretical and that few vaccines had met these requirements before introduction into public health use.

At CDC, the AIDS division began to look at diverse biomedical approaches to prevention. Bill Heyward, after returning from Projet SIDA's untimely demise in Kinshasa, spent some years in Geneva working with WHO on HIV vaccine issues. Alan Greenberg, returned from Projet RETRO-CI in Abidjan to become the division's Epidemiology Branch Chief, and invested in HIV vaccine preparedness, and later, pre-exposure prophylaxis (PrEP) with anti-retroviral drugs (Chapter 19).

The Bangkok vaccine trial, involving 2,546 IDUs and thirty-six months of follow-up, began in early 1999, finished enrollment in mid-2000, and was completed in 2003.[59] CDC was a partial funder and its staff participated in running the study. It was an operational success but a scientific disappointment. HIV incidence was similar in the group that had received the vaccine as in the control group receiving a placebo.[60] Comparable results of lack of efficacy were obtained in the North American trial in MSM.[61] Many commentaries described these studies as failures, which, though understandable, was incorrect; the vaccine was a failure, the trials were a success because they answered the question of whether AIDSVAX was protective or not. It was unfortunately not the answer wanted.

The AIDSVAX and VaxGen stories did not end there. A later trial, RV144, also in Thailand, involved a "prime boost" approach, one product given first and followed later by boosting with another agent.[62] The AIDSVAX B/E product was the boost part of the regimen, with the initial injections involving a canarypox virus encompassing several HIV genes. Initial efficacy (the reduction in HIV incidence in persons receiving the active vaccine compared to placebo recipients) was estimated at 31 percent. These results were considered interesting and encouraging, but also controversial[63] and insufficient to take the product forward for public health implementation. The search for an HIV vaccine is covered more fully in Chapter 19.

Tuberculosis and Opportunistic Infections

The prevention-oriented cohort studies inevitably yielded participants whose HIV infections evolved to disease. An OI in Thailand that had been known to cause diagnostic consternation elsewhere was disseminated penicilliosis, an infection with the fungus now called *Talaromyces marneffei*).[64,65] However, as elsewhere, no opportunistic disease was more important than TB,[66,67,68] and because HIV prevalence was highest in northern Thailand the Chiang Rai site was especially affected.

At CDC, Curran along with Ken Castro (Chapters 3 and 6), who would later become head of CDC's Division of Tuberculosis Elimination, used to say that TB and HIV hang out together in populations and are a bad influence on each other. HIV-associated immune deficiency increases the risk of latent TB infection progressing to active disease. It also renders people more susceptible to TB infection. Congregate settings such as hospitals and prisons can suffer outbreaks of TB among HIV-infected persons, including with drug-resistant organisms.

Programmatically, tension existed between TB and HIV professionals, just as it had in sub-Saharan Africa and, indeed, in the world's leading public health agencies. The TB establishment had fixed, structured ways of addressing the disease through a strategy called DOTS (directly observed therapy, short course) that treated every patient the same, a different approach from the individualism emphasized by the HIV community. The HIV and TB camps were equally suspicious of each other. However, HIV disrupted the established rules because DOTS simply did not control TB in HIV-infected populations.[69]

CDC staff and colleagues analyzed provincial and hospital records in Chiang Rai and demonstrated TB trends similar to those reported from African sites.[66] After years of decline, TB incidence began steadily increasing after about 1991. The proportion of TB patients who were HIV-infected increased to almost half over a five-year period. Patients with HIV-associated TB were younger than HIV-negative TB patients, had an increased frequency of extrapulmonary or disseminated disease, and were more likely to die: after one year, two thirds of the HIV-positive TB patients had died, compared with 10 percent of seronegative patients. These data were a warning to other countries in the region of inevitable trends if HIV was not contained.

TB has long been recognized to have an increased incidence among IDUs. Nonadherence to treatment, the greatest risk factor for drug resistance in patients with TB, is common among drug users. Injection drug use, HIV, and poor TB treatment adherence were a potent combination for driving resistance to TB medicines. Especially dangerous is multidrug resistant tuberculosis (MDR-TB), which indicates resistance to at least two critical TB medicines, rifampin and isoniazid.

The Thailand researchers found that MDR-TB was indeed more prevalent in HIV-infected patients in Bangkok (5.4% versus 0.4% in HIV-negative patients).[67] A persistent problem worldwide wherever TB is prevalent is the risk of infection in healthcare workers exposed to patients. Although Thailand recognized this problem[68] and implemented interventions that reduced TB incidence in health staff, it remains a widespread challenge deserving more attention.

2000 and Beyond

Mastro returned to the United States in 2000 after a highly productive seven-year tenure as the collaboration's director (Figure 16.4). Unlike CDC sites in Kinshasa and Abidjan, the Thailand collaboration has not been overtaken by political and social strife and celebrated its fortieth anniversary in July 2020. Although AIDS was not the primary focus in the FETP's first decade, the subsequent AIDS investment made by the collaboration has had long-lasting impact.

Nonetheless, the new millennium has brought profound change. From early focus on field epidemiology and then HIV research, the collaboration has expanded to encompass diverse research priorities and program implementation, including in the realm of health security, emerging infectious diseases, and influenza. The HIV focus has shifted—partly because the Thai epidemic has lessened and is no longer the overriding health priority that it was but also because of the increased complexity and expense of the world of HIV research.

For CDC, it became apparent that clinical trials in HIV/AIDS were becoming ever more demanding, requiring high-level funding and large study populations. Descriptive and analytic epidemiologic studies had answered most of the questions concerning risk factors and transmission,

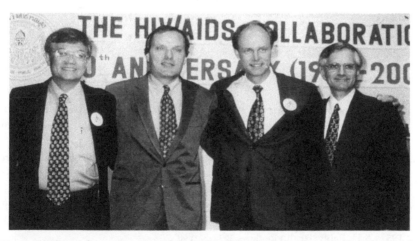

Figure 16.4. 10th anniversary of the HIV/AIDS Collaboration, 2000. Pictured (l–r): Khanchit Limpakarnjanarat, Tim Mastro, Jordan Tappero, Bruce Weniger. (Kevin De Cock, personal collection)

and the new priorities concerned program implementation following the advent of PEPFAR and The Global Fund to Fight AIDS, Tuberculosis and Malaria ("The Global Fund," Chapter 22). CDC later supported trials of PrEP in IDUs in Thailand[70] and heterosexual persons in Botswana,[71] as well as a trial of combination ART to prevent mother-to-child transmission in breastfeeding women in Kenya (Chapter 22).[72] Increasingly, however, the pressing questions could only be answered through multisite studies. The intervention research portfolio was largely taken over by major global research funders, especially NIH and European entities, and implemented through academia in multiple countries. The Bangkok collaboration supported by CDC remains part of the NIH-supported networks for HIV research.

Weniger worked in the vaccine area at CDC after returning from Thailand. He retired in 2010 and has remained in academia. Mastro, who had been overseeing HIV vaccine research in Greenberg's HIV Epidemiology Branch after his return to the United States in 2000, moved to leadership positions in global HIV work and retired from CDC in 2008. Like the sites in Kinshasa and Abidjan, the Thailand project had contributed substantially to understanding and combating HIV's global impact. Mastro, Weniger, and many of their colleagues remained involved in AIDS research and public health activities domestically and globally in their subsequent careers. The Thailand HIV/AIDS collaboration has been an eminently successful venture in which the host country has taken leadership, strengthened other national institutions, and enhanced its capacity to address other infectious health threats.

Notes

1. Thacker SB, Stroup DF, Sencer DJ. Epidemic assistance by the Centers for Disease Control and Prevention: role of the Epidemic Intelligence Service, 1946–2005. Am J Epidemiol 2011;174(Suppl):S4–S15.
2. Langmuir DA. The Epidemic Intelligence Service of the Center for Disease Control. Public Health Rep 1980;95:470–477. https://www.ncbi.nlm.nih.gov/pmc/articles/PMC1422746/pdf/pubhealthrep00127-0062.pdf
3. Schneider D, Evering-Watley M, Walke H, Bloland PB. Training the global public health workforce through applied epidemiology training programs: CDC's experience, 1951–2011. Public Health Reviews 2011;33:190–203.
4. Frieden TR, De Cock KM. The CDC's Center for Global Health. Lancet 2012;379:986–988.

5. "WENIGER, BRUCE," *The Global Health Chronicles*, accessed January 2, 2023, https://www.globalhealthchronicles.org/items/show/7735.
6. Weniger BG, Limpakarnjanarat K, Ungchusak K, et al. The epidemiology of HIV infection and AIDS in Thailand. AIDS 1991;5(Suppl 2):S71–S85.
7. Weniger BG. History of the early HIV/AIDS epidemic in Thailand and highlights of the country's key contributions to global prevention. Siam Society, May 2, 2019. https://www.youtube.com/watch?v=H4QCczw-tvc
8. "GAYLE, HELENE," *The Global Health Chronicles*, accessed December 12, 2022. https://globalhealthchronicles.org/items/show/7957
9. Piot P, Plummer FA, Mhalu FS, Lamboray J-L, Chin J, Mann JM. AIDS: an international perspective. Science 1988;239:573–579.
10. Ou CY, Takebe Y, Luo CC, et al. Wide distribution of two subtypes of HIV-1 in Thailand. AIDS Res Hum Retroviruses 1992;8:1471–1472.
11. Kalish ML, Baldwin A, Raktham S, et al. The evolving molecular epidemiology of HIV-1 envelope subtypes in injecting drug users in Bangkok, Thailand: implications for HIV vaccine trials. AIDS 1995;9:851–857.
12. Limpakarnjanarat K, Ungchusak K, Mastro TD, et al. The epidemiologic evolution of HIV 1 subtypes B and E among heterosexuals and injecting drug users in Thailand, 1992–1997. AIDS 1998;12:1108–1109.
13. Mastro TD, Kunanusont C, Dondero TJ, Wasi C. Why do HIV-1 subtypes segregate among persons with different risk behaviors in South Africa and Thailand? AIDS 1997;11:113–116.
14. Kitayaporn D, Vanichseni S, Mastro TD, et al. Infection with HIV 1 subtypes B and E in injecting drug users screened for enrollment into a prospective cohort in Bangkok, Thailand. J Acquir Immune Defic Syndr Hum Retrovirol 1998;19:289–295. doi: 10.1097/00042560-199811010-00012.
15. Choopanya K, Des Jarlais DC, Vanichseni S, et al. Incarceration and risk for HIV infection among injection drug users in Bangkok. J Acquir Immune Defic Syndr 2002;29:86–94.
16. Choopanya K, Des Jarlais DC, Vanichseni S, et al. HIV risk reduction in a cohort of injecting drug users in Bangkok, Thailand. J Acquir Immune Defic Syndr 2003;33:88–95.
17. Mastro TD, Kitayaporn D, Weniger BG, et al. Estimating the number of HIV-infected injection drug users in Bangkok: a capture-recapture method. Am J Public Health 1994;84:1094–1099.
18. Weniger BG, Brown T. The march of AIDS through Asia. N Engl J Med 1996;335:343–345.
19. Nopkesorn T, Mastro TD, Sangkharomya S, et al. HIV-1 infection in young men in northern Thailand. AIDS 1993;7:1233–1239.
20. Nelson KE, Celentano DD, Eiumtrakol S, et al. Changes in sexual behavior and a decline in HIV infection among young men in Thailand. N Engl J Med 1996;335:297–303.
21. "OU, CHIN-YIH," *The Global Health Chronicles*, accessed January 29, 2023. https://globalhealthchronicles.org/items/show/7956.

22. "SCHOCHETMAN, GERALD," *The Global Health Chronicles*, accessed January 3, 2023, https://globalhealthchronicles.org/items/show/6486.

23. Ou C-Y, Kwok S, Mitchell SW, et al. DNA amplification for direct detection of HIV-1 in DNA of peripheral blood mononuclear cells. Science 1988;239:295–297.

24. Schochetman G, Ou C-Y, Jones WK. Polymerase chain reaction. J Infect Dis 1988;158:1154–1157.

25. Ou C-Y, Ciesielski CA, Myers G, et al. Molecular epidemiology of HIV transmission in a dental practice. Science 1992;256:1165–1171.

26. Rogers MF, Ou C-Y, Rayfield M, et al. Use of the polymerase chain reaction for early detection of the proviral sequences of human immunodeficiency virus in infants born to seropositive mothers. N Engl J Med 1989;320:1649–1654.

27. Hu DJ, Vanichseni S, Mastro TD, Raktham S, et al. Viral load differences in early infection with two HIV-1 subtypes. AIDS 2001;15:683–691.

28. Amornkul PN, Thansuphasawadikul S, Limpakarnjanarat K, et al. Clinical disease associated with HIV-1 subtype B' and E infection among 2104 patients in Thailand. AIDS 1999;13:1963–1969. doi: 10.1097/00002030-199910010-00020.

29. Mastro TD, Satten GA, Nopkesorn T, Sangkharomya S, Longini IM Jr. Probability of female-to-male transmission of HIV-1 in Thailand. Lancet 1994;343:204–207.

30. Satten GA, Mastro TD, Longini IM Jr. Modelling the female-to-male per-act HIV transmission probability in an emerging epidemic in Asia. Stat Med 1994;13:2097–2106. doi: 10.1002/sim.4780131918.

31. Bunnell RE, Yanpaisarn S, Kilmarx PH, et al. HIV-1 seroprevalence among childbearing women in northern Thailand: a rapidly evolving epidemic. AIDS 1999;13:509–515.

32. Siriwasin W, Shaffer N, Roongpisuthipong A, et al. HIV prevalence, risk factors and partner serodiscordance among pregnant women, Bangkok, Thailand. JAMA 1998;280:49–54.

33. Bennetts A, Shaffer N, Phophong P, et al. Differences in sexual behaviors between HIV-infected pregnant women and their husbands, Bangkok, Thailand. AIDS Care 1999;11:649–661.

34. Kilmarx PH, Limpakarnjanarat K, Mastro TD, et al. HIV-1 seroconversion in a prospective study of female sex workers in northern Thailand: continued high incidence among brothel-based women. AIDS 1998;12:1889–1898.

35. Kilmarx PH, Supawitkul S, Wankrairoj M, et al. Explosive spread and effective control of human immunodeficiency virus in northernmost Thailand: the epidemic in Chiang Rai province, 1988–99. AIDS 2000;14:2731–2740.

36. Kilmarx PH, Palanuvej T, Limpakarnjanarat K, et al. Seroprevalence of HIV among female sex workers in Bangkok: evidence of ongoing infection risk after the "100% condom program" was implemented. J Acquir Immune Defic Syndr 1999;21:313–316.

37. Kilmarx PH. Text message from the Congo. https://www.astmh.org/ASTMH/media/Documents/Text-message-from-the-Congo.pdf.

38. Kilmarx PH, van de Wijgert JH, Chaikummao S, et al. Safety and acceptability of the candidate microbicide Carraguard in Thai Women: findings from a Phase II Clinical Trial. J Acquir Immune Defic Syndr 2006;43:327–334. doi: 10.1097/01.qai.0000243056.59860.c1.

39. van Griensven F, Kilmarx PH, Jeeyapant S, et al. The prevalence of homosexual and bisexual orientation and related health risks among adolescents in northern Thailand. Arch Sex Behav 2004:33:137–147.

40. Connor EM, Sperling RS, Gelber R, et al. Reduction of maternal-infant transmission of human immunodeficiency virus type 1 with zidovudine treatment. N Engl J Med 1994;331:1173–1180.

41. Adjorlolo-Johnson G, De Cock KM, Ekpini E, et al. Prospective comparison of mother-to-child transmission of HIV-1 and HIV-2 in Abidjan, Ivory Coast. JAMA 1994;272:462–466. Erratum in JAMA 1994;272:1482.

42. Shaffer N, Chuachoowong R, Mock P, et al. Short course zidovudine for perinatal HIV-1 transmission in Bangkok, Thailand: a randomized controlled trial. Lancet 1999;353:773–780.

43. Wiktor SZ, Ekpini E, Karon JM, et al. Short-course oral zidovudine for prevention of mother-to-child transmission of HIV-1 in Abidjan, Côte d'Ivoire: a randomised trial. Lancet 1999;353:781–785.

44. "SHAFFER, NATHAN," The Global Health Chronicles, accessed January 29, 2023, https://www.globalhealthchronicles.org/items/show/8131.

45. Shaffer N, Roongpisuthipong A, Siriwasin W, et al. Maternal viral load and perinatal HIV-1 subtype E transmission, Thailand. Bangkok Collaborative Perinatal HIV Transmission Study Group. J Infect Dis 1999;179:590–599. doi: 10.1086/314641

46. "SIMONDS, RJ," The Global Health Chronicles, accessed January 29, 2023, https://www.globalhealthchronicles.org/items/show/8139.

47. Chuachoowong R, Shaffer N, Siriwasin W, et al. Short-course antenatal zidovudine reduces both cervicovaginal human immunodeficiency virus type 1 RNA levels and risk of perinatal transmission. J Infect Dis 2000;181:99–106.

48. Lurie P, Wolfe SM. Unethical trials of interventions to reduce perinatal transmission of the human immunodeficiency virus in developing countries. N Engl J Med 1997;337:853–856.

49. Angell M. The ethics of clinical research in the Third World. N Engl J Med 1997;337:847–849.

50. De Cock KM. Publicity, politics, and public health: the case of placebo-controlled trials for the prevention of mother-to-child transmission of HIV in resource-poor countries. International AIDS Society Newsletter 1997;8:9–10.

51. Varmus H, Satcher D. Ethical complexities of conducting research in developing countries. N Engl J Med 1997;337:1003–1005.

52. The conduct of clinical trials of maternal–infant transmission of HIV supported by the United States Department of Health and Human Services in developing countries. Washington, DC: Department of Health and Human Services, July 1997. http://www.columbia.edu/cu/musher/AIDS_case/nimh_cdc_review.htm.

53. Hudgens MG, Longini IM, Halloran ME, et al. Estimating the transmission probability of human immunodeficiency virus in injecting drug users in Thailand. Appl Statist 2001;50:1–14.

54. Hudgens MG, Longini IM, Vanichseni S, et al. HIV-1 subtype-specific transmission probabilities among injecting drug users in Bangkok, Thailand. Am J Epidemiol 2002;155:159–168.

55. MacQueen KM, Vanichseni S, Kitayaporn D, et al. Willingness of injection drug users to participate in an HIV vaccine efficacy trial in Bangkok, Thailand. J Acquir Immune Defic Syndr 1999;21:243–251.

56. Vanichseni S, Kitayaporn D, Mastro TD, et al. Continued high HIV-1 incidence in a vaccine trial preparatory cohort of injection drug users in Bangkok, Thailand. AIDS 2001;15:397–405.

57. Esparza J. A brief history of the global effort to develop a preventive HIV vaccine. Vaccine 2013;31:3502–3518.

58. Cohen J. Shots in the dark: the wayward search for an AIDS vaccine. New York: WW Norton and Co; 2001.

59. Vanichseni S, Tappero JW, Pitisuttithum P, et al. Recruitment, screening and characteristics of injecting drug users participating in the AIDSVAX B/E HIV vaccine trial, Bangkok, Thailand. AIDS 2004;18:311–316.

60. Pitisuttithum P, Gilbert P, Gurwith M, et al. Randomized, double-blind, placebo-controlled efficacy trial of a bivalent recombinant glycoprotein 120 HIV-1 vaccine among injection drug users in Bangkok, Thailand. J Infect Dis 2006;194:1661–1671.

61. Flynn NM, Forthal DN, Harro CD, et al. Placebo-controlled phase 3 trial of a recombinant glycoprotein 120 vaccine to prevent HIV-1 infection. J Infect Dis 2005;191:654–665.

62. Rerks-Ngarm S, Pitisuttithum P, Nitayaphan S, et al. Vaccination with ALVAC and AIDSVAX to prevent HIV-1 infection in Thailand. N Engl J Med 2009;361:2209–2220.

63. Desrosiers RC. Protection against HIV acquisition in the RV144 trial. J Virol 2017;91:e00905–e009017.

64. Kaufman L, Standard PG, Jalbert M, Kantipong P, Limpakarnjanarat K, Mastro TD. Diagnostic antigenemia tests for penicilliosis marneffei. J Clin Microbiol 1996;34:2503–2505.

65. Imwidthaya P, Sekhon AS, Mastro TD, Garg AK, Ambrosie E. Usefulness of a microimmunodiffusion test for the detection of *Penicillium marneffei* antigenemia, antibodies, and exoantigens. Mycopathologia 1997;138:51–55.

66. Yanai H, Uthaivoravit W, Panich V, et al. Rapid increase in HIV-related tuberculosis, Chiang Rai, Thailand, 1990–1994. AIDS 1996;10:527–531.

67. Punnotok J, Shaffer N, Naiwatanakul T, et al. Human immunodeficiency virus-related tuberculosis and primary drug resistance in Bangkok, Thailand. Int J Tuberc Lung Dis 2000;4:537–543.

68. Do AN, Limpakarnjanarat K, Uthaivoravit W, et al. Increased risk of *Mycobacterium tuberculosis* infection related to the occupational exposures of health care workers in Chiang Rai, Thailand. Int J Tuberc Lung Dis 1999;3:377–381.

69. De Cock KM, Chaisson RE. Will DOTS do it? A reappraisal of tuberculosis control in countries with high rates of HIV infection. Int J Tuberc Lung Dis 1999;3:457–465.

70. Choopanya K, Martin M, Suntharasamai P, et al. Antiretroviral prophylaxis for HIV infection in injecting drug users in Bangkok, Thailand (the Bangkok Tenofovir Study): a randomised, double-blind, placebo-controlled phase 3 trial. Lancet 2013;381:2083–2090. doi:10.1016/S0140-6736(13)61127-7.

71. Thigpen MC, Kebaabetswe PM, Paxton LA, et al. Antiretroviral preexposure prophy-laxis for heterosexual HIV transmission in Botswana. N Engl J Med. 2012;367:423–434. doi:10.1056/NEJMoa1110711.
72. Thomas TK, Masaba R, Borkowf CB, et al. Triple-antiretroviral prophylaxis to pre-vent mother-to-child HIV transmission through breastfeeding—the Kisumu Breastfeeding Study, Kenya: a clinical trial. PLoS Med 2011;8:e1001015. doi:10.1371/journal.pmed.1001015.

SECTION III
THE MODERN AIDS ERA

17

Advances in Science and Public Health

Kevin M. De Cock

The first two sections of this book describe the recognition of AIDS in the United States, CDC's investigations into the growing US epidemic, and the agency's early international activities on the global AIDS front, including its involvement with WHO. This final section updates the story in relation to the scientific advances on the virus and its disease course, CDC's domestic and international work on HIV/AIDS, and the global response to the pandemic, all from a vantage point more than forty years after the first case reports appeared in the *MMWR*.[1,2]

In the early 1980s, public health investigations focused on the nature, extent, and cause of this new syndrome. Painstaking science bridging diverse disciplines subsequently uncovered HIV's now widely accepted nonhuman primate origin. This work highlighted the importance of molecular epidemiology and phylogenetics in understanding the origins and spread of infectious pathogens and drew attention to the reality that the majority of emerging infections have a zoonotic (animal) origin.[3]

The elucidation of AIDS epidemiology, the discovery of the causative virus, and the introduction of HIV diagnostics formed the foundation for subsequent understanding of HIV pathogenesis and natural history along with the development of major biomedical interventions. Recognition of the benefits of ART in 1996 transformed AIDS from an inevitably fatal disease to a medically manageable condition. Research subsequently clarified the role of ART in HIV prevention: suppressing viral load in persons with HIV and thus limiting transmission, as well as acting as PrEP in HIV-negative persons. Another important research advance, after years of debate, was demonstration of the protective efficacy of male circumcision against heterosexual acquisition of HIV in men.

Science does not progress in linear fashion, and HIV research and program implementation have also suffered setbacks and frustration. The promise that control of STIs might contain population-level HIV transmission was

Kevin M. De Cock, *Advances in Science and Public Health* In: *Dispatches from the AIDS Pandemic*. Kevin M. De Cock, Harold W. Jaffe, and James W. Curran and Edited by: Robin Moseley, Oxford University Press.
© Oxford University Press 2023. DOI: 10.1093/oso/9780197626528.003.0017

not fulfilled, and aspirations for a vaccine to prevent and treatment to cure HIV remain unrealized. With emphasis on biomedical interventions, the continued relevance of behavioral factors is too easily forgotten, including for promoting treatment adherence and preventing risk compensation, as evidenced by escalating rates of other STIs, especially among MSM.[4] HIV prevention among people who inject drugs remains challenged by incomplete promotion and uptake of harm reduction interventions.

In the history of AIDS, the advent of ART was a "before and after" moment. Domestically, CDC had to reprioritize its surveillance efforts from AIDS to HIV—the "front-end" of the epidemic. Internationally, the unequal access to ART emerged as a dominant theme soon after its clinical impact was demonstrated. This section also examines WHO's changing role in the epidemic: the instability of the organization's AIDS work over the 1990s; the establishment of a new entity, UNAIDS, to coordinate the world's AIDS response; and WHO's subsequent recommitment to the AIDS field. While CDC remained engaged with WHO and UNAIDS through provision of technical assistance and secondment of staff, the agency's global role increased exponentially with President George W. Bush's announcement of PEPFAR in 2003.

One of the enduring frustrations about AIDS is that we will not know how the story ends—AIDS will still be here when we are not. Nonetheless, the remarkable scientific and programmatic advances detailed in the final chapters of this book resulted in altered perceptions and attitudes. Henceforth, there was hope as well as determination that the future would be different.

Notes

1. CDC. *Pneumocystis* pneumonia—Los Angeles. MMWR Morb Mortal Wkly Rep 1981;30:250–252.
2. De Cock KM, Jaffe HW, Curran JW. Reflections on 40 Years of AIDS. Emerg Infect Dis 2021;27:1553–1560. doi: 10.3201/eid2706.210284.
3. Jones KE, Patel NG, Levy MA, Storeygard A, Balk D, Gittleman JL, Daszak P. Global trends in emerging infectious diseases. Nature 2008;451:990–993. doi: 10.1038/nature06536.
4. CDC. Sexually Transmitted Disease Surveillance 2019. https://www.cdc.gov/std/statistics/2019/default.htm

18

Origins

Kevin M. De Cock

As discussed in Chapter 9, LAV, the novel retrovirus isolated by Françoise Barré-Sinoussi and colleagues at the Institut Pasteur in 1983, became accepted as the definitive cause of AIDS ([1,2,3,4]) and was later renamed as HIV. Once the viral etiology of AIDS was clear, obvious questions arose: Where did the virus come from, and how did it cause a pandemic?

Africa

I first heard suggestion of an African origin for the AIDS agent in the fall of 1983, after the publication on LAV[1] but before it was universally recognized as the cause of AIDS. James (Jim) Maynard, head of the viral hepatitis group at CDC, was visiting my boss, Alan Redeker, on the liver unit at Los Angeles County–University of Southern California (LAC-USC) Medical Center where I was a fellow. The unit had extensive experience with all forms of viral hepatitis, including hepatitis B and D, which were frequent in gay men in Los Angeles.[5] I asked Maynard what the thinking was at CDC about the cause of AIDS. He replied that he thought it likely that AIDS was due to a virus from Africa with similar epidemiology to that of hepatitis B.

The large hepatitis patient population at LAC-USC Medical Center shared many features with persons at risk for AIDS.[5] Having recently spent three years teaching internal medicine at the University of Nairobi in Kenya, I was intrigued by Maynard's suggestion. Several different viral infections, such as Lassa fever and Ebola, had been newly described in Africa, showing that infectious agents could exist undetected until unusual circumstances brought them to attention. Often this meant infection in an expatriate or missionary who could access sophisticated diagnosis and care unavailable to the local population. As described earlier (Chapters 5 and 13), by 1983 case reports of Africans with AIDS-like illness seeking care in Europe were

Kevin M. De Cock, *Origins* In: *Dispatches from the AIDS Pandemic*. Kevin M. De Cock, Harold W. Jaffe, and James W. Curran and Edited by: Robin Moseley, Oxford University Press. © Oxford University Press 2023.
DOI: 10.1093/oso/9780197626528.003.0018

frequent. A hypothetical African origin might also explain AIDS in Haiti; after Congolese independence in 1960, numerous francophone Haitians went to work in the former Belgian Congo (Zaire/Democratic Republic of Congo [DRC]) to replace Belgian administrators.

I wrote a paper titled "AIDS: an old disease from Africa?" that was published in the *British Medical Journal* in 1984.[6] The response to the paper surprised me for two reasons: first, because of the interest aroused and, second, for the controversy generated. It was my first exposure to the sensitivity around the topic of AIDS origins. African sentiment toward AIDS was one of disdain because of the ingrained association between the disease and homosexuality, a widespread taboo on the African continent. At the "International Symposium on African Aids" (sic) in late 1985, held, ironically, in Brussels, a group of African scientists coordinated by the Ugandan microbiologist Herbert Nzanze (whom I had known in Nairobi) issued a strong statement rejecting the concept of an African origin. Later, the book *AIDS, Africa and Racism* by Richard and Rosalind Chirimuuta[7] argued that proposing an African origin was based on racism. From its earliest days, AIDS was seen not as a disease but as a disgrace.

In addition to the stigma attached to the disease, African countries were afraid that admitting to even having AIDS cases would negatively affect tourism and exports. Some countries suppressed information and failed to report cases to WHO. The topic of AIDS in Haitians (Chapter 6) had provoked similarly angry discussions as to whether HIV had been introduced to Haiti by American tourists or whether the virus had jumped to mainland America from the island of Hispaniola. In his book *AIDS and Accusation: Haiti and the Geography of Blame*,[8] Paul Farmer, the late anthropologist, physician, and founder of the organization Partners in Health, refuted the putative Haitian source for HIV in the United States, attributing such a view to racial and ethnic prejudice. Bill Pape (Chapter 6), one of Haiti's most respected physicians and medical researchers, emphasized the negative impact that discussions of HIV's origin had had on his country.

The question of HIV's origin caused so much controversy that many suggested it be ignored. The political position of WHO and others was that HIV's origin was of no importance, that what mattered was not where the virus came from but where it was going. These attitudes were expedient but unsustainable. First, science would do what science does, inevitably pursuing research questions as intriguing as where HIV came from. Second, AIDS posed the greatest infectious disease challenge of the late twentieth century.

It was imperative to understand how this pandemic had come about if we were to address similar events in the future.

Early and Alternative Hypotheses: HIV and Polio Vaccines

Suggestions appeared early on that HIV was a human creation. The British venereologist John Seale was prolific in claiming that HIV had been genetically engineered in a biological warfare laboratory. Similar views were echoed by eastern European communist propaganda that blamed the US government. Rumors circulated that HIV was artificially created to decimate homosexuals and people of color. Other speculations were that AIDS emerged following the smallpox eradication campaign's use of injection needles. However, the hypothesis of a man-made pandemic that attracted the most attention concerned oral polio vaccination.

Tom Curtis, reporting for *Rolling Stone*, was the first to suggest that AIDS might have arisen from human exposure in Central Africa to oral polio virus vaccine contaminated with a simian retrovirus.[9] Curtis wrote that under the direction of Hilary Koprowski, then a virologist with the Wistar Institute in Philadelphia, oral polio virus vaccine was given to close to half a million people in parts of Zaire (DRC), Rwanda, and Burundi in 1957–1960 over the course of polio vaccination trials. The vaccine had been grown in monkey kidney cells and tested in chimpanzees in a laboratory facility near Stanleyville (today called Kisangani) near the end of the River Congo. Early AIDS cases were described in approximately the same geographic areas as those where the polio vaccine studies were conducted. Koprowski bitterly contested the suggestions made by Curtis, rejecting the possibility of simian immunodeficiency virus (SIV) contamination, and disagreeing about the geographic overlap.

The hypothesis was subsequently taken up with vigor by the English journalist Edward Hooper in *The River*, a 1,000-page book published in 1999.[10] This was Hooper's second AIDS book; the first, *Slim*, gave an account of his personal relationships and investigations surrounding AIDS in East Africa a decade earlier.[11] Hooper maintained that the oral polio vaccine was grown in chimpanzee tissues, which provided the route for retroviral entry into humans. His prestige and that of the hypothesis was enhanced by the interest expressed by William Hamilton, a renowned evolutionary biologist and fellow of the United Kingdom's Royal Society. Hamilton died in early 2000 from complications of gastrointestinal bleeding following a field expedition to DRC to pursue the issue of SIV in chimpanzees. A meeting on the origins of AIDS that Hamilton had lobbied for was held at the Royal Society later in 2000. Various presentations at the meeting saw support for the oral polio virus vaccine hypothesis erode, although Hooper has continued defending it zealously up to the present day. I was one of the presenters at the Royal Society's meeting and described the epidemiologic principles underpinning proof of causation, requirements that the oral polio vaccine hypothesis did not meet.[12]

The hypothesis is based on a weak ecologic association between the areas where some early AIDS cases were seen[13] and where oral polio vaccine was administered, taking no account of bias or incompleteness in the reporting of a small number of possible AIDS cases in a country as large as DRC. Because transport and communications routes there were limited and often centered around the River Congo, many unrelated but reported events will inevitably appear geographically associated. By contrast, all manner of occurrences in the country's vast interior could have easily gone unrecognized, including potential AIDS cases. These factors alone make the strength of the putative ecologic association uncertain.

Later, testing of remnant materials from the Wistar Institute used in oral poliovirus vaccine preparation showed no evidence of SIV, HIV, or chimpanzee cells[14,15]—refuting, inter alia, Hooper's contention that the polio vaccine had been grown in chimpanzee material. Subsequent field work near Kisangani yielded an SIV isolate from fecal specimens taken from wild-living chimpanzees; this virus was distinct from the HIV-1 lineage clustering with viruses from central African chimpanzees, now considered the origin of the HIV-1 pandemic, and instead clustered with distinct viruses from the eastern chimpanzee subspecies in Tanzania.[16] In other words, the virus of chimpanzees from the area of DRC where the polio vaccine studies were done was not at all closely related to pandemic HIV—further evidence against the oral polio vaccine as a source.

The most important factor in epidemiologic discussions of causation, however, is the element of time: if causal, exposures must occur before outcomes. Meticulous work on viral phylogenetics and molecular clocks has convincingly shown that human AIDS viruses evolved from their simian ancestors before Koprowski's oral polio activities in Central Africa.[17,18,19] The diversity of HIV-1 subtypes present for many years in DRC is also inconsistent with a point-source epidemic that putatively would have started in the late 1950s, when the polio vaccine trials took place.

Simian Immunodeficiency Viruses and HIV

As AIDS cases increased in the United States in the early 1980s, workers at several American nonhuman primate colonies described an AIDS-like illness in Asian macaques from which a simian retrovirus, SIVmac, was later isolated[20,21] This macaque virus was genetically distant from HIV-1. Extensive research subsequently identified several dozen other genetically diverse simian retroviruses specific to different types of African primates in the wild. These viruses were occurring at widely varying prevalence and, importantly, appeared not associated with illness in their simian hosts.[22] Genetically, the simian viruses and human viruses clustered within one lineage (or sector) of the overall phylogenetic tree of lentiviruses, the genus of retroviruses that infects a wide variety of mammals and to which HIV belongs. Put simply, the human AIDS viruses were more closely related to the simian viruses than to other lentiviruses infecting horses, cattle, and cats, indicating that human and simian viruses had evolved over time from common ancestors.[23]

After the description in 1986 of the second human AIDS virus, HIV-2, in patients from West Africa (Chapter 15),[24] it was shown that HIV-2 and the viruses in captive macaques were closely related to a virus of sooty mangabeys, SIVsmm.[25] Asian primates in the wild did not harbor SIV so the primate lentiviruses must have developed after the evolutionary separation of African and Asian monkeys. The finding of SIVsmm in captive Asian macaques that had been imported over many years into the United States implied that they had been infected from African sooty mangabeys in captivity. The startling conclusion was that both SIVmac and HIV-2 were derived from the sooty mangabey virus SIVsmm, which had jumped species to establish these new infections.

Apes are humans' closest genetic and biological relatives. They include chimpanzees and gorillas and differ from monkeys in having greater intelligence, an appendix, and no tail. SIV infection in chimpanzees, therefore, would be relevant to studies of HIV in humans. Martine Peeters and her husband Eric Delaporte had worked at ITM in Antwerp with Peter Piot before commencing field work in Gabon in the 1980s. There, they began screening wild-caught chimpanzees, finding just two SIV-infected animals from fifty that were tested, and designating the viruses as SIVcpzGAB1 and SIVcpzGAB2.[26]

They also isolated another virus from a chimpanzee called Noah who was residing in the Antwerp zoo after having been illegally imported into Belgium from DRC.[27] Surprisingly, Noah's virus, SIVcpzANT, was about twice as divergent from HIV-1 and both SIVcpzGAB isolates as the human and Gabonese chimpanzee viruses were from each other. In other studies, Beatrice Hahn at the University of Alabama at Birmingham accessed material from a deceased US primate center chimpanzee (Marilyn) and found an SIVcpz infection that was close to the Gabonese chimpanzee viruses.[28] (Intriguingly, it was later shown that SIVcpz itself is a result of cross-species transmission and of recombination of simian viruses from red-capped mangabeys [SIVrcm]—a type of monkey hunted by chimpanzees—and SIVs of different *Cercopithecus* species.[23,29])

The apparent low prevalence of SIVcpz in chimpanzees and the genetic diversity of these isolates questioned their relevance to HIV-1. However, synergistic research across chimpanzee and human retroviral genetics, laboratory diagnostics, and animal ecology clarified the discrepancies.[23,28,30] Chimpanzees are divided into four subspecies (Figure 18.1) based on their mitochondrial DNA. For HIV, the two of relevance are the central and eastern chimpanzees, *Pan troglodytes troglodytes* (Ptt) and *Pan*

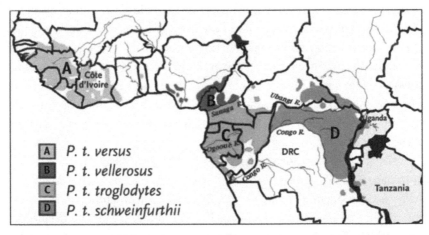

Figure 18.1. Geographic distribution of *Pan troglodytes* subspecies. (Adapted from Sharp PM, Shaw GM, Hahn BH. Simian immunodeficiency virus infection of chimpanzees. J Virol 2005;79(7):3891-3902).

troglodytes schweinfurthii (*Pts*), respectively. The ranges of these apes are nonoverlapping: chimpanzees of the *Ptt* subspecies are concentrated centrally in Cameroon, the Republic of Congo, and Gabon, and those of *Pts* are from locations in Central to East Africa. The infected animals from Gabon, as well as Marilyn in the United States, were of the subspecies *Ptt*, while Noah in Antwerp belonged to *Pts*. A conclusion was that the different SIVcpz agents had coevolved with their natural ape hosts. Furthermore, the absence of SIVcpz infection in the large number of chimpanzees tested in American primate colonies reflected that those animals were mostly of subspecies other than *Ptt* or *Pts*, and therefore were not naturally infected.

In 1999, I met Beatrice Hahn at the University of Alabama at Birmingham where she expressed interest in our Yambuku work showing HIV had been present in remote Zaire in 1976 (Chapter 13). She asked advice about epidemiologic principles concerning diagnostic test performance, and we discussed public health implications of cross-species transmission of different viruses. A paper, "AIDS as a zoonosis: scientific and public health implications," resulted and was published in 2000 in *Science*, summarizing the then-available knowledge.[31]

HIV-1 in humans is differentiated into various groups, M (the main pandemic form), N, O, and P. Infections with N are very rare, and with P, vanishingly so. Groups N and P infections have been restricted to persons in or from Cameroon, while group O infections, estimated to number about 100,000, have occurred all over west central Africa. Hahn and colleagues developed techniques for identifying SIV infections noninvasively by detecting SIV antibodies and viral nucleic acids directly in chimpanzee and gorilla fecal material collected in the forest.[32,33] Their studies have given unique insight, not only into further phylogenetic linkages between human and simian viruses, but also into the epidemiology of SIVcpz and the gorilla virus SIVgor in the wild.

In the phylogenetic tree (Figure 18.2), human viruses from the different groups (M, N, O and P) are interspersed between chimpanzee and gorilla viruses, indicating that the different HIV groups cannot have evolved from a common single ancestral human virus but instead resulted from four different, cross-species transmission events. By sequencing endemic SIVcpz strains in wild-living chimpanzee populations, it was possible to trace the origins of HIV-1 groups M and N to distinct, geographically isolated chimpanzee communities in Cameroon that harbor their closest viral relatives.

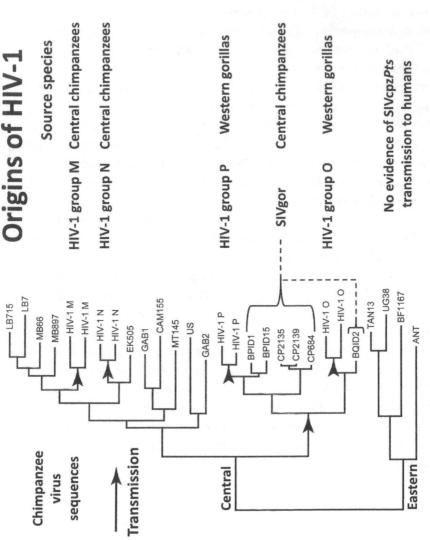

Figure 18.2. Phylogenetic tree of human and simian immunodeficiency viruses. Different groups of HIV-1 are closer to simian viral relatives than to each other, indicative of cross-species transmission. (Courtesy of Beatrice Hahn)

Viruses from the human groups O and P are closely related to SIV isolates from western gorillas in Cameroon. Molecular studies found that SIVgor clustered phylogenetically within strains of SIVcpz, indicating that western gorillas originally acquired their SIV through cross-species transmission from chimpanzees. SIVgor in western gorillas occurs at lower prevalence than SIVcpz in chimpanzees. Human group P viruses were traced to a localized area of western Cameroon, but group O viruses are not especially closely related to any one gorilla strain, and their specific geographic origin cannot be pinpointed. It is only in Cameroon, however, that gorillas have been shown to be infected with SIVgor and the conclusion is that all four human HIV-1 groups emerged in Cameroon (B. Hahn, personal communications).

From work in Gombe National Park (home to habituated *Pts*) in northwestern Tanzania in East Africa, as well as other observations, it has also been shown that SIVcpz is not a benign infection in its natural host.[34] Molecular epidemiological studies have shown that SIVcpz is transmitted sexually in chimpanzees, can be passed from mother to infant, causes immune deficiency with AIDS like illness, and can reduce chimpanzee population size.[35,36]

Early HIV and AIDS

When AIDS was first described in patients in Los Angeles in 1981, an immediate question was whether similar cases had been seen earlier. When a blood test for HIV became available in 1985, serum banks proved their utility by allowing retrospective testing, the equivalent of viral archeology. Fortuitously, collections of serum were available from New York City and San Francisco from studies on HBV and its vaccine in gay men and from the hepatitis clinic at LAC–USC Medical Center in Los Angeles. HIV was shown to have been present in gay men in both New York[37] and San Francisco[38] as early as 1978 and in gay men with hepatitis B in Los Angeles in 1979.[5]

A concerted effort was undertaken to trawl through medical records, publications, and other biologic repositories to look for other early examples of HIV infection. The overwhelming conclusions were that earlier cases of proven HIV or probable AIDS were in Africans or were associated with exposure in Africa. A paper by Belgian authors in the *Scandinavian Journal of Infectious Diseases* documented three cases of probable AIDS and four of proven HIV infection most likely acquired in Central Africa, all between the years 1962 and 1976.[13] Another study found that a Norwegian sailor and truck driver, his wife, and his daughter had died of AIDS in

1976—all infected with HIV-1 group O, presumably acquired initially by the male in Cameroon.[39] A Danish surgeon who had worked in Zaire died in 1977 and was retrospectively shown to have been infected with HIV.[40] In her book, *Virus Hunt*, investigating the origin of HIV, Dorothy Crawford, former Professor of Virology at the London School of Hygiene and Tropical Medicine, recalls talking to Bila Kapita (Chapter 13) in Kinshasa.[41] Kapita recounted to her that his first memory of what he would later recognize as an AIDS case was in a Haitian nurse in Kinshasa in 1978.

Retrospective testing of several biologic specimens from Kinshasa documented the presence of HIV-1 even earlier—in a serum specimen from 1959[42] and a lymph node biopsy in 1960.[19] As described in Chapter 13, CDC scientists found evidence of HIV infection in five serum samples that had been collected in northern Zaire during the 1976 Ebola outbreak[43] and a virus was isolated from one.[44]

Early cases of HIV-2 infection were also diagnosed retrospectively. A Portuguese man died with HIV-2 in London in 1978, likely infected in Guinea Bissau two decades earlier.[45] The age distribution of HIV-2 in Guinea Bissau showed higher prevalence in older people, unusual for an STI and probably indicating exposure long before.

HIV-1 group M, the pandemic form of the virus, has diversified over time and currently is known to exist in nine different subtypes (also referred to as clades, identified by a letter), with sub-subtypes and recombinants between them complicating matters further. HIV-1 has a high mutation rate, but as with other viruses, that rate is relatively constant. Comparing differences between sequences from the same gene from different isolates gives some indication of how long they have been diverging: the closer they are, the more recent their divergence. This simplistic explanation illustrates the concept of a "molecular clock" that allows timing of viral evolution.

Applying advanced computer analyses to data on viral sequences from around the world allowed Bette Korber and colleagues at the Los Alamos National Laboratory to propose a time for entry of HIV-1 into the human population of around 1931.[17] Working with the Congolese sequences from 1959 and 1960, Michael Worobey and colleagues proposed a somewhat earlier time range for the most recent common ancestor of the HIV-1 group M—between 1884 and 1924.[19] The Congolese specimens from 1959 and 1960 are most closely related, respectively, to subtypes D and A, indicating clade divergence was already established in Kinshasa at that time. Extensive subtyping work has shown Kinshasa and DRC to have the greatest degree of

HIV-1 clade diversity in the world. This suggests a local "starburst" of evolution from a common ancestor, while later dissemination of specific subtypes and then local founder effects resulted in distribution and establishment of individual subtypes across different parts of the globe.

Worobey and colleagues further looked at molecular evolution in the Americas.[46] With genetic material from eight retrospectively identified HIV-1-positive specimens collected in 1978–1979 in New York and San Francisco, they produced additional genetic trees incorporating North American and Caribbean viral sequences. By the time of specimen collection, considerable HIV-1 diversity was already apparent across the American sequences. Molecular clock analyses suggested a common subtype B viral ancestor in the Caribbean, presumably Haiti, in 1967, with entry into New York City, the origin of the subsequent American epidemic, around 1971 and spread to San Francisco around 1976.

Expansion of the Epidemic

Understanding viral origins is not the same as understanding why or when epidemic spread occurs. Mere origin in itself is insufficient to predict an epidemic. Today, Cameroon has a low-level epidemic and HIV prevalence in DRC has not increased substantially since the 1980s. By contrast, rapid spread of HIV in southern Africa from the 1990s onward led to population prevalence levels over 20 percent, the highest in the world, yet this region is distant from where HIV originated. Also, prevalence can change over time, and, to interpret trends, "peak prevalence," whenever it occurs, needs to be considered along with current prevalence.

Drawing conclusions about interacting factors causing pandemic spread or its timing is necessarily speculative. First the virus had to cross the species barrier, which presumably occurred in a remote location through human mucosal exposure to chimpanzee blood or other infectious secretions. The likeliest scenario for such exposure would have been through hunting, butchering, or other handling of infected chimpanzees but this is unproven. Next, the virus would have to propagate in human populations, requiring biological adaptation as well as epidemic spread.

Molecular epidemiologic and phylogenetic analyses linked to Congolese sociodemographic and historical data, published in *Science* in 2014,[18] have suggested that amplification and dissemination of infection occurred in the early twentieth century, with Kinshasa the epicenter and source of further spread (Figure 18.3). The principal early mode of transport was along the

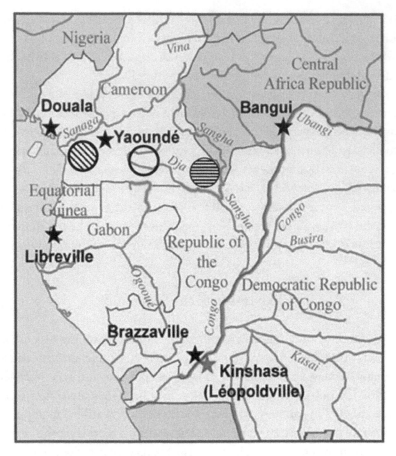

HIV-1 group M (⊜ ~1920): spread to Kinshasa, and
from there throughout the DRC to eastern and
southern Africa, Haiti, and beyond; millions of cases

HIV-1 group O (origin site not known, ~1926):
spread within Cameroon and neighboring countries;
hundreds of thousands of cases

HIV-1 group N (○ ~1950s): restricted to Cameroon;
~20 cases

HIV-1 group P (⊘ no origin date estimate):
restricted to Cameroon; 2 cases

Figure 18.3. Locations and timing of HIV-1 emergence. (Courtesy of
Beatrice Hahn)

rivers of the region; a railway network was also developed in the first half of the twentieth century. Dramatically rapid social and economic change, population movement, separation from family, prostitution, and high rates of other STIs were plausible factors for promoting epidemic expansion.

An alternative proposed hypothesis envisaged transmission by the very extensive use of injections in medical campaigns for diseases such as sleeping sickness. The Canadian physician Jacques Pepin strongly promoted this view in his book, *The Origins of AIDS*.[47] The virologist and primate researcher Preston Marx and colleagues have argued that mutation rates in any one individual infected with SIVcpz would have been inadequate to develop into HIV-1, and they proposed the "serial passage theory of HIV emergence."[48] This entailed serial and rapid passage between individuals through extensive use of medical injections, which, it was argued, would drive adaptation and pathogenicity in the new host. The ability of a virus to cross species and adapt to a new host is of major basic science interest, and it is not fully understood how SIVcpz adapted to evolve into HIV-1 in humans.

The origins of the HIV-2 epidemic seem inextricably linked to Portuguese colonial history, specifically Guinea Bissau and the war of liberation that led to independence in 1974. The great majority of cases of HIV-2 have some link to West Africa or Portugal. Many epidemiologic observations suggest this is a receding rather than emerging infection whose epidemiologic drivers, albeit incompletely understood, have lessened since the height of the struggle for independence and have been overtaken by forces promoting spread of HIV-1.

Conclusions

Extraordinary science has clarified the simian origins of what in 1981 presented as a mysterious new human syndrome. HIV-1 groups M and N are derivatives of SIVcpz in west-central African chimpanzees, specifically from Cameroon; in contrast, HIV-1 groups O and P originated as the result of transmissions from western gorillas, which in turn acquired their SIVgor infection from chimpanzees; HIV-2 is derived from a West African sooty mangabey virus; and cross-species transmission to humans occurred decades before recognition of AIDS. There is a continuing risk of cross-species transmissions as exemplified, among others, by SARS (severe acute respiratory syndrome), MERS (Middle East respiratory syndrome), Ebola and Marburg virus diseases, avian influenza, and COVID-19. Further spill-over events must be anticipated and prepared for in a globalized world.

Notes

1. Barre-Sinoussi F, Chermann JC, Rey F, et al. Isolation of a T-lymphotropic retrovirus from a patient at risk for acquired immune deficiency syndrome (AIDS). Science 1983;220:868–871.
2. Gallo RC, Salahuddin SZ, Popovic M, et al. Frequent detection and isolation of cyto-pathic retroviruses (HTLV-III) from patients with AIDS and at risk for AIDS. Science 1984;224:500–503.
3. Levy JA, Hoffman AD, Kramer SM, Landis JA, Shimabukuro JM, Oshiro LS. Isolation of lymphocytopathic retroviruses from San Francisco patients with AIDS. Science 1984;225:840–842.
4. Feorino PM, Kalyanaraman VS, Haverkos HW, et al. Lymphadenopathy associated virus infection of a blood donor–recipient pair with acquired immunodeficiency syn-drome. Science 1984;225:69–72.
5. De Cock KM, Niland JC, Lu HP, et al. Experience with human immunodeficiency virus infection in patients with hepatitis B virus and hepatitis delta virus infection in Los Angeles, 1977–1985. Am J Epidemiol 1988;127:1250–1260.
6. De Cock KM. AIDS: An old disease from Africa? BMJ 1984;289:306–308.
7. Chirimuuta RC, Chirimuuta RJ. AIDS, Africa and racism. Free Association Books; 1989.
8. Farmer P. AIDS and accusation: Haiti and the geography of blame. Berkeley: University of California Press; 2006.
9. Curtis T. The Origin of AIDS. A startling new theory attempts to answer the question "was it an act of God or an act of man?" Rolling Stone, 1992;626:54–59, 61, 106, 108.
10. Hooper E. The river. A journey to the source of HIV and AIDS. New York: Little Brown and Company; 1999.
11. Hooper E. Slim: reporter's own story of AIDS in east Africa. London: Bodley Head; 1990.
12. De Cock KM. Epidemiology and the emergence of human immunodeficiency virus and aquired immune deficiency syndrome. Philos Trans R Soc Lond B Biol Sci 2001;356:795–798. doi: 10.1098/rstb.2001.0857.
13. Sonnet J, Michaux JL, Zech F, Brucher JM, de Bruyere M, Burtonboy G. Early AIDS cases originating from Zaïre and Burundi (1962–1976). Scand J Infect Dis 1987;19:511–517.
14. Plotkin SA. CHAT oral polio vaccine was not the source of human immunodeficiency virus type 1 group M for humans. Clin Infect Dis 2001;32:1068–1084. doi: 10.1086/319612.
15. Blancou P, Vartanian JP, Christopherson C., et al. Polio vaccine samples not linked to AIDS. Nature 2001;410:1045–1046. doi: 10.1038/35074171.

16. Worobey M, Santiago ML, Keele BF, et al. Origin of AIDS: contaminated polio vaccine theory refuted. Nature 2004;428:820. doi: 10.1038/428820a.
17. Korber B, Muldoon M, Theiler J, et al. Timing the ancestor of the HIV-1 pandemic strains. Science 2000;288:1789–1796.
18. Faria NR, Rambaut A, Suchard MA, et al. The early spread and epidemic ignition of HIV-1 in human populations. Science 2014;346:56–61.
19. Worobey M, Gemmel M, Teuwen D, et al. Direct evidence of extensive diversity of HIV-1 in Kinshasa by 1960. Nature 2008;455:661–664.
20. Letvin NL, Eaton KA, Aldrich WR, et al. Acquired immunodeficiency syndrome in a colony of macaque monkeys. Proc Natl Acad Sci U S A 1983;80:2718–2722.
21. Daniel MD, Letvin NL, King NW, et al. Isolation of T-cell tropic HTLV-III-like retrovirus from macaques. Science 1985;228:1201–1204.
22. Chakrabarti L, Guyader M, Alizon M, et al. Sequence of simian immunodeficiency virus from macaque and its relationship to other human and simian retroviruses. Nature 1987;328:543–547.
23. Sharp PM, Hahn BH. Origins of HIV and the AIDS pandemic. Cold Spring Harb Perspect Med 2011;1:a006841.
24. Clavel F, Brun-Vezinet F, Chamaret S, et al. Isolation of a new human retrovirus from West African patients with AIDS. Science 1986;233:343–346.
25. Hirsch VM, Olmsted RA, Murphey-Corb M, Purcell RH, Johnson PR. An African primate lentivirus (SIVsm) closely related to HIV-2. Nature 1989;339:389–392.
26. Peeters M, Honoré C, Huet T, et al. Isolation and partial characterization of an HIV-related virus occurring naturally in chimpanzees in Gabon. AIDS 1989;3:625–630.
27. Peeters M, Fransen K, Delaporte E, et al. Isolation and characterization of a new chimpanzee lentivirus (simian immunodeficiency virus isolate cpz-ant) from a wild-captured chimpanzee. AIDS 1992;6:447–451.
28. Gao F, Bailes E, Robertson DL, et al. Origin of HIV-1 in the chimpanzee Pan troglodytes troglodytes. Nature 1999; 397:436–441.
29. Bailes E, Gao F, Bibollet-Ruche F, et al. Hybrid origin of SIV in chimpanzees. Science 2003;300:1713.
30. Sharp PM, Shaw GM, Hahn BH. Simian immunodeficiency virus infection of chimpanzees. J Virol 2005;79:3891–3902.
31. Hahn BH, Shaw GM, De Cock KM, Sharp PM. AIDS as a zoonosis: scientific and public health implications. Science 2000;287;607–614.
32. Santiago ML, Rodenburg CM, Kamenya S, et al. SIVcpz in wild chimpanzees. Science 2002;295:465. doi: 10.1126/science.295.5554.465.
33. Keele BF, Van Heuverswyn F, Li Y, et al. Chimpanzee reservoirs of pandemic and nonpandemic HIV-1. Science 2006;313:523–526. doi: 10.1126/science.1126531.
34. Bibollet-Ruche F, Russell RM, Weimin L, et al. CD4 receptor diversity in chimpanzees protects against SIV infection. Proc Natl Acad Sci U S A 2019;116:3229–3238. doi: 10.1073/pnas.1821197116.
35. Keele BF, Jones JH, Terio KA, et al. Increased mortality and AIDS-like immunopathology in wild chimpanzees infected with SIVcpz. Nature 2009;460:515–519. doi:10.1038/nature08200

36. Rudicell RS, Jones JH, Wroblewski E, et al. Impact of simian immunodeficiency virus infection on chimpanzee population dynamics. PLoS Pathog 2010;6:e1001116. doi: 10.1371/journal.ppat.1001116.
37. Stevens CE, Taylor PE, Zang EA, et al. Human T-cell lymphotropic virus type III infection in a cohort of homosexual men in New York City. JAMA 1986;255:2167–2172.
38. Jaffe HW, Darrow WW, Echenberg DF, et al. The acquired immunodeficiency syndrome in a cohort of homosexual men: a six-year follow-up study. Ann Intern Med 1985;103:210–214. doi: 10.7326/0003-4819-103-2-210
39. Frøland SS, Jenum P, Lindboe CF, Wefring KW, Linnestad PJ, Böhmer T. HIV-1 Infection in Norwegian Family before 1970. Lancet 1988;1:1344–1345. doi: 10.1016/s0140-6736(88)92164-2.
40. Bygbjerg IC. AIDS in a Danish surgeon (Zaire, 1976). Lancet 1983;1:925. doi: 10.1016/s0140-6736(83)91348-x.
41. Crawford D. Virus hunt. Oxford: Oxford University Press; 2013.
42. Nahmias AJ, Weiss J, Yao X, et al. Evidence for human infection with an HTLV III/LAV- like virus in Central Africa, 1959. Lancet 1986;327:1279–1280.
43. Nzilambi N, De Cock KM, Forthal DN, et al. The prevalence of infection with human immunodeficiency virus over a 10-year period in rural Zaire. N Engl J Med 1988;318:276–279. doi: 10.1056/NEJM198802043180503.
44. Getchell JP, Hicks DR, Svinivasan A, et al. Human immunodeficiency virus isolated from a serum sample collected in 1976 in Central Africa. J Infect Dis 1987;156:833–836.
45. Bryceson ADM, Tomkins AM, Ridley D, et al. HIV-2 associated AIDS in the 1970s. Lancet, 1988;2:221. doi: 10.1016/s0140-6736(88)92325-2.
46. Worobey M, Watts T, McKay R, et al. 1970s and 'Patient 0' HIV-1 genomes illuminate early HIV/AIDS history in North America. Nature 2016;539:98–101.
47. Pepin J. The origins of AIDS. Cambridge: Cambridge University Press; 2011.
48. Marx PA, Drucker EM, Schneider WH. The serial passage theory of HIV emergence. Clin Infect Dis 2011;52:421–422.

19

Increased Understanding,
Improved Outcomes

Kevin M. De Cock

Diagnostics, Viral Load, and HIV Epidemiology

HIV is a lifelong infection. Except for infants who may carry antibodies from their mothers for eighteen months of life, HIV antibody in a person's blood indicates infection with HIV. Although the HIV antibody test introduced in 1985[1] was primarily intended to protect the blood supply, it also allowed for individual diagnosis of HIV and immediately provided enormous prevention and research opportunities.[2] Previously, epidemiologic insights had come from studies of persons meeting the AIDS case definition or having what was called AIDS-related complex (Chapter 3). Blood tests for HIV also allowed study of its natural history, risk factors for transmission, and spread in various populations over time. HIV antibody testing opened a new era for clinical diagnosis, surveillance, prevention, treatment, and research.

Two other tests had widespread implications. As described earlier, CD4+ T-lymphocytes ("CD4 cells") play a central role in the immune system and are progressively depleted during HIV infection. Failure of the immune system, with loss of CD4 cells, opens the floodgates to opportunistic pathogens and malignancies normally kept in check. CD4 cells are measured either in absolute numbers (number of cells per cubic millimeter of blood) or as a percentage of all lymphocytes. This testing gives an indication of the severity of immune damage: the lower the CD4 count the more severe the immune deficiency. Repeat testing can show the rapidity of immune decline. CD4 cell thresholds were defined, indicating levels below which the risk of specific opportunistic diseases was greatly increased.[3] Certain "opportunists" were more aggressive, occurring earlier and at relatively higher CD4 counts compared to others. PCP, for example, became a threat at CD4 counts below

Kevin M. De Cock, *Increased Understanding, Improved Outcomes* In: *Dispatches from the AIDS Pandemic*. Kevin M. De Cock, Harold W. Jaffe, and James W. Curran and Edited by: Robin Moseley, Oxford University Press.
© Oxford University Press 2023. DOI: 10.1093/oso/9780197626528.003.0019

200 per cubic millimeter (cu mm).[*] By contrast, *Mycobacterium avium* infection was rare in persons with CD4 counts higher than 100/cu mm. TB, which was not included in the original case definition for AIDS, shows increased incidence from earliest HIV infection. It becomes ever more frequent as immune function declines, with a greater tendency to spread throughout the body.[4] All these observations had implications for guidance about preventive and therapeutic options.

The third important test was for HIV viral load, measuring the amount of virus in the blood. Viral load is measured in numbers of viral copies per milliliter (ml) of blood. Viral load came to widespread notice at the 1996 international AIDS conference in Vancouver, which drew the world's attention to the benefit of ART[5] and a new class of drugs, protease inhibitors.[6] There, the clinical virologist John Mellors depicted outcomes in persons with HIV, stratified by their viral load.[7] The more virus there was in their blood, the more rapid their progression to AIDS and death. Also at the conference, John Coffin, a retrovirologist then at NIH's National Cancer Institute, combined CD4 cell count and viral load in an insightful analogy. He likened HIV infection to a train heading toward a cliff edge. The virus represented the force propelling the train, an increased amount of virus portraying greater speed. CD4 cell count was a surrogate for the distance to the inevitable crash, the onset of opportunistic diseases and death.

A simple and unifying concept explained pathogenesis. Immune deficiency was caused by the virus, and viral load drove disease progression. Treatment suppressed the virus, and viral load was a surrogate for measuring treatment impact. CD4 testing measured the severity of immune deficiency and allowed estimation of the risk of disease and timing for preventive treatments. CD4 cell trends showed how well the immune system was recovering in response to ART.

Viral load also gave crucial insights into HIV transmission. It had long been known that sex partners of persons with advanced HIV disease were more likely to be infected than partners of those with less severe immune deficiency.[8,9] Another observation was that the recipients of HIV-positive blood transfusions invariably acquired the infection.[10,11] Surveillance of healthcare workers with needle stick injuries and studies of postexposure prophylaxis with zidovudine (also called azidothymidine [AZT]) identified risk factors

---

[*] The normal CD4 count is in the range of about 500–1500 per cu mm. CD4 cells can also be measured as a percentage of all lymphocytes, the normal being about 25 percent to 65 percent. CD4 percentages may be less susceptible to spontaneous variation.

for infection, including exposures from patients with terminal AIDS, deep injuries, and injuries with sharp objects visibly contaminated with blood.[12] These observations suggested exposure to higher amounts of virus was more likely to transmit infection.

Studies of HIV in mothers and infants and in discordant heterosexual couples showed viral load to be the dominant risk factor for transmission. CDC's Nathan Schaffer and colleagues in Thailand (Chapter 16) showed that mothers who transmitted HIV to their infants had viral loads more than four times higher than nontransmitting mothers, and a dose-response association was observed.[13] Mothers with the lowest viral loads did not transmit.

Collaborative field sites had been established in Uganda in the heavily affected area around Lake Victoria in association with Johns Hopkins University and the British Medical Research Council.[14] It was in this area that David Serwadda and Nelson Sewankambo, young physicians from Uganda's Makerere University, had led early research efforts describing the HIV wasting syndrome called "slim disease" (Chapter 15).[15] These sites followed entire populations over time, monitoring demography, HIV trends, transmission dynamics, and impact of prevention efforts. The Rakai investigators later reported on their three years of follow-up among discordant couples, where one partner was infected with HIV and the other not.[16] About one fifth of the 415 initially negative participants became infected, with an annual infection rate of about 12 percent. HIV viral load was significantly higher in partners who transmitted compared to those who did not, and a dose-response association existed. Persons with the lowest viral loads did not transmit. A threshold could be suggested below which HIV transmission was exceptionally rare. Viral load thus became the critical focus for both prevention and treatment.

Opportunistic Infection Prophylaxis

In the decade following the first AIDS reports, clinical research clarified the spectrum of disease in patients with HIV infection. Research into the treatment of OIs set up a tense atmosphere between clinicians who believed interventions should be evaluated in placebo-controlled trials (the orthodox view) and those who felt any hopeful measures should be tried. Community activism challenged medical orthodoxy. The NIH-sponsored AIDS Clinical Trials Group (ACTG) was established in 1987 through NIH's National

Institute of Allergy and Infectious Diseases (NIAID), whose director was Anthony (Tony) Fauci. This collaborative network, later to be emulated for HIV prevention, vaccines, and microbicides, brought together leading clinical scientists who collaborated on a broad agenda that included the evaluation of therapies aimed at HIV itself as well as its opportunistic complications.

PCP has been the most common life-threatening or fatal infectious complication of HIV in the United States. Long recognized as a risk for other immunosuppressed patients such as those receiving cancer chemotherapy or treatment to prevent transplant rejection, PCP was amenable to treatment and prevention,[17] and simple therapies such as cotrimoxazole were available. In addition, the concept of primary and secondary prophylaxis was well accepted; primary prophylaxis referred to provision of therapy to prevent an infection while secondary prevention described maintenance treatment to prevent recurrence. Both primary and secondary prophylaxis for PCP became rapidly and widely adopted.

CDC's Jon Kaplan (Chapter 3) played a central role in the agency's work in this area. Kaplan observed that experience with individual antiretroviral drugs in the early 1990s was not saving lives. Along with colleagues from NIH and academia, CDC published guidance in 1992 on the prevention of PCP[18] and extended this advice to children the following year. Kaplan and his then-supervisor Harold Jaffe recognized the need to address OIs more methodically. "There are over 20 of these AIDS-defining conditions," Kaplan said. "So okay . . . can we look at all of them in a systematic way to see how we can prevent these infections in our patients with HIV?"[19] A collaboration between CDC, NIH, the Infectious Diseases Society of America (IDSA), and others resulted in publication of comprehensive guidelines for both treatment and prevention, first published in the *MMWR*[20] and then elsewhere.[21,22] After five editions over the next seventeen years, the publication went online,[23] facilitating regular updating.

As described in Section II, CDC's international work made important contributions to elucidating the spectrum of disease associated with HIV in lower-income settings, through studies of living patients as well as decedents. Two papers were published in the *American Journal of Tropical Medicine and Hygiene* in 1996[24] and 2001[25] summarizing knowledge and providing recommendations to extend the success of OI prophylaxis experienced in high-income settings to other areas.

The era of OI treatment and prevention began to fade after 1996 with expansion of ART. With patients' CD4 counts rising above the threshold for initiation of preventive treatment against PCP and other infections, an urgent question was whether prophylaxis was still needed or could be stopped. For low-income countries, access to ART became a more pressing issue than trying to treat and prevent HIV's complications. Debates about preventive therapy for TB were to play out much later. In retrospect, the countries of the southern hemisphere largely missed out on the real, albeit incomplete, benefits of opportunistic prophylaxis. The knowledge and experience gained from this therapy remain relevant today in view of the surprisingly large number of persons everywhere still presenting with advanced immunosuppression. Nonetheless, the realization after 1996 was that the best prophylaxis against OIs in adults as well as children was ART.

HIV Treatment

A decade earlier, I was an EIS officer when Jim Curran sent a memo around CDC announcing that a randomized, placebo-controlled trial of the antiviral drug zidovudine, a compound developed years before but abandoned as an anticancer agent, had been stopped by the Data and Safety Monitoring Board. HIV-infected patients treated with the active drug had better survival and reduced incidence of OIs compared to placebo recipients. When the trial was halted, all study subjects were offered zidovudine therapy. In March 1987, FDA approved zidovudine for the treatment of AIDS.

Zidovudine belongs to a class of drugs called nucleoside reverse transcriptase inhibitors (NRTIs). These agents act by interrupting a key feature of retroviruses, the reading ("transcription") of HIV RNA to form DNA, which then is integrated into the genome of the host CD4 cell. The introduction of zidovudine, at the time the only approved antiviral for HIV, led to furious debates about pricing (up to $10,000 per patient per year) set by Burroughs Wellcome, the pharmaceutical manufacturer, and about patent ownership. The results of the trial, sponsored by Burroughs Wellcome, that led to fast-track FDA approval of zidovudine were published in the *New England Journal of Medicine* in 1987.[26] Subsequent encouraging studies examined lowering zidovudine dose to reduce toxicity, especially anemia, and to treat patients with less severe immunodeficiency.[27,28,29]

Zidovudine had short-term benefits, but long-term outcomes were unknown and here differences in philosophic approaches to medicine in the United States and the United Kingdom emerged. Medicine in Britain was more conservative in adopting new interventions, adhering more closely to the Hippocratic maxim "Do no harm." The American medical mindset favored doing something rather than nothing. The British medical community dealing with early AIDS cases, heavily concentrated in London, was relatively small. Individuals and groups particularly influential were Ian Weller (now Sir Ian), Janet Darbyshire, and the Medical Research Council's HIV Clinical Trials Centre.

A study with major impact was the Concorde trial, a joint Anglo-French study comparing early with deferred treatment with zidovudine.[30] After three years of follow-up, clinical endpoints of AIDS or death were equally distributed across the two study groups. Early treatment with zidovudine yielded no long-term clinical benefit. Presented at the international AIDS conference in Berlin in 1993, with the definitive paper appearing in the *Lancet* a year later, the results caused disappointment, consternation, and debate. The fundamental challenge was that monotherapy with zidovudine inevitably led to drug resistance and treatment failure.

Weller was one of the founding organizers of "The Glasgow Conference," the HIV drug therapy meeting held biannually in Glasgow since the early 1990s. I recall differences of opinion between US and UK investigators at the 1994 conference, the British heavily influenced by results of the Concorde Trial while Americans such as Doug Richman were confident about more powerful drugs in development. I also recall the lack of interest in AIDS in low-income countries at that time. When I was introduced at the conference to speak on AIDS care in such settings, the large hall completely emptied.

Slow progress included efforts to combine different NRTI drugs as well as development of different drug classes with varied modes of action, the most important being protease inhibitors. A paper in the *New England Journal of Medicine* described CDC-funded clinical surveillance in sentinel settings following the introduction of protease inhibitor-containing regimens.[6] A figure from the article (Figure 19.1) became one of the most widely used pictures for teaching and conference presentations, deaths declining as protease inhibitor usage increased. Over the course of 1996, especially after the iconic conference in Vancouver, triple drug therapy became accepted as standard of care in high-income countries.[5] At a national level, CDC surveillance data showed precipitous declines in AIDS mortality as ART uptake increased (Figure 19.2), and AIDS lost its place as the leading cause of death in young persons.

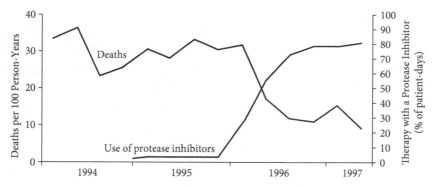

Figure 19.1. Mortality and frequency of use of antiretroviral therapy that included a protease inhibitor among HIV-infected patients with CD4+ counts <100 per cu mm, January 1994–June 1997. (Palella FJ Jr., Delaney KM, Moorman AC, et al. Declining morbidity and mortality among patients with advanced human immunodeficiency virus infection. N Engl J Med 1998;338;853–860).

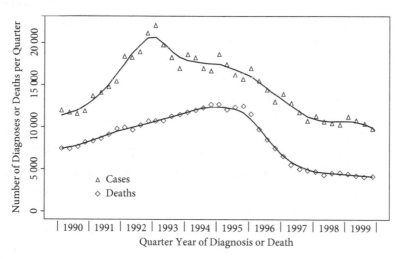

Figure 19.2. AIDS cases and deaths among adults and adolescents in the United States by quarter year, 1990–1999. (Karon JM, Fleming PL, Steketee RW, De Cock KM. HIV in the United States at the turn of the century: an epidemic in transition. Am J Public Health 2001;91:1060-1068.)

Steady progress has continued since these early events. Although not all are extensively used, over two dozen antiretroviral drugs from eight different classes have received FDA approval. Different international bodies have issued and continually revise treatment guidelines, the most influential being those coordinated by NIH.[31] Pharmacologic advances resulted in different drugs being combined into one preparation, so that AIDS is now treatable with a once-daily pill.

After the introduction of combination ART, questions persisted about when to initiate treatment.[32] Therapy as soon as possible was intuitively logical, while drug toxicity, treatment fatigue, and the possibility of drug resistance were arguments promoted for waiting. Sequential changes to guidelines, mostly based on expert opinion with imperfect supporting data, progressively recommended earlier treatment. Finally, in 2015, results were published of two trials, START and TEMPRANO, that randomized patients to immediate or deferred treatment.[33,34] Unequivocally, immediate therapy resulted in better overall and disease-free survival. Why that question took so long to answer merits discussion, but the science is now clear: persons with HIV should initiate ART as soon as possible, the aim being suppression of the virus to undetectable levels.[35]

ART can restore near normal or full lifespan in persons with HIV. Nonetheless, lifelong treatment poses diverse challenges. Resources may not be available to initiate and maintain treatment for the tens of millions worldwide requiring antiretrovirals. Adherence is challenging, drug resistance a threat, and toxicity and drug interactions are possible. The noninfectious complications of HIV may not fully respond to ART. Lifelong ART for children or adolescents is daunting. "Pill fatigue" is a reality, as are mental illness and addiction issues that patients may face but that ART does not address. For all these reasons, research on a cure for HIV is a priority.[36]

Distinction is made between a sterilizing cure, meaning eradication of HIV from the body, and a functional cure that results in undetectable viremia without ART, even if virus persists in sanctuary sites not reached by treatment, or as latent infection. A broad research agenda is examining the biology and immunology of latency, as well as agents to reverse it or target HIV DNA that is integrated into the host genome.[36]

To date, five persons are thought to have been cured of HIV through stem cell transplants from donors who were homozygous (had inherited the gene from both parents) for the delta 32 mutation on the chemokine CCR5 receptor.[37,38,39] This receptor is generally necessary for HIV cell entry, and persons homozygous for this mutation have a natural resistance to HIV. The first, "the Berlin Patient," Timothy Brown, had been on ART for his HIV infection since 1996 but developed acute myeloid leukemia a decade later.[37] He underwent two stem cell transplants in 2007 and 2008 from a donor with the homozygous CCR5 delta 32 mutation and subsequently remained off ART without HIV being detectable. He died in 2020 from a recurrence of leukemia. The second, "the London Patient," and the third had been in HIV-1 remission for thirty and fourteen months, respectively, after stopping ART when their respective case reports were published in 2020 and 2022.[38,39]

HIV Prevention

Early CDC recommendations for HIV prevention relied exclusively on behavior change (including condom use), but behavior change—especially in relation to sex and drug use—is difficult. Advances in biomedical interventions for HIV prevention have yielded greater impact than progress in the behavioral sciences, but the distinction between behavioral and biomedical issues is somewhat artificial. Uptake and adherence to medically prescribed interventions can determine success or failure. Recommendations on structural and behavioral interventions are provided in the CDC Compendium of Evidence-Based Interventions and Best Practices for HIV Prevention.[40]

Treatment as Prevention

Experience with antiretroviral prevention of mother-to-child transmission of HIV introduced the concept of HIV treatment as prevention.[41] Early prevention guidance such as for correct and consistent condom use had been HIV serostatus-neutral, yet HIV is only transmitted from people living with HIV. CDC promoted "prevention for positives" including through what was called the "SAFE Initiative," the Serostatus Approach to Fighting the Epidemic.[42]

Several later papers contributed to the argument that treatment was an important prevention tool. In 2006, Julio Montaner from Vancouver published an opinion piece in *The Lancet* arguing that ART scale-up, through its suppressive effect on HIV viral load and therefore on HIV transmission, was the essential intervention to control the AIDS pandemic.[43] Brian Williams developed a mathematical model based on the South African epidemic, suggesting HIV could, in theory, be eliminated by universal and repeated HIV testing and treating of persons already infected[44] (Chapter 21). If HIV-infected persons were identified and treated as soon as possible (with perfect programmatic implementation), then transmission would cease, and HIV-infected persons would eventually die without new infections being generated. NIH scientists coined the term "Test and Treat" for this approach.[45] Most important were results from the HIV Prevention Trials Network (HPTN) 052 study, designated by the journal *Science* as the scientific breakthrough of the year in 2011.[46] Myron (Mike) Cohen and colleagues showed that provision of ART to the infected partner in discordant couples reduced HIV transmission by 96 percent, confirming earlier observational data.[47] Reviews comparing the efficacy of various interventions indicated ART to be the most potent form of prevention available.[48,49]

Four ambitious evaluations of "Universal Test and Treat" (UTT) were undertaken in southern and East Africa between 2012 and 2017. These randomized studies compared UTT to standard of care in almost one quarter of a million people across different communities, with HIV incidence as primary outcome. If the scientific questions were "Does UTT reduce community HIV incidence?" and "If so, by how much?" the political question was "Will UTT end the AIDS epidemic?" Expectations were high.

The results, published in *The Lancet* and the *New England Journal of Medicine* in 2018[50] and 2019,[51,52,53] respectively, were controversial, somewhat disappointing, but generally explicable. The study in Botswana[51] showed a statistically significant 30 percent reduction in HIV incidence in the UTT communities. The trials in East Africa[52] and South Africa[50] showed no difference between UTT and control communities. The fourth and more complex study, conducted in Zambia and South Africa, showed a significant 30 percent reduction in one of the two intervention arms but, surprisingly, not in the one with the most intense treatment and prevention package.[53] Despite these efforts, HIV incidence overall remained high across all the studies. Three of the four studies achieved the "90:90:90" targets (90% of people living with HIV diagnosed; 90% of the diagnosed on ART; 90% of the treated virally suppressed) that had been defined by UNAIDS in 2014 (Chapter 21) and adopted globally.[54]

Debate ensued as to whether these expensive studies were worthwhile and why UTT did not reduce HIV incidence more.[55] To an extent, the research had been overtaken by events, since universal treatment had become recommended over the course of the trials, and differences between comparison groups may have been eroded. If it had been known at the beginning that every individual with HIV needs ART as soon as possible, then the UTT trials might not have been undertaken.

We did learn that 90:90:90 does not equate with HIV elimination and that "Test and Treat" alone will not control the pandemic under realistic field conditions. Nonetheless, ART is key to HIV prevention. The collective research has shown that HIV-infected individuals who are virally suppressed do not transmit HIV to their sex partners, leading to the advice that "U=U" (undetectable equals untransmittable).[56]

Prevention of Mother-to-Child Transmission

Without intervention, 15 percent to 40 percent of infected pregnant women transmit HIV to their infants.[57] The higher range applies to those who breastfeed, who have approximately twice the transmission rate of nonbreastfeeding mothers. ACTG 076, the original trial that showed two thirds reduction in HIV transmission from infected mothers to infants, involved a complex regimen of zidovudine.[41] After this advance, priorities included scale-up of this intervention, defining remediable risk factors for perinatal transmission, and evaluation of more potent as well as simpler regimens. CDC's Martha Rogers (Chapter 4) and later Mary-Glenn Fowler, who came to CDC from NIH, were especially influential in overseeing CDC's involvement in this specialized area of work, both in the United States (Figure 19.3) and internationally.

Studies in West Africa and Thailand following the 076 study were described in Section II.[58,59,60] Subsequent and sequential research aimed to identify the best antiretroviral regimen in the simplest, most practical dosing schedule for low-income settings. The PETRA study in South Africa compared shorter regimens of zidovudine and lamivudine with placebo in a complex four-arm study.[61] The lowest transmission rate at six weeks was 5.7 percent. However, following extensive breastfeeding, infant infection rates at eighteen months ranged from 15 percent to 22 percent. Another especially influential early trial was the HIVNET 012 study, examining single-dose intrapartum nevirapine, a non-nucleoside reverse transcriptase inhibitor (NNRTI), given to the mother and a single postpartum dose to the infant.[62] At fourteen to sixteen weeks the rate of infection was 13.1 percent

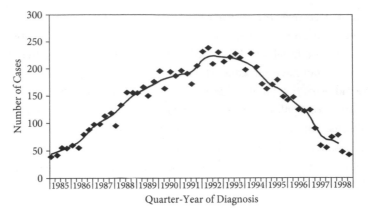

Figure 19.3. Estimated incidence of AIDS among children aged <13 years who were infected with HIV perinatally by quarter year of diagnosis—United States, 1985–1998. (MMWR Morb Mortal Wkly Rep 1999;48[RR13]:1–28.)

in the nevirapine group, almost half that of the comparison group receiving a short zidovudine regimen.

The study generated enthusiasm because single-dose treatment presented a simple intervention that could be widely used in lower-income settings. However, such a short regimen did not address HIV transmission through breastfeeding, which in the African context could last for up to two years. Moreover, single-dose nevirapine predisposed women to viral resistance not only to that specific drug but to agents across the whole class of NNRTIs, thus jeopardizing their own future treatment options.

The breastfeeding conundrum was particularly controversial because of the history of western companies promoting formula feeding for commercial gain. Lack of access to clean water made formula feeding a risk for diarrhea, a leading cause of infant death in low-income settings, second only to respiratory infections. The awful choice that faced policymakers and healthcare workers, but especially HIV-positive mothers, was whether to adopt formula to avoid HIV transmission but risk diarrheal disease and potential death or choose breastfeeding but risk death from AIDS.[63]

The University of Nairobi in Kenya and the University of Washington in the United States have had a productive collaboration extending back to the earliest days of AIDS. With Ruth Nduati as lead field investigator, their group undertook a courageous, sometimes criticized trial that randomized HIV-infected, delivering women into breast- or formula-feeding groups.[64]

Published in the *Journal of the American Medical Association* in 2000, the study showed that breastfed infants did indeed have a higher rate of HIV infection, almost 37 percent compared with about 20 percent in the formula-fed infants. However, a similar proportion of infants in both study arms, over one fifth, had died by two years of age. The debates and the polarization sometimes forgot the true goal, to have an infant who not only was free of HIV but also survived.

In the early 2000s, when global guidelines still advocated that ART be deferred until advanced immunodeficiency, CDC initiated a trial of triple ART throughout pregnancy and breastfeeding in Kenya, the "Kisumu Breastfeeding Study," under the field leadership of Timothy (Tim) Thomas.[65] Nduati's group from the University of Nairobi conducted the "Kesho Bora Study" ("a better tomorrow" in Swahili).[66] Continuous ART seemed the most potent intervention to suppress viral load in pregnant women while allowing breastfeeding and thus avoiding the negative consequences of formula feeding in poor settings. The collective results from these and several other combination ART studies showed that transmission rates could be brought down to well below 10 percent while still maintaining breastfeeding.

Global health developments gradually overtook the methodical research planned, as well as the complex WHO guidelines that required CD4 testing and distinguished between treatment of women for their own health and prevention of vertical transmission.[67] Workers in Malawi challenged WHO with a new approach (initially called "Option B+").[68] They recommended that HIV-positive pregnant women, irrespective of CD4 count, simply start lifelong triple ART during pregnancy. In view of later research and changes to treatment practice, this was prescient advice. When treatment recommendations changed to initiate ART as early as possible, pregnant women were included under the revisions. In all updates of WHO guidelines since 2010, advice on treatment and prevention of mother-to-child transmission has been consolidated and not viewed or published separately from other treatment recommendations. In addition, focus on preventing transmission of HIV from mothers to infants has broadened to also include prevention of congenital syphilis and infant HBV infection, an approach referred to as "triple elimination."[69]

Prior to ART availability, Cesarean section was of interest as an intervention. With full viral suppression, it is not indicated, but it may reduce transmission in women who present late or have high viral loads at delivery.[70] The last perinatal HIV transmission trial to be completed was the NIH-sponsored

PROMISE study, which compared combination ART with an older regimen of combined zidovudine and single dose nevirapine.[71] Although transmission of HIV was lower in the combination ART group (now the standard of care), the study nonetheless showed that mothers had more side effects from full therapy and their infants had lower birth weights and increased risk for being premature.

Microbicides and Pre-Exposure Prophylaxis

Over half of people living with HIV worldwide are women. In sub-Saharan Africa, the rate of new HIV infections in girls and young women is often twice that in adolescent boys and young men. In view of this female vulnerability to HIV infection, there has long been demand for research and development of female-controlled preventive measures. Initial interest was in vaginal microbicides, products women could introduce into the vagina prior to intercourse. These products had to be safe, easy to use, not interfere with sexual pleasure, and not be obvious to the male partner.

The research was discouraging until the results of the CAPRISA 004 study in South Africa were presented at the 2010 international AIDS conference in Vienna by South African Quarraisha Abdool Karim, who received a standing ovation. This randomized controlled trial compared HIV incidence in women who were provided vaginal applicators filled with tenofovir gel (an antiretroviral) or a placebo. Overall, women receiving the tenofovir gel had a 39 percent reduction in HIV incidence compared to controls.[72] Proof of concept was established for a female-controlled HIV preventive intervention, but it was antiretroviral based.

Applicators and gels are not easy to use or dispose of discreetly, and there has been interest in more convenient devices. Two trials in sub-Saharan Africa examined use of a self-inserted vaginal ring, replaced monthly, that releases the antiviral drug dapivirine on a slow and continuous basis.[73,74] HIV incidence in ring users was reduced by about one third, and efficacy increased with higher adherence.

After animal studies had shown antiretroviral drugs offered protection against infection with simian immunodeficiency viruses (SIV) following diverse challenges, human efficacy trials of oral PrEP had an inauspicious start in the early 2000s.[75] Planned trials in Cambodia and West Africa aroused concerns regarding community engagement. Activists mounted fierce demonstrations, leading to the studies being abandoned amidst controversy, misunderstanding, and missed opportunities for all concerned.

Results of the first randomized controlled trial of oral PrEP in men and transgender women who have sex with men were published in the *New England Journal of Medicine* in late 2010, with Robert (Bob) Grant from the University of California San Francisco the lead investigator.[76] Almost 2,500 study participants were followed internationally for a median period of just over one year. HIV incidence in persons receiving the active intervention, a combination of the antiretrovirals tenofovir and emtricitabine, was 44 percent lower than in placebo recipients.

A large body of research followed these early efforts, with available knowledge synthesized and public health guidelines issued.[77,78,79] Almost 20,000 persons have been studied in over a dozen randomized controlled trials. Most involved the use of tenofovir with or without emtricitabine, and both continuous and on-demand PrEP were examined. Over half of the trials were conducted in Africa involving persons at risk for heterosexual transmission, and one trial examined persons using injection drugs in Thailand.[80] Trials in high-income countries mostly focused on MSM. Further knowledge has come from observational data, including from trials that were switched to open-label use of the drugs when newly available information required placebos to be terminated.

PrEP unquestionably reduced HIV incidence. An analysis across the available studies showed an overall reduction of 54 percent.[78] However, a consistent observation has been that efficacy is correlated with the degree of adherence; PrEP obviously does not work if the drugs are not taken. Preventive efficacy exceeded 70 percent in persons with 70 percent or greater adherence, and PrEP was efficacious in all risk categories. Side effects from the drugs have mostly been transient. A danger is the development of drug resistance if the preventive, but nontherapeutic, regimens are inadvertently administered to persons already infected or in their incubation period, emphasizing the importance of excluding active HIV infection before starting PrEP.

The most recent research concerns different preparations of PrEP, including long-acting compounds. The HPTN studies 083 and 084 examined the long-acting drug cabotegravir, delivered by monthly injection, which obviates the requirement of short-term adherence.[81,82] Efficacy was greater than that of oral tenofovir, offering new prevention possibilities. Comparing HIV incidence in cabotegravir recipients and the recipients of placebos in other prevention trials in similar time periods and regions suggested a protective efficacy of 96 percent.[83] Reminiscent of the reproductive health research experience that yielded diverse contraceptive options, future work will likely include examination of depot (slow-release) and other long-acting preparations of PrEP such as implants, increasing PrEP choices for persons at risk of HIV. There is also increasing interest in multipurpose technologies combining HIV prevention modalities with contraception for women wishing to prevent not only HIV but also pregnancy.

CDC guidelines on use of PrEP, issued in 2017, are regularly reviewed and updated.[79] Evidence is emerging that PrEP can reduce HIV incidence at a population level when there is high coverage with ART of persons already infected, as was demonstrated in MSM in Sydney and London.[84,85] The promise that PrEP might reduce HIV incidence in highly vulnerable adolescents in sub-Saharan Africa and elsewhere remains to be studied and realized.

A unifying view would be recognition that all populations require the highest possible coverage with ART to minimize the prevalence of persons with uncontrolled virus in a community, and that PrEP for at-risk individuals can add to this foundation to achieve universal protection against HIV. In this way, HIV transmission is blocked by treatment of infected persons and the most highly susceptible are protected by PrEP. Nonetheless, PrEP should be viewed within the overall context of sexual and reproductive health, recognizing that the risk of unwanted pregnancy and potential exposure to other STIs remains relevant at the population level. There is more to PrEP than efficacy in controlled trials.

HIV Vaccines

The ultimate prize for HIV research would be development of an efficacious HIV vaccine. The history of HIV vaccine research illustrates the difficulty in developing vaccines for chronic infections in which natural immunity does not itself provide complete protection. Examples include diseases such as malaria and TB for which available vaccines are limited in efficacy. Longstanding debate has focused on what level of basic understanding of correlates of immunity against HIV is required before proceeding to clinical trials of potential candidates, and what public health benefit might accrue from a partially effective vaccine. A theoretical concern about partially effective vaccines, including for HIV, is that they could drive mutations promoting viral escape from the vaccine concerned.

Of the eight randomized, placebo-controlled trials of HIV vaccine candidates conducted to date, seven gave negative results.[86,87] The much-awaited STEP trial of an adenovirus-vectored vaccine stimulating cellular immunity actually increased the risk of infection in MSM who were un-circumcised and already had antibodies to adenovirus type 5.[88] The only positive study, the Thai RV144 trial suggested an efficacy of 26 percent to 31 percent but was criticized by some in its analyses.[89,90] A trial of an anal-ogous regimen targeted at subtype C virus in South Africa showed no effi-cacy.[91] Two trials of a "mosaic" vaccine aimed at protecting against multiple global strains of HIV, "Imbokodo" in women in South Africa and "Mosaico" in MSM and transgender persons in Europe and North America, were begun in 2017 and 2019, respectively. The Imbokodo trial was halted in August 2021 after primary analysis showed lack of protective efficacy;[87] the Mosaico study was halted prematurely in early 2023.

For the time being, a vaccine against HIV remains frustratingly elusive. It would be tempting to attribute these negative results to lack of funding or commitment, but close to three quarters of annual funding for HIV research and development goes toward work relevant to vaccines.[92] In an environ-ment of greatly increased access to other efficacious preventive interventions, considerations of how to assess vaccine efficacy, and which populations should be prioritized if we had a vaccine, have become more complex.

Immunology research has led to development of broadly neutralizing antibodies (bNAbs) against HIV characterized by greater potency and broader activity than previous preparations. "Passive immunization" through administration of potent antibody preparations has been a long-established approach to prevention of various infections including HBV . Specific mono-clonal antibody compounds have entered other therapeutic practice, such as for the treatment of Ebola or COVID-19. These advances have led to the con-cept of antibody-mediated prevention (AMP). NIH-sponsored trials in the Americas and sub-Saharan Africa (HVTN 704/HPTN 085 and HVTN 703/ HPTN 081, respectively) examined passive immunity from a bNab prepara-tion, VRC01, as a prevention intervention.[93] Relative protection was shown against sensitive HIV-1 strains, but overall incidence was not reduced. Nonetheless, this line of research is considered encouraging as proof of prin-ciple that adequately broad antibodies, whether from active or passive im-munization, could prevent HIV infection.

Male Circumcision

Suggestions that male circumcision might protect men against heterosexual acquisition of HIV date back to the 1980s.[94,95] A strong ecologic association was found across Africa between higher HIV prevalence and lack of circumcision in men.[96] Case control and cohort studies subsequently demonstrated an increased frequency of HIV in uncircumcised compared with circumcised African men,[16,97,98] and this association held for both HIV-1 and HIV-2.[99] In the Rakai study of viral load and risk of heterosexual transmission described earlier, HIV-negative men who were uncircumcised had an annual incidence of HIV of approximately 17 percent, while no new HIV infections occurred in the fifty circumcised, HIV-negative men.[16]

A study comparing two high-HIV-prevalence African cities with two lower prevalence ones found few differences in sexual behavior but did find associations between HIV and lack of male circumcision, as well as HIV and genital ulcer disease.[100] An early systematic review of twenty-seven African studies concluded that male circumcision was associated with at least a halving of the risk of HIV acquisition in men.[101]

In the face of the several dozen studies suggesting male circumcision was protective, pressure grew to introduce it as an HIV prevention strategy. Concern persisted, however, that the protective association could be spurious, perhaps explained by differences in social, cultural, or religious factors influencing sexual behavior and networks. To definitively address the concern about residual confounding, three intervention trials were conducted in Uganda, Kenya, and South Africa, actively circumcising men and comparing their subsequent course to that of an uncircumcised control group. Circumcision reduced new HIV infections in men by about 60 percent.[102,103,104] Voluntary medical male circumcision was subsequently introduced as an intervention against HIV in sub-Saharan Africa (Chapter 21). The close-to-universal practice of male circumcision in West Africa is likely a principal reason for the lesser severity of the HIV pandemic there than in eastern and southern parts of the continent.

Earlier research on circumcision in MSM had given conflicting results about protective efficacy. The most recent and largest systematic review of global data, encompassing sixty-two observational studies and over 100,000 men, found a protective efficacy of 42 percent in low- and middle-income countries, but not in high-income countries.[105] Biological plausibility suggests the intervention could only be protective in men practicing insertive anal intercourse. Male circumcision protects against several other STIs in heterosexual and homosexual men. Guidelines do not currently recommend male circumcision as a prevention strategy for MSM, but the topic deserves more research.[106]

Blood Safety

AIDS in recipients of blood or blood-product transfusions and the work of CDC AIDS Task Force member Bruce Evatt and his Division of Host Factors were discussed in Chapter 8. Evatt has written about the devastating impact of the HIV epidemic on the hemophilia population.[107] The recommendation to use only heat-treated clotting factor preparations appeared in the *MMWR* in late 1984 and was widely implemented by early 1985,[108,109] with CDC the first to show the efficacy of this procedure.[108] Molecular biology would later allow production of recombinant clotting factor.[110] Evatt observed that no person with hemophilia born in the United States in 1985 or later became infected with HIV.[107]

Also as described in Chapter 8, the most important interventions to prevent HIV transmission through blood transfusion were the deferral of "high-risk" donors followed by the introduction of HIV testing of donated blood. Controversy concerning patents and commercial interests, as well as blame and litigation around blood safety, played out around the world.[111,112] Measures instituted in high-income countries proved to be highly effective, while many low- and middle-income countries lacked infrastructure for safe collection, storage, and distribution of blood; quality control; and a pool of regular, safe donors.[113] A first requirement is avoidance of unnecessary blood transfusions, which requires education of medical providers.[114] Great progress has been made in low-income settings through development assistance,[115] but this area of medicine remains relatively neglected and protection against HIV and other bloodborne agents, including hepatitis viruses, malaria, and syphilis, is far from assured.

Since 1999, blood banks in the United States have required nucleic acid testing of blood donations to detect HIV RNA in case the donation was made during the "window period" before antibody has developed. This still leaves the so-called "eclipse period" between infection and RNA detectability in blood, estimated to be around nine days. FDA requires US donors to complete a questionnaire to screen for risk factors associated with HIV infection.

Recommendations concerning deferral of individuals for donation have been made less restrictive since CDC's original guidance.[116] The US blood supply is now exceptionally safe, but occasional transfusion-associated HIV infections have still occurred, with the risk estimated at around one in 1.5 million.[117]

Control of Other Sexually Transmitted Infections

It had long been known that other STIs, especially ulcerative conditions such as chancroid and syphilis but also nonulcerative ones such as gonorrhea, facilitate transmission and acquisition of HIV.[118] Researchers from the London School of Hygiene and Tropical Medicine and their colleagues in Tanzania published results of a community randomized trial in *The Lancet* in 1994.[119] Intensified STI treatment throughout the intervention communities reduced new HIV infections by about 40 percent. These results were met with great acclaim—STI treatment seemed to offer an affordable approach to HIV prevention in African settings, and these findings were of relevance worldwide. Unfortunately, another study, in Uganda's Rakai District, failed to replicate these results.[120] No other subsequent work has shown that control of STIs reduces population-level incidence of HIV infection, and debate ensued about reasons for these diverse trial results.[121] A randomized controlled trial of suppressive therapy for genital herpes, an ulcerative viral condition strongly associated with HIV acquisition and transmission, likewise failed to show protection against HIV infection in women and MSM.[122]

Although there is general acknowledgment, including by CDC, that untreated STIs can enhance HIV transmission and acquisition and STI consultation offers patients an opportunity for HIV prevention services,[123] the reality is starker. STI treatment and research remain underfunded and inadequately prioritized everywhere, despite their adverse consequences, which include infertility, congenital infections, and ectopic pregnancy. In the United States, rates of STIs, including syphilis and gonorrhea, have increased substantially from their historic lows in the early 2000s, especially among MSM.[124] CDC issued revised STI treatment guidelines in 2021,[125] and several influential bodies have more recently released reports and plans.[126,127] STI services are important for drawing individuals into HIV prevention and care, but STI treatment alone will not contain HIV transmission at the population level.

Interventions for People who Inject Drugs

Official CDC guidance for individuals who inject drugs continues to state that the best way to keep from acquiring or transmitting HIV is to stop injecting.[128] For the many persons unable or unwilling to do this, syringe services programs can offer evidence-based interventions to limit harm. These services can include provision and disposal of safe injection equipment, vaccination against HBV, skin and wound care, STI and TB prevention and treatment, addiction services, and, of course, HIV treatment and prevention. Syringe services programs can also provide naloxone to reduce deaths from opioid overdoses. There is no evidence that such programs increase illicit drug use or crime. Some countries such as Switzerland have taken pragmatism further to provide heroin on prescription and supervised, safe injection sites, and have subsequently documented reduced mortality in the drug injection populations.[129]

Despite abundant evidence of the health benefits of these initiatives,[128,130] US federal funds cannot generally be used for procuring needles and syringes for drug injectors, and many state and local jurisdictions have interdictions in place for such programs. United Nations agencies including WHO, the United Nations Office on Drugs and Crime, and UNAIDS have endorsed a harm-reduction approach for reducing HIV in people who inject drugs.[131] Needle- and syringe-exchange programs have sometimes been used in emergency situations such as the highly publicized outbreak of HIV in Indiana that resulted from widespread injection of the opioid oxymorphone.[132]

Conclusions

In the four decades since AIDS was described, effective interventions against all modes of HIV transmission have been developed, and what was an invariably fatal infection has become a manageable disease. Persons infected with HIV can now live a normal or near-normal lifespan if they have access to early ART and are able to adhere to its use, yet many persons with HIV still present late or with advanced disease, even in high-income countries. Despite ART and effective preventive interventions, hundreds of thousands of AIDS deaths still occur annually worldwide, as well as more than one and a half million new HIV infections. Theoretically, it should be possible to control the HIV pandemic with the prevention tools available but practical experience shows the stringent and widespread implementation required is challenging. The greatest research goals—an HIV cure and vaccine—remain out of reach.

The emergence of antiretroviral drugs as central to the management and prevention of HIV has implications for the pandemic and how it is perceived and addressed. HIV has become another disease for which biomedical approaches are available to reduce its individual and societal impact, lessening the attention from other sectors and disciplines. By drawing AIDS into the mainstream of infectious disease practice, science has robbed the disease of some of its mystique from the earliest years and certainly the widespread attention it received. AIDS nonetheless remains a pandemic, a leading scientific and social priority, and a paradigm of a global health challenge.

Notes

1. CDC. Provisional Public Health Service inter-agency recommendations for screening donated blood and plasma for antibody to the virus causing acquired immunodeficiency syndrome. MMWR Morb Mortal Wkly Rep 1985;34:1–5.
2. CDC. Additional recommendations to reduce sexual and drug abuse-related transmission of human T-lymphotropic virus type III / lymphadenopathy-associated virus. MMWR Morb Mortal Wkly Rep 1986;35:152–155.
3. Crowe SM, Carlin JB, Stewart KI, Lucas CR, Hoy JF. Predictive value of CD4 lymphocyte numbers for the development of opportunistic infections and malignancies in HIV-infected persons. J Acquir Immune Defic Syndr 1991;4:770–776.
4. De Cock KM, Soro B, Coulibaly IM, Lucas SB. Tuberculosis and HIV infection in sub-Saharan Africa. JAMA 1992;268:1581–1587.
5. Williams IG, De Cock KM. The XI International Conference on AIDS. Vancouver, 7–12 July 1996. A review of Clinical Science Track B. Genitourin Med 1996;72:365–369.
6. Palella FJ Jr, Delaney KM, Moorman AC, et al. Declining morbidity and mortality among patients with advanced human immunodeficiency virus infection. HIV Outpatient Study Investigators. N Engl J Med 1998;338:853–860.
7. Mellors JW, Rinaldo CR Jr, Gupta P, White RM, Todd JA, Kingsley LA. Prognosis in HIV-1 infection predicted by the quantity of virus in plasma. Science 1996;272:1167–1170. doi:10.1126/science.272.5265.1167 [published correction appears in Science 1997;275:14].
8. Berkley SF, Widy-Wirski R, Okware SI, et al. Risk factors associated with HIV infection in Uganda. J Infect Dis. 1989;160:22–30. doi:10.1093/infdis/160.1.22.
9. De Vincenzi I. A longitudinal study of human immunodeficiency virus transmission by heterosexual partners. N Engl J Med 1994;331:341–346.

10. Donegan E, Stuart M, Niland JC, et al. Infection with human immunodeficiency virus type 1 (HIV-1) among recipients of antibody-positive blood donations. Ann Intern Med. 1990;113:733–739. doi:10.7326/0003-4819-113-10-733.

11. Colebunders R, Ryder R, Francis H, et al. Seroconversion rate, mortality, and clinical manifestations associated with the receipt of a human immunodeficiency virus-infected blood transfusion in Kinshasa, Zaire. J Infect Dis. 1991;164:450–456. doi:10.1093/infdis/164.3.450.

12. Cardo DM, Culver DH, Ciesielski CA, et al. A case-control study of HIV seroconversion in health care workers after percutaneous exposure. Centers for Disease Control and Prevention Needlestick Surveillance Group. N Engl J Med 1997;337:1485–1490. doi: 10.1056/NEJM199711203372101.

13. Shaffer N, Roongpisuthipong A, Siriwasin W, et al. Maternal virus load and perinatal human immunodeficiency virus type 1 subtype E transmission, Thailand. Bangkok Collaborative Perinatal HIV Transmission Study Group. J Infect Dis 1999;179:590–599. doi: 10.1086/314641.

14. Mulder DW, Nunn AJ, Wagner HU, Kamali A, Kengeya-Kayondo JF. HIV-1 incidence and HIV-1-associated mortality in a rural Ugandan population cohort. AIDS 1994;8:87–92. doi: 10.1097/00002030-199401000-00013.

15. Serwadda D, Mugerwa RD, Sewankambo NK, et al. Slim disease: a new disease in Uganda and its association with HTLV-III infection. Lancet 1985;2:849–852. doi: 10.1016/S0140-6736(85)90122-9.

16. Quinn TC, Wawer MJ, Sewankambo N, et al. Viral load and heterosexual transmission of human immunodeficiency virus type 1. Rakai Project Study Group. N Engl J Med 2000 Mar 30;342(13):921–929. doi: 10.1056/NEJM200003303421303.

17. Masur H. Prevention and treatment of Pneumocystis pneumonia. New Engl J Med 1992;327:1853–1860.

18. CDC. Recommendations for prophylaxis against Pneumocystis carinii pneumonia for adults and adolescents infected with human immunodeficiency virus. MMWR Morb Mortal Wkly Rep 1992;41(RR-4).

19. "KAPLAN, JOHN," *Global Health Chronicles*, accessed January 29, 2023. https://glo balhealthchronicles.org/items/show/8137.

20. CDC. USPHS/IDSA guidelines for the prevention of opportunistic infections in persons infected with human immunodeficiency virus: a summary. MMWR 1995;44:1–34.

21. USPHS/IDSA Prevention of Opportunistic Infections Working Group. USPHS/IDSA guidelines for the prevention of opportunistic infections in persons infected with human immunodeficiency virus: disease-specific recommendations. Clin Infect Dis 1995;21(Suppl 1):S32–S43.

22. USPHS/IDSA Prevention of Opportunistic Infections Working Group. USPHS/IDSA guidelines for the prevention of opportunistic infections in persons infected with human immunodeficiency virus: a summary. Ann Intern Med 1996;124:349–368.

23. Guidelines for the prevention and treatment of opportunistic infections in adults and adolescents with HIV. Available at https://clinicalinfo.hiv.gov/en/guidelines/

adult-and-adolescent-opportunistic-infection/whats-new-guidelines. Accessed September 13, 2021.

24. Kaplan JE, Hu DJ, Holmes KK, Jaffe HW, Masur H, De Cock KM. Preventing opportunistic infections in human immunodeficiency virus-infected persons: implications for the developing world. Am J Trop Med Hyg 1996;55:1–11.

25. Grant AD, Kaplan JE, De Cock KM. Preventing opportunistic infections among HIV-infected adults in African countries. Am J Trop Med Hyg 2001;65:810–821.

26. Fischl MA, Richman DD, Grieco MH, et al. The efficacy of azidothymidine (AZT) in the treatment of patients with AIDS and AIDS-related complex. A double-blind, placebo-controlled trial. N Engl J Med 1987;317:185–191. doi: 10.1056/NEJM198707233170401.

27. Richman DD, Fischl MA, Grieco MH, et al. The toxicity of azidothymidine (AZT) in the treatment of patients with AIDS and AIDS-related complex. A double-blind, placebo-controlled trial. N Engl J Med 1987;317:192–197. doi: 10.1056/NEJM198707233170402.

28. Fischl MA, Richman DD, Hansen N, et al. The safety and efficacy of zidovudine (AZT) in the treatment of subjects with mildly symptomatic human immunodeficiency virus type 1 (HIV) infection. A double-blind, placebo-controlled trial. The AIDS Clinical Trials Group. Ann Intern Med 1990;112:727–737. doi: 10.7326/0003-4819-112-10-727.

29. Volberding, PA, Lagakos SW, Koch MA, et al. Zidovudine in asymptomatic human immunodeficiency virus infection. A controlled trial in persons with fewer than 500 CD4-positive cells per cubic millimeter. The AIDS Clinical Trials Group of the National Institute of Allergy and Infectious Diseases. N Engl J Med 1990;322:941–949.

30. Concorde Coordinating Committee. Concorde: MRC/ANRS randomised double-blind controlled trial of immediate and deferred zidovudine in symptom-free HIV infection. Lancet 1994;343:871–881.

31. Panel on Antiretroviral Guidelines for Adults and Adolescents. Guidelines for the use of antiretroviral agents in adults and adolescents with HIV. Department of Health and Human Services. Available at https://clinicalinfo.hiv.gov/sites/default/files/inline-files/AdultandAdolescentGL.pdf. Accessed September 13, 2021.

32. De Cock KM, El-Sadr WM. When to start ART in Africa—an urgent research priority. N Engl J Med 2013;368:10:886–889.

33. INSIGHT START Study Group, Lundgren JD, Babiker AG, et al. Initiation of antiretroviral therapy in early asymptomatic HIV infection. N Engl J Med 2015;373:795–807.

34. TEMPRANO ANRS 12136 Study Group, Danel C, Moh R, et al. A trial of early antiretroviral and isoniazid preventive therapy in Africa. N Engl J Med 2015;373:808–822.

35. De Cock KM, El-Sadr WM. From START to finish: implications of the START study. Lancet Infect Dis 2016;16:13–14.

36. Deeks SG, Anchen N, Cannon C, et al. Research priorities for an HIV cure: International AIDS Society Global Scientific Strategy 2021. Nature Medicine 2021;27:2085-2098.

37. Brown TR. I am the Berlin patient: a personal reflection. AIDS Res Hum Retroviruses 2015;31:2–3. doi: 10.1089/aid.2014.0224.

38. Gupta RK, Peppa D, Hill AL, et al. Evidence for HIV-1 cure after CCR5Δ32/Δ32 allogeneic haemopoietic stem-cell transplantation 30 months post analytical treatment interruption: a case report. Lancet HIV 2020;7:e340–e347.

39. Hsu JM, Van Besien K, Glesby JM, et al. HIV-remission with CCR5Δ32Δ32 haplocord transplant in a US woman: IMPAACT P1007. Abstract 65. Conference on Retroviruses and Opportunistic Infections (CROI), February 12–16, 2022.

40. CDC. HIV/AIDS prevention research synthesis project. Compendium of evidence-based interventions and best practices for HIV prevention. Available at https://www.cdc.gov/hiv/research/interventionresearch/compendium/index.html.   Accessed September 13, 2021.

41. Connor EM, Sperling RS, Gelber R, et al. Reduction of maternal-infant transmission of human immunodeficiency virus type 1 with zidovudine treatment. N Engl J Med 1994;331:1173–1180.

42. Janssen RS, Holtgrave DR, Valdiserri RO, Shepherd M, Gayle HD, De Cock KM. The serostatus approach to fighting the HIV epidemic: prevention strategies for HIV-infected individuals. Am J Public Health 2001;91:1019–1024.

43. Montaner JS, Hogg R, Wood E, Kerr T, Tyndall M, Levy AR, Harrigan PR. The case for expanding access to highly active antiretroviral therapy to curb the growth of the HIV epidemic. Lancet 2006;368:531–536. doi: 10.1016/S0140-6736(06)69162-9.

44. Granich RM, Gilks CF, Dye C, De Cock KM, Williams BG. Universal voluntary HIV testing with immediate antiretroviral therapy as a strategy for elimination of HIV transmission: a mathematical model. Lancet 2009;373:48–57. doi: 10.1016/S0140-6736(08)61697-9.

45. Dieffenbach CW, Fauci AS. Universal voluntary testing and treatment for prevention of HIV transmission. JAMA 2009;301:2380–2382.

46. Cohen MS, Chen YQ, McCauley M, et al. Prevention of HIV-1 infection with early antiretroviral therapy. N Engl J Med 2011;365:493–505. doi: 10.1056/NEJMoa1105243.

47. Donnell D, Baeten JM, Kiarie J, et al. Heterosexual HIV-1 transmission after initiation of antiretroviral therapy: a prospective cohort analysis. Lancet 2010;375:2092–2098. doi: 10.1016/S0140-6736(10)60705-2.

48. Abdool Karim SS, Abdool Karim Q. Antiretroviral prophylaxis: a defining moment in HIV control. Lancet 2011;378:e23–e25.

49. Dabis F, Newell ML, Hirschel B. HIV drugs for treatment, and for prevention. Lancet 2010;375:2056–2057. doi: 10.1016/S0140-6736(10)60838-0.

50. Iwuji CC, Orne-Gliemann J, Larmarange J, et al. Universal test and treat and the HIV epidemic in rural South Africa: a phase 4, open-label, community cluster randomised trial. Lancet HIV 2018;5:e116–e125. doi: 10.1016/S2352-3018(17)30205-9.

51. Makhema J, Wirth KE, Pretorius Holme M, et al. Universal testing, expanded treatment, and incidence of HIV infection in Botswana. N Engl J Med 2019;381:230–242. doi: 10.1056/NEJMoa1812281.

52. Havlir DV, Balzer LB, Charlebois ED, et al. HIV testing and treatment with the use of a community health approach in rural Africa. N Engl J Med 2019;381:219–229. doi: 10.1056/NEJMoa1809866.

53. Hayes RJ, Donnell D, Floyd S, et al. Effect of universal testing and treatment on HIV Incidence—HPTN 071 (PopART). N Engl J Med 2019;381:207–218. doi: 10.1056/NEJMoa1814556.

54. UNAIDS. 90-90-90. An ambitious treatment target to help end the AIDS epidemic. Geneva, Switzerland; 2014.

55. Havlir D, Lockman S, Ayles H, et al. What do the Universal Test and Treat trials tell us about the path to HIV epidemic control? J Int AIDS Soc 2020;23:e25455. doi: 10.1002/jia2.25455.

56. Eisinger RW, Dieffenbach CW, Fauci AS. HIV viral load and transmissibility of HIV infection: undetectable equals untransmittable. JAMA 2019;321:451–452. doi: 10.1001/jama.2018.21167.

57. De Cock KM, Fowler MG, Mercier E, et al. Prevention of mother-to-child HIV transmission in resource-poor countries: translating research into policy and practice. JAMA 2000;283:1175–1182. doi: 10.1001/jama.283.9.1175.

58. Wiktor SZ, Ekpini E, Karon JM, Nkengasong J, et al. Short-course oral zidovudine for prevention of mother-to-child transmission of HIV-1 in Abidjan, Côte d'Ivoire: a randomised trial. Lancet 1999;353:781–785.

59. Dabis F, Msellati P, Meda N, et al. 6-month efficacy, tolerance, and acceptability of a short regimen of oral zidovudine to reduce vertical transmission of HIV in breastfed children in Côte d'Ivoire and Burkina Faso: a double-blind placebo-controlled multicentre trial. DITRAME Study Group. DIminution De La Transmission Mère-Enfant. Lancet 1999;353:786–792.

60. Shaffer N, Chuachuuwong R, Mock PA, et al. Short course zidovudine for perinatal HIV-1 transmission in Bangkok, Thailand: a randomized controlled trial. Lancet 1999;353:773–780.

61. Petra Study Team. Efficacy of three short-course regimens of zidovudine and lamivudine in preventing early and late transmission of HIV-1 from mother to child in Tanzania, South Africa, and Uganda (Petra study): a randomised, double-blind, placebo-controlled trial. Lancet 2002;359:1178–1186.

62. Guay LA, Musoke P, Fleming T, et al. Intrapartum and neonatal single-dose nevirapine compared with zidovudine for prevention of mother-to-child transmission of HIV-1 in Kampala, Uganda: HIVNET 012 randomised trial. Lancet. 1999;354:795–802.

63. Kourtis AP, Bulterys M. Eds. Human immunodeficiency virus type 1 (HIV-1) and breastfeeding. Science, research advances, and policy. Springer, 2012.

64. Nduati R, John G, Mbori-Ngacha D, et al. Effect of breastfeeding and formula feeding on transmission of HIV-1: a randomized clinical trial. JAMA 2000;283:1167–1174. doi: 10.1001/jama.283.9.1167.

65. Thomas TK, Masaba R, Borkowf CB, et al. Triple-antiretroviral prophylaxis to prevent mother-to-child HIV transmission through breastfeeding—the Kisumu Breastfeeding Study, Kenya: a clinical trial. PLoS Med 2011;8:e1001015. doi:10.1371/journal.pmed.1001015.

66. Kesho Bora Study Group, de Vincenzi I. Triple antiretroviral compared with zidovudine and single-dose nevirapine prophylaxis during pregnancy and breastfeeding for prevention of mother-to-child transmission of HIV-1 (Kesho Bora study): a randomised controlled trial. Lancet Infect Dis 2011;11:171–180.

67. WHO. Antiretroviral drugs for treating pregnant women and preventing HIV infection in infants: recommendations for a public health approach (2010 version).
Geneva: World Health Organization; 2010.

68. Schouten PEJ, Jahn A, Midiani D, et al. Prevention of mother-to-child transmission of
HIV and the health-related Millennium Development Goals: time for a public health
approach. Lancet 2011;378: 282–284.

69. Cohn J, Owiredu MN, Taylor MM, et al. Eliminating mother-to-child transmission of
human immunodeficiency virus, syphilis and hepatitis B in sub-Saharan Africa. Bull
World Health Organ 2021;99:287–295.

70. Caitlin E. Kennedy CE, Yeh PT, Pandey S, Betran AP, Narasimhan M. Elective cesarean section for women living with HIV: a systematic review of risks and benefits.
AIDS 2017;31:1579–1591.

71. Fowler MG, Qin M, Fiscus SA, et al. Benefits and risks of antiretroviral therapy
for perinatal HIV prevention. N Engl J Med 2016;375:1726–1737. doi: 10.1056/
NEJMoa1511691.

72. Abdool Karim Q, Abdool Karim SS, Frohlich JA, et al. Effectiveness and safety of
tenofovir gel, an antiretroviral microbicide, for the prevention of HIV infection in
women. Science 2010;329:1168–1174.

73. Baeten JM, Palanee-Phillips T, Brown ER, et al. Use of a vaginal ring containing
dapivirine for HIV-1 prevention in women. N Engl J Med 2016;375:2121–2132.

74. Nel A, van Niekerk N, Kapiga S, et al. Safety and efficacy of a dapivirine vaginal ring
for HIV prevention in women. N Engl J Med 2016;375:2133–2143.

75. Singh JA, Mills EJ. The abandoned trials of pre-exposure prophylaxis for HIV: what
went wrong? PLoS Med 2005;2(9):e234.

76. Grant RM, Lama JR, Anderson PL, et al. Preexposure chemoprophylaxis for HIV prevention in men who have sex with men. N Engl J Med 2010;363:2587–2599.

77. Cáceres CF, Mayer KH, Baggaley R, O'Reilly KR. PrEP implementation science: state-
of-the-art and research agenda. J Int AIDS Soc 2015;18(Suppl 3):20527. doi: 10.7448/
IAS.18.4.20527.

78. Chou R, Evans C, Hoverman A, et al. Preexposure prophylaxis for the prevention of
HIV infection. Evidence report and systematic review for the US Preventive Services
Task Force. JAMA 2019;321:2214–2230.

79. CDC. US Public Health Service: Preexposure prophylaxis for the prevention of HIV
infection in the United States—2017 update: a clinical practice guideline. Available at
https://www.cdc.gov/hiv/pdf/risk/prep/cdc-hiv-prep-guidelines-2017.pdf. Accessed
August 22, 2021.

80. Choopanya K, Martin M, Suntharasamai P, et al. Antiretroviral prophylaxis for
HIV infection in injecting drug users in Bangkok, Thailand (the Bangkok Tenofovir
Study): a randomised, double-blind, placebo-controlled phase 3 trial. Lancet
2013;381:2083–2090. doi: 10.1016/S0140-6736(13)61127-7.

81. Landovitz RJ, Donnell D, Clement ME, et al. Cabotegravir for HIV prevention in cisgender men and transgender women. N Engl J Med 2021;385:595–608.
doi:10.1056/NEJMoa2101016.

82. Eshleman SH, Fogel JM, Piwowar-Manning E, et al. Characterization of human
immunodeficiency virus (HIV) infections in women who received injectable

cabotegravir or tenofovir disoproxil fumarate/emtricitabine for HIV prevention: HPTN 084 [published online ahead of print, 2022 Mar 18]. J Infect Dis 2022;jiab576. doi:10.1093/infdis/jiab576.

83. Donnell D, Gao F, Hughes J, et al. Counterfactual estimation of CAB-LA efficacy against placebo using external trials. Abstract 86. Conference on Retroviruses and Opportunistic Infections (CROI), February 12–16, 2022.

84. Grulich AE, Guy R, Amin J, et al. Population-level effectiveness of rapid, targeted, high-coverage roll-out of HIV pre-exposure prophylaxis in men who have sex with men: the EPIC-NSW prospective cohort study. Lancet HIV 2018;11:e629–e637. doi: 10.1016/S2352-3018(18)30215-7.

85. Nwokolo N, Hill A, McOwan A, Pozniak A. Rapidly declining HIV infection in MSM in central London. Lancet HIV 2017;4:e482–e483. doi: 10.1016/S2352-3018(17)30181-9.

86. Esparza J. A brief history of the global effort to develop a preventive HIV vaccine. Vaccine 2013;31:3502–3518.

87. NIH. HIV vaccine candidate does not sufficiently protect women against HIV infection. News releases, August 31, 2021. https://www.nih.gov/news-events/news-releases/hiv-vaccine-candidate-does-not-sufficiently-protect-women-against-hiv-infection

88. Buchbinder SP, Mehrotra DV, Duerr A, et al. Efficacy assessment of a cell-mediated immunity HIV-1 vaccine (the Step Study): a double-blind, randomised, placebo-controlled, test-of-concept trial. Lancet 2008;372:1881–1893. doi: 10.1016/S0140-6736(08)61591-3.

89. Rerks-Ngarm S, Pitisuttithum P, Nitayaphan S, et al. Vaccination with ALVAC and AIDSVAX to prevent HIV-1 Infection in Thailand. N Engl J Med 2009;361:2209–2220.

90. Desrosiers RC. Protection against HIV acquisition in the RV144 trial. J Virol 2017;91:e00905-17. https://doi.org/10.1128/JVI.00905-17.

91. Gray GE, Bekker LG, Laher F, et al. Vaccine efficacy of ALVAC-HIV and bivalent subtype C gp120-MF59 in adults. N Engl J Med 2021;384:1089–1100. doi:10.1056/NEJMoa2031499.

92. Resource Tracking for HIV Prevention Research & Development Working Group. HIV Prevention Research & Development Investments. https://www.hivresourcetracking.org/

93. Corey L, Gilbert PB, Juraska M, et al. Two randomized trials of neutralizing antibodies to prevent HIV-1 acquisition. N Engl J Med 2021:384(11):1003–1014. doi:10.1056/NEJMoa2031738.

94. Alcena V. AIDS in third world countries. NY State J Med 1986;86:446.

95. Fink AJ. A possible explanation for heterosexual male infection with AIDS. New Engl J Med 1986;315:1167.

96. Bongaarts J, Reining P, Way P, Conant F. The relationship between male circumcision and HIV infection in African populations. AIDS 1989;3:373-377.

97. Simonsen JN, Cameron DW, Gakinya MN, et al. Human immunodeficiency virus infection among men with sexually transmitted diseases. Experience from a center in Africa. N Engl J Med 1988;319:274–278. doi: 10.1056/NEJM198808043190504.

98. Cameron DW, Simonsen JN, D'Costa LJ, et al. Female to male transmission of human immunodeficiency virus type 1: risk factors for seroconversion in men. Lancet 1989;2:403–407. doi: 10.1016/s0140-6736(89)90589-8.

99. Diallo MO, Ackah AN, Lafontaine MF, et al. HIV-1 and HIV-2 infections in men attending sexually transmitted disease clinics in Abidjan, Côte d'Ivoire. AIDS 1992;6:581–585. doi: 10.1097/00002030-199206000-00010.

100. Auvert B, Buvé A, Lagarde E. Male circumcision and HIV infection in four cities in sub-Saharan Africa. AIDS 2001;15(Suppl):S31–S40. doi: 10.1097/00002030-200108004-00004.

101. Weiss HA, Quigley MA, Hayes RJ. Male circumcision and risk of HIV infection in sub-Saharan Africa: a systematic review and meta-analysis. AIDS 2000;14:2361–2370.

102. Auvert B, Taljaard D, Lagarde E, Sobngwi-Tambekou J, Sitta M, Puren A. Randomized, controlled intervention trial of male circumcision for reduction of HIV infection risk: the ANRS 1265 trial. Plos Medicine 2005;2:1112–1122.

103. Bailey RC, Moses S, Parker CB, Agot K, Maclean I, Krieger JN, et al. Male circumcision for HIV prevention in young men in Kisumu, Kenya: a randomised controlled trial. Lancet 2007;369:643–656.

104. Gray RH, Kigozi G, Serwadda D, et al. Male circumcision for HIV prevention in men in Rakai, Uganda: a randomised trial. Lancet 2007;369:657–666.

105. Yuan T, Fitzpatrick T, Ko NY, et al. Circumcision to prevent HIV and other sexually transmitted infections in men who have sex with men: a systematic review and meta-analysis of global data. Lancet Global Health 2019;7:e436–e47.

106. Pintye J et al. Benefits of male circumcision for MSM: evidence for action. Lancet Global Health 2019;7:e388–e389.

107. Evatt BL. The tragic history of AIDS in the hemophilia population, 1982–1984. J Thromb Haemost 2006;4:2295–2301.

108. McDougal JS, Martin LS, Cort SP, Mozen M, Heldebrant CM, Evatt BL. Thermal inactivation of the acquired immunodeficiency syndrome virus, human T lymphotropic virusIII/lymphadenopathy associated virus, with special reference to antihemophilic factor. J Clin Invest 1985;76:875–877.

109. CDC. Update: acquired immunodeficiency syndrome (AIDS) in persons with hemophilia. MMWR Morb Mortal Wkly Rep 1984;33:589–591.

110. White GC. Hemophilia: an amazing 35-year journey from the depths of HIV to the threshold of cure. Trans Am Clin Climatol Assoc 2010;121:61–75.

111. Feldman E, Bayer R, Eds. Blood feuds: AIDS, blood, and the politics of medical disaster. New York: Oxford University Press; 1999.

112. Harden VA. AIDS at thirty. A history. Washington, DC: Potomac Books; 2012.

113. Moore A, Herrera G, Nyamongo J, et al. Estimated risk of HIV transmission by blood transfusion in Kenya. Lancet 2001;358:657–660. doi: 10.1016/S0140-6736(01)05783-X.

114. Lackritz EM, Campbell CC, Ruebush TK 2nd, et al. Effect of blood transfusion on survival among children in a Kenyan hospital. Lancet 1992;340:524–528. doi: 10.1016/0140-6736(92)91719-o.

115. Basavaraju SV, Mwangi J, Nyamongo J, et al. Reduced risk of transfusion-transmitted HIV in Kenya through centrally co-ordinated blood centres, stringent donor selection and effective p24 antigen-HIV antibody screening. Vox Sang 2010;99:212–219. doi: 10.1111/j.1423-0410.2010.01340.x.

116. FDA. Revised recommendations for reducing the risk of human immunodeficiency virus transmission by blood and blood products. Guidance for industry. Available at https://www.fda.gov/media/92490/download. Accessed August 22, 2021.

117. CDC. HIV transmission through transfusion—Missouri and Colorado, 2008. MMWR Morbid Mortal Wkly Rep 2010;59;1335–1339.

118. Fleming DT, Wasserheit JN. From epidemiological synergy to public health policy and practice: the contribution of other sexually transmitted diseases to sexual transmission of HIV infection. Sex Transm Infect 1999;75:3–17. doi: 10.1136/sti.75.1.3.

119. Grosskurth H, Todd J, Mwijarubi E, et al. Impact of improved treatment of sexually transmitted diseases on HIV infection in rural Tanzania: randomised controlled trial. Lancet 1995;346:530–536.

120. Wawer MJ, Sewankambo NK, Serwadda D, et al. Control of sexually transmitted diseases for AIDS prevention in Uganda: a randomised community trial. Rakai Project Study Group. Lancet 1999;353:525–535. doi: 10.1016/s0140-6736(98)06439-3.

121. Grosskurth H, Gray R, Hayes R, Mabey D, Wawer M. Control of sexually transmitted diseases for HIV-1 prevention: understanding the implications of the Mwanza and Rakai trials. Lancet 2000;355:1981–1987.

122. Celum C, Wald A, Hughes J, et al. Effect of aciclovir on HIV-1 acquisition in herpes simplex virus 2 seropositive women and men who have sex with men: a randomised, double-blind, placebo-controlled trial. Lancet. 2008;371:2109–2119. doi:10.1016/S0140-6736(08)60920-4.

123. St Louis ME, Levine WC, Wasserheit JN, et al. HIV prevention through early detection and treatment of other sexually transmitted diseases, United States. MMWR Morbid Mortal Wkly Rep 1998;47:1–24.

124. CDC. Sexually transmitted disease surveillance 2019. Atlanta: US Department of Health and Human Services; 2021. Available at https://www.cdc.gov/std/statistics/2019/default.htm. Accessed August 22, 2021.

125. CDC. Sexually transmitted diseases treatment guidelines, 2021. MMWR Morbid Mortal Wkly Rpt 2021;70(RR-04):1–187.

126. US Department of Health and Human Services. Sexually transmitted infections national strategic plan for the United States: 2021–2025. Washington, DC; 2020. Available at https://www.hhs.gov/sites/default/files/STI-National-Strategic-Plan-2021-2025.pdf. Accessed August 22, 2021.

127. National Academies of Sciences, Engineering, and Medicine. Sexually transmitted infections: adopting a sexual health paradigm. Washington, DC: The National Academies Press; 2021. https://doi.org/10.17226/25955.

128. CDC. Summary of information on the safety and effectiveness of syringe services programs (SSPs). Available at https://www.cdc.gov/ssp/syringe-services-programs-summary.html. Accessed August 22, 2021.

129. Wolf M, Herzig M. Inside Switzerland's radical drug policy innovation. Stanford Social Innovation Review. July 22, 2019. Available at https://ssir.org/articles/entry/inside_switzerlands_radical_drug_policy_innovation#bio-footer. Accessed August 22, 2021.

130. Aspinall EJ, Nambiar D, Goldberg DJ, et al. Are needle and syringe programmes associated with a reduction in HIV transmission among people who inject drugs: a systematic review and meta-analysis. Int J Epidemiol 2014;43:235–248. doi:10.1093/ije/dyt243.

131. WHO, UNODC, UNAIDS technical guide for countries to set targets for universal access to HIV prevention, treatment and care for injecting drug users. World Health Organization; 2009. Available at https://apps.who.int/iris/handle/10665/44068. Accessed August 22, 2021.

132. Peters PJ, Pontones P, Hoover KW, et al. HIV infection linked to injection use of oxymorphone in Indiana, 2014-2015. N Engl J Med 2016;375:229–239. doi: 10.1056/NEJMoa1515195.

20

CDC in the Modern AIDS Era

Kevin M. De Cock

The CDC of the twenty-first century is larger and more complex than the agency confronting AIDS in 1981, greatly increased in its workforce, organizational units, focus, and global reach.[1] Despite the breadth of its expertise, CDC's work in infectious diseases continues to attract the most attention, not least because these can rapidly threaten the health of the population at large and even national security. Although CDC has extended its global footprint—currently working in more than sixty countries—it remains primarily a domestic agency with the priority of protecting the health of the American people. And core to that mission, outbreak investigation and disease surveillance are key. These same activities—surveillance and response to new clusters of infections—remain central to CDC's current strategy for combating AIDS.

HIV and AIDS Surveillance and Case Definitions

CDC's early experience with case definitions and surveillance for AIDS is described in Chapter 3. Initially, surveillance was driven by the need to describe the extent of this new disease, define groups at risk, and determine its geographic extension. Once AIDS had been established as an ongoing, national public health challenge and not just a self-limited outbreak, surveillance served to monitor trends, guide prevention and other programs, and evaluate the impact of interventions.[2,3] Apart from the name itself, which comes from another era and has an admittedly jarring overtone of government control, one would expect the generally dry topic of disease surveillance to arouse little political or community concern. With AIDS, this was not so.

CDC epidemiologist Richard Selik (Chapter 3) continued to play an important role in later revisions of the AIDS case definition and surveillance

Kevin M. De Cock, *CDC in the Modern AIDS Era* In: *Dispatches from the AIDS Pandemic*. Kevin M. De Cock, Harold W. Jaffe, and James W. Curran and Edited by: Robin Moseley, Oxford University Press. © Oxford University Press 2023. DOI: 10.1093/oso/9780197626528.003.0020

system.[4] Meade Morgan (Chapters 3 and 11) was the lead statistician for these efforts and wrote code for computerization of the data, which initially was based on DOS. This system was maintained for many years after DOS had generally been left behind. A running joke in the surveillance group was that the DOS-based system was kept because CDC wanted to ensure "this Windows thing" was not just a passing fad; it was an example of the attitude "if it ain't broke, don't fix it," as well as an early indicator of national underinvestment in electronic public health data infrastructure.

The case definition that was introduced in 1982 served its purpose, but, with recognition that AIDS was the late-stage manifestation of HIV after years of infection, expectations and interpretations of AIDS surveillance changed. Persons with AIDS were recognized as having severe disability, relevant to provision of health care and other services and benefits. Deeper understanding of HIV pathogenesis and disease led to revisions of the case definition in both 1985[5] and 1987.[6]

The first revision was modest but, importantly, acknowledged the spectrum of HIV-related disease. Several additional conditions were now considered AIDS-defining if the person's HIV test was positive; a negative HIV test precluded an AIDS diagnosis and report. The 1987 revision was more extensive and complex. Indicator diseases were expanded, consideration was given as to whether they were diagnosed definitively or presumptively, and HIV test results were taken into account if available. Importantly, TB in an HIV-infected person was now considered AIDS-defining, but only if disseminated or extrapulmonary—both generally indicative of an impaired immune response.

By the early 1990s, CDC was under pressure to adapt reporting still further. Experts wanted their own special interest diseases to be AIDS-defining. Community representatives demanded to be heard. Women's health advocates contended that CDC surveillance missed conditions that affected HIV-infected women, such as pelvic inflammatory disease and cancer of the cervix. People of color and those injecting drugs argued that HIV in their populations was often associated with bacterial infections and pulmonary TB. CDC epidemiologists countered that surveillance estimates would not be substantially altered by such inclusions and wished to avoid endless pressure to further expand the definition of AIDS.

The problem with AIDS indicator diseases was captured in the very term—they were indicators of HIV-related immunodeficiency, but not a direct measure of immune function. Selik commented, "In the beginning, not only did we not have a test for HIV, even the tests for the immunodeficiency were not widely available. If they had been widely available at the beginning, we might have based the case definition solely on a test for immunodeficiency."[7] I recall a conversation with Jim Curran in the early 1990s wherein he mused on what surveillance would entail if, somehow, we could start again, but with updated knowledge. Perhaps the essentials to report would be persons infected with HIV; those immunosuppressed to a certain level; and those dying from HIV. Indicator diseases could be tracked if they were of public health importance in their own right, such as with TB.

An additional problem concerned widespread failure to distinguish between a surveillance system intended for public health and a disease staging system to be used for clinical management of individual patients. And, linkages with resources were at play. In the United States, access to social and health services for HIV-infected persons was sometimes predicated on whether individuals met the AIDS case definition. So it was that CDC undertook an extensive but controversial revision of the case definition in 1992 that became almost as much a political issue as a technical one.

The 1992 international AIDS conference was originally scheduled to be held in Boston but was switched to Amsterdam because of US restrictions on free travel of people living with HIV. Jonathan Mann played an organizing role. Activism was in the air, and this was still the time when some conference attendees displayed evident illness. CDC's Ruth Berkelman, who had been leading AIDS surveillance, was there watching senior staff member James (Jim) Buehler give a technical presentation on the anticipated case definition changes. Neither seemed to expect the activist criticism that engulfed the presentation, and Buehler looked stunned and dismayed that he, a forward-thinking epidemiologist, could be the object of such aggression. At home, CDC was soon inundated from all sides with political pressures, community inputs, letter-writing campaigns (Figure 20.1), and other attempts to influence how AIDS should be defined.

Key additions to the revised case definition that was published in January 1993 included cervical cancer, recurrent pneumonia, and pulmonary TB, all in the presence of a positive test for HIV.[8] Although focused on the United States, the discussions on case definitions also had international impact. Over time, CDC staff, including Selik, Buehler, myself, and others had turned attention to international practices for AIDS case surveillance.[9,10,11,12] The association of all forms of TB with HIV was especially important; not including TB in international case definitions for AIDS (many of which were based on

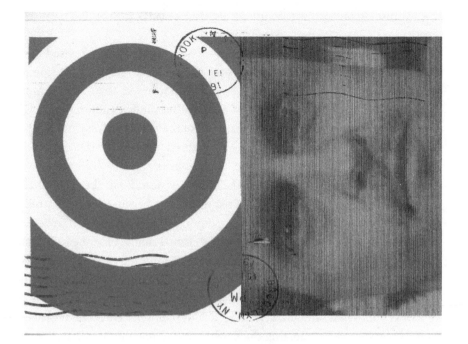

HEY CURRAN:
  We will no longer be placated by your use-
less meetings. We've already met with you
twice, demonstrated at your headquarters
and taken over your boss's office. Then we
exposed and shamed you at the Women and
HIV Conference. What does it take to get you
to act? For the last time, Curran, here's our list
of demands...

  • **WE DEMAND** that the CDC expand its
    AIDS definition to include the opportunis-
    tic infections that affect women including
    gynecological disease like cervical cancer,
    PID and vaginal thrush.
  • **WE DEMAND** that the CDC collect and
    interpret data according to routes of trans-
    mission rather than using the misleading
    and murderous "risk group" label.
  • **WE DEMAND** that the CDC document all
    modes of woman-to-woman transmission.
  • **WE DEMAND** that the CDC publicly and
    financially support the existence of anony-
    mous test sites that ensure the anonymity
    of those who choose to test.

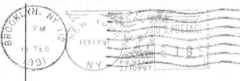

James Curran
Center for Disease Control
1600 Clifton Road N.E.
26 Executive Park
Atlanta, GA 30333

Figure 20.1. AIDS postcard, 1991. Thousands of these cards were sent to Jim Curran's home. (Jim Curran, personal collection)

the US case definition) was to miss the predominant cause of ill health and death in HIV-infected persons worldwide.

Perhaps the most controversial decision about CDC's 1993 revised case definition for AIDS, yet in some ways the most logical, was the inclusion of any HIV-infected person with a CD4+ cell count of less than 200/cu mm. Such persons were at high risk for PCP and other illnesses and required OI prophylaxis. On the other hand, at least half of them were still asymptomatic and living normal lives and may not have wanted to have an AIDS diagnosis or to be caught up in a national surveillance system.

Two further issues complicated the 1993 revision. First, the CD4 criterion hugely increased the number of reported cases because previously only people with indicator diseases had been reported. Expanding the number of reportable conditions certainly reduced the comparability of sequential data, but only to a limited degree because the most common manifestations of AIDS were already captured. Now, however, a surge of asymptomatic or only mildly unwell people were being newly reported. This made interpretation of trends impossible, and CDC was faced with the rather embarrassing need to interpret trends by adjusting the new reports to the old case definition so that "like" could be compared with "like." Second, the rest of the world did not go along with the inclusion of the CD4 count threshold as an indicator of AIDS. Other high-income countries that had largely followed CDC surveillance practice and guidance since the earliest days of the epidemic now parted ways.

The latest revision to the case definition, which consolidated a revision from 2008,[13] was made in 2014 after extensive consultation.[14] It amalgamated into one definition adult as well as pediatric definitions (not discussed here), eliminated the need to distinguish between presumptive and definitive diagnosis of specific infections, and clarified requirements for laboratory diagnosis of HIV infection, including with HIV-2 (Chapter 15). It also included guidance on HIV disease staging, all while emphasizing that the categorization and definition were intended for public health surveillance, not clinical care.

While scientific advances on the understanding of HIV infection played a major role in the evolution of AIDS case definitions, the advent of ART forced fundamental reappraisal of surveillance practice. Tracking HIV, and not just AIDS, was clearly necessary but was to be enormously controversial politically and socially.

HIV Reporting

In the mid-1990s, CDC established a new center to address AIDS, sexually transmitted diseases (STDs), and TB, a major organizational change consolidating multiple programs. CDC Director David Satcher appointed Helene Gayle as the founding Director of the new Center. Today, the National Center for HIV, Viral Hepatitis, STD, and TB Prevention (NCHHSTP) is one of CDC's largest Centers with about 1,700 employees and an annual budget of approximately $1.3 billion. In 1997, Gayle appointed me to oversee CDC's Division of HIV/AIDS Prevention—Surveillance and Epidemiology. When I sought advice from Curran, who had for several years been serving as Dean of the Rollins School of Public Health at Emory University, he commented that surveillance was perhaps the most important thing CDC did; decisions about targeting of interventions and allocation of resources depended on surveillance data, and only CDC was positioned to collect the required information. At least three quarters of the $100 million annual budget allocated for HIV epidemiology was devoted to various surveillance activities.

AIDS case surveillance, implemented and funded in all states and territories for active case finding, was extraordinarily complete and representative. The relentless progression of immune deficiency meant that virtually all HIV-infected persons would develop AIDS and come to the attention of public health surveillance. This gave a comprehensive picture of AIDS across the country and allowed detailed analyses of the essentials of descriptive epidemiology: time, place, and person. However, AIDS cases represented HIV transmissions that had occurred a decade earlier, reflecting the median incubation period for disease. An analogy was that we were looking in the rearview mirror as we tried to understand what was happening in front of us. The HIV epidemic was changing, with more infections in young people, more heterosexual transmission, and deeper reach into communities of color. AIDS case surveillance in the 1990s was reflecting what had happened in the 1980s.

An even greater and sudden challenge was the effect of ART. With rapid expansion of treatment, the predictable link between HIV infections and AIDS cases was interrupted. If AIDS cases declined, it was uncertain whether this reflected treatment access and success or reduced HIV transmission.[15,16,17] If AIDS cases increased, we would not know whether transmission had escalated, access had been reduced, or treatment had failed. CDC and the communities that depended on accurate data suddenly faced being unable to interpret HIV epidemiology and trends. For all these reasons, an absolute priority was to begin national reporting of HIV infection rather than just AIDS, and this was Gayle's charge to me as the incoming surveillance and epidemiology division director.

Within the division, our Surveillance Branch Chief was John Ward,[18] who had joined CDC in 1984 as an EIS officer working on AIDS. He recalled being told on arrival, "John, your job is to protect the nation's blood supply," and added that "At CDC, epidemiology is perceived to be a mobile skill, and you're to move around and apply it as needed."[18] The early 1980s were characterized by reticence regarding explicit wording of HIV prevention messages. Ward led a hilarious skit at the end of the 1986 EIS conference where a whistle or other noise replaced every potentially sensitive word in a message that would never have received official approval.

In October 1997, the New England Journal of Medicine had published an influential paper by Larry Gostin (Chapter 14), now at Georgetown University, Cornelius Baker from the National Association of People with AIDS, and Ward.[15] This unusual coalition of authors bridged different constituencies but together made the case for moving to nationwide HIV case reporting. At the time, twenty-six states required HIV as well as AIDS case reporting, but they accounted for less than a quarter of the nation's AIDS cases. They also did not include the cities with the highest AIDS numbers and most intense activism. Arguments in favor of HIV reporting were that the HIV epidemic would be viewed in real time, a more accurate burden would be measured, and prevention and treatment services could be better targeted, including for women and children. Funding allocations would be rationalized and no longer tied to outdated AIDS data.

The lightning rod for community opposition was what identifier would be used for reporting. Although AIDS surveillance had worked well and confidentiality of reported cases had been maintained, HIV reporting was viewed differently. Three themes lay behind the vehement opposition from communities. First, there was concern about stigma and discrimination if confidentiality of data, specifically people's names, were compromised. Many persons with HIV were healthy and working, and breaches of privacy could potentially threaten their employment. Second, some argued that people would be deterred from seeking testing and care if they knew their names were to be reported. And finally, there was a more visceral, unarticulated concern among HIV-infected people amounting to "I just don't want the government to have my name," despite privacy protections.

CDC was committed to protecting confidentiality but also had to prioritize data quality. Critically important was to avoid duplicate reporting of cases; for this reason, each case had to have a unique identifier. CDC epidemiologists felt strongly that names were essential to assure this accuracy. Many community members wanted codes for initial reporting, not names, and different systems were proposed. Some CDC staff, especially in our complementary AIDS division that funded prevention programs, felt conflicted or even opposed our intent. Curran warned me that CDC risked goodwill from the community and wastage of political capital if the agency insisted on HIV reporting by name.

Patricia Fleming, a PhD epidemiologist with strong connections in state health departments, succeeded Ward as head of the AIDS Surveillance Branch when the latter became editor of the *MMWR*. Under Fleming's leadership, community concerns were systematically addressed with study results and other data. Individual studies showed that HIV testing was not reduced where cases were reported by name. Evaluations of code-based systems and their comparison with named reporting showed the latter to be superior in data quality. Confidentiality of name-based reports was shown to be stringent. Anonymous testing was still widely available for persons who did not wish to be linked with official services or surveillance. Increasingly, community leaders came around to accept CDC's proposals.

I was surprised, late in the process, at the approvals required and intense scrutiny that our guidance document attracted. While this was ostensibly a technical publication, it was viewed almost exclusively as political at higher levels. With strong support from Center Director Gayle and her deputy, Ronald (Ron) Valdiserri, we submitted the document to leadership at CDC; then to HHS, including to Donna Shalala, the HHS Secretary; and to Sandy Thurman, Director of the Office of National AIDS Policy at The White House. All these steps required in-person presentations and discussion, reflecting greater than usual concerns about CDC recommendations.

I recall a final, tense phone call with Deborah von Zinkernagel, Deputy Director of the Office of HIV/AIDS Policy at HHS.* Numerous senior CDC staff were gathered around a speakerphone in Atlanta. When von Zinkernagel

---

* The Director of the Office of HIV/AIDS Policy at HHS was Eric Goosby, later Global AIDS Coordinator in the Obama administration (Chapter 22).

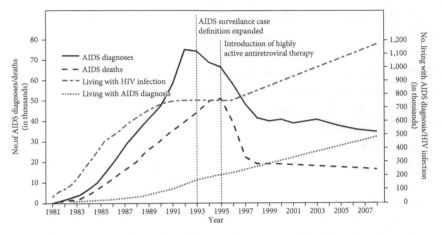

Figure 20.2. Estimated number of AIDS diagnoses and deaths and estimated number of persons living with AIDS diagnosis and living with diagnosed or undiagnosed HIV infection among persons aged ≥13 years—United States, 1981–2008. (MMWR Morb Mortal Wkly Rep 2011;60[21]:689–693).

asked for the specific language concerning identifiers, I replied that CDC recommended that HIV reporting be conducted by name. "That's not going to work," she said gently. After a moment's silence, I asked whether the word "advise" rather than "recommend" was acceptable. The final language in the document is "CDC advises that state and local surveillance programs use the same confidential name-based approach for HIV surveillance as is currently used for AIDS surveillance nationwide."[19] I refrained from commenting that the title of the *MMWR* series under which the document would be published was "Recommendations and Reports." With time, sensitivities resolved and by April 2008 all fifty states, the District of Columbia, and Puerto Rico had implemented name-based HIV infection surveillance without adverse consequences (Figure 20.2).

Ending the HIV Epidemic in the United States?

Depressingly, annual US incidence remained stable for many years at about 40,000–50,000 new HIV infections, despite a federal commitment of approximately $20 billion annually for combating the epidemic. (In comparison, the first *five-year* allocation for PEPFAR dealing with the global epidemic was $15 billion.) Key populations, especially MSM, accounted for the great majority of new HIV infections. The highest rate of new infections was in young, Black MSM. As mentioned in Chapter 19, a worrying separate epidemic, the opioid crisis, which started in the early 2000s, generated several outbreaks of injecting drug use-associated HIV and hepatitis C.[20]

The HIV epidemic also shifted geographically, moving more into the southern United States, including its rural areas.[21] Most strikingly, surveillance data in the second decade of the new century clarified the intensely focal nature of HIV transmission. Over 50 percent of new HIV infections were diagnosed in just forty-eight counties, San Juan (Puerto Rico), and Washington, DC. Another seven states had a substantial rural HIV burden. Clearly, prevention of HIV transmission needed to be focused on where HIV transmission was actually occurring. A theme of modern prevention emerged: to focus more sharply on disproportionately affected populations and local transmission sites, rather than on the broad categories of age, sex, race/ethnicity, and risk group by which traditional surveillance data were stratified.

In February 2019, President Trump made an unexpected announcement in his State of the Union address—a commitment to end the domestic HIV epidemic. A *JAMA* editorial published one month after the speech gave details of the plan.[22] The authors included the heads of NIH's National Institute for Allergy and Infectious Diseases, CDC, the Substance Abuse and Mental Health Services Administration (SAMHSA), the Indian Health Service (IHS), and the Office of the Assistant Secretary at HHS.[23] Reminiscent of the specificity of global aspirations set forth by the UN and PEPFAR, the domestic HIV elimination initiative had defined targets: to reduce new HIV infections by 75 percent by 2025 and by 90 percent by 2030. With commitment to these aims, the ability to measure progress would be essential, highlighting again the need for surveillance.

The influence of the global experience on the domestic situation was striking. NIH's Tony Fauci, the major spokesperson for the *JAMA* editorial, highlighted this, and CDC scientists published articles assessing US progress toward the 90:90:90 targets (Chapter 19) espoused by UNAIDS.[24] CDC estimated that in 2016, 86 percent of HIV-infections in the United States were diagnosed, 74 percent of persons with diagnosed HIV were in care, and 83 percent of persons in care were virally suppressed. For the United States, the "second and third" target estimates were lower than in some low- or middle-income countries.

The new HIV elimination initiative built upon the scientific developments over the past decade, particularly the therapeutic and prevention benefit of viral suppression through ART, the proven efficacy of PrEP, and the capacity for molecular detection of HIV clusters and chains of transmission. The strategic initiative was based on four pillars: to maximize early diagnosis of HIV infection; to achieve viral suppression in persons with HIV through ART as early as possible; to prevent new HIV infections, including and especially through use of PrEP; and to detect and curtail clusters of new HIV infections. An important determination of the initiative was to direct resources to the localities most heavily affected by HIV; as Jonathan (Jono) Mermin,[25] now overall director of CDC's HIV work, described it: "Put your money where your epidemic is."[26]

The initiative draws on the comparative advantages of the various agencies involved, including the Health Resources and Services Administration (HRSA), IHS, SAMHSA, NIH, and CDC. HRSA implements the Ryan White HIV/AIDS Program (Chapter 10), which supports more than half of the 1.1 million people living with HIV/AIDS in the United States. The IHS focuses on Native American populations who have long been medically underserved. SAMHSA provides expertise and services for substance users, including medication-assisted treatment programs, behavioral and counseling support, and, within existing laws or with special exemptions, needle and syringe programs for drug injectors. NIH provides advice and updates on scientific research to refine best practices.

CDC's role in the initiative is implemented through its traditional and most important national partners, state and local health departments and civil sector organizations. Increasing HIV testing and rapidly linking HIV-infected persons to care are primary objectives. The focus of the initiative on hotspots of infection and the emphasis on targets highlight the essential character of CDC as the "data agency" and its core institutional priorities of surveillance, monitoring of program impact, and epidemiologic investigations.

Surveillance in the Modern Era

The increased reliance on HIV case reporting evolved in parallel with an increase in electronic communications, explosion of social media, decreased use of printed materials, and greatly increased power of information retrieval. A cursory look at NCHHSTP's website shows the complexity of materials available, ranging from specialized scientific reports, including *MMWR* articles, to slide sets, infographics, pocket guides, videos, and other products.[27]

For HIV surveillance, the most important communication is the annual report, which summarizes data to the end of a calendar year and accounts for a twelve-month reporting delay.[21] Because HIV epidemiology changes slowly, data are presented for multiple years. The data remain extraordinarily comprehensive and cover all states, the District of Columbia, and six US territories, including Puerto Rico. The analyzed data are used by public health partners, academia, and others to monitor trends for policy formulation, program planning, allocation of resources, and communication and advocacy. They provide the roadmap for addressing the US HIV epidemic and reflect continuous efforts to identify sites and populations of active transmission. It must be accepted, however, that unlike AIDS case reporting, which is essentially complete by virtue of disease progression, HIV case reporting cannot capture the untested. Modeling is therefore used to extrapolate from reported CD4 test results and their distribution to assess the incidence and prevalence of HIV infections and the number that are undiagnosed.[28]

Surveillance data show the US epidemic is slowly declining, with just under 40,000 new HIV diagnoses reported annually since 2014, and HIV deaths dropping.[29] Almost four fifths of reported HIV infections are in males. The largest risk category remains MSM, who account for about 70 percent of reports; heterosexual contact is responsible for about a quarter of HIV infections. Although the proportion attributable to injection drug use is small, approximately 7 percent, there has been a slight rate increase in this transmission category since 2014. Drug overdoses nationally have continued to increase, approaching an annual figure of 100,000 for the year 2020,[30] all illustrative of the public health challenge of drug injection and its associated consequences, including HIV and hepatitis C, as described above. Surveillance highlights national inequalities: rates of HIV are highest in the South, and racial/ethnic minorities are disproportionately affected. Blacks/African Americans have rates of HIV eight times higher than Whites, and Hispanics/Latinos about three-and-a-half times higher.

An additional advance in CDC's recent surveillance practice is use of HIV phylogenetic data to recognize and address clusters, as highlighted under the US HIV elimination initiative. Persons with new HIV diagnoses routinely have specimens submitted for viral load measurements and antiretroviral drug-resistance analyses. The sequencing data from these specimens are submitted to CDC's surveillance system. Comparison of sequences allows construction of phylogenetic trees and identification of linked infections. This provides an important addition to standard partner services, which aim to identify at-risk contacts of infected persons, identify sexual or needle-sharing networks, and provide prevention and treatment services.

Phylogenetic sequencing has given insight into linkages between risk groups, clarifying, for example, the high proportion of HIV-infected women whose source of infections were MSM.[31] Phylogenetic sequencing can determine both who is in a cluster and the cluster size, allowing rapid follow-up to recognize infected persons as early as possible—important because of the high viral load and infectiousness during recent infection. Sequencing can also show that infected persons are not part of a cluster, which can save unnecessary investigations. Phylogenetic surveillance requires careful consideration of confidentiality and ethical issues. Directionality of transmission—from whom to whom—cannot be established with certainty from sequencing data alone, although affected communities have expressed concern about potential use of these types of data for criminalization of transmission from persons with HIV.

Social determinants, the social, economic, environmental, and structural factors that can profoundly influence health outcomes, are also gaining more attention.[32] So it is that people living within a few city blocks of each other can have widely different health indicators. Traditional surveillance stratification in the United States—age, sex, race/ethnicity, and behavioral risk—does not give full understanding of health disparities.

Concerning social determinants, CDC examined reports of adult HIV diagnoses in 2018 geocoded to the census tract level in relation to social determinant data from the US Census Bureau's American Community Survey. The five specific indicators examined were the federal poverty status, education level, median household income, health insurance coverage, and Gini index (a measure of income inequality). In summary, all measures of deprivation, including adverse educational levels, were associated with increased HIV reports, and these associations applied largely across race/ethnicity and transmission categories. Importantly, within income categories, differences by race/ethnicity persisted and were even more marked at higher levels of privilege. The results deserve wide communication and discussion and indicate how much remains to be done to understand and reduce health disparities across the US population.

HIV is a complex infection, and no single indicator adequately captures the state of the epidemic. Three approaches are applicable in general to all diseases: reporting of new cases, population-based surveys, and special studies. CDC supports all of these in various ways, including, for example, special studies of risk behaviors, youth, and others. Together, these studies and reporting systems describe the American HIV epidemic in more detail than for any disease anywhere in the world. The story told is one of inequality—inequality affecting risk and access, both more complex than just individual choice. The HIV epidemic will not be controlled without, first, the most affected populations having access to the most effective interventions. Other persistent barriers, including health disparities and stigma and discrimination across multiple levels, must also be addressed. And ultimately, addressing the epidemic must a shared responsibility between society as a whole and those most affected, especially MSM.

Epidemiology and surveillance have been foundational for understanding and responding to the HIV epidemic. Even as we must resist premature declarations of victory over HIV, there is ample evidence that the epidemic can be substantially contained. Surveillance, the conscience of any epidemic, as Curran tellingly described it years ago, will remain essential as the arbiter of our efforts.

Notes

1. CDC official mission statements & organizational charts. https://www.cdc.gov/about/organization/cio-orgcharts/index.html
2. CDC. Updated guidelines for evaluating public health surveillance systems: recommendations from the guidelines working group. MMWR Morbid Mortal Wkly Rep 2001;50(RR13):1–35.
3. Lee LM, Teutsch SM, Thacker SB, Eds. Principles and practice of public health surveillance. Third Edition. New York: Oxford University Press, 2010.
4. Selik RM, Haverkos HW, Curran JW. Acquired immune deficiency syndrome (AIDS) trends in the United States, 1978–1982. Am J Med 1984;76:493–500. doi: 10.1016/0002-9343(84)90669-7.
5. CDC. Revision of the case definition of acquired immunodeficiency syndrome for national reporting—United States. MMWR Morbid Mortal Wkly Rep 1985;34:373–375.
6. CDC. Revision of the CDC surveillance case definition for acquired immunodeficiency syndrome. MMWR 1987;36(Suppl 1S):1S–15S.

7. "SELIK, RICHARD," *The Global Health Chronicles*, accessed December 28, 2022, https://globalhealthchronicles.org/items/show/6869.
8. CDC. 1993 revised classification system for HIV infection and expanded surveillance case definition for AIDS among adolescents and adults. MMWR Morbid Mortal Wkly Rep 1992;41(No. RR-17).
9. De Cock KM, Selik RM, Soro B, Gayle H, Colebunders RL. For debate. AIDS surveillance in Africa: a reappraisal of case definitions. BMJ 19919;303(6811):1185–1188. doi: 10.1136/bmj.303.6811.1185.
10. Buehler JW, De Cock KM, Brunet J-B. Surveillance definitions for AIDS. AIDS 1993;7:S73–S81.
11. De Cock KM, Lucas SB, Coulibaly D, Coulibaly I-M, Soro B. Expansion of surveillance case definition for AIDS in resource-poor countries. Lancet 1993;342:437–438.
12. Diaz T, De Cock KM, Brown T, Ghys P, Boerma JT. New strategies for HIV surveillance in resource-constrained settings: an overview. AIDS 2005;19(Suppl 2):S1–S8.
13. CDC. Revised surveillance case definitions for HIV infection among adults, adolescents, and children aged <18 months and for HIV infection and AIDS among children aged 18 months to <13 years. MMWR 2008;57(No. RR-10).
14. CDC. Revised surveillance case definition for HIV infection—United States, 2014. MMWR Morbid Mortal Wkly Rep 2014;63(RR03):1–10.
15. Gostin LO, Ward JW, Baker C. National HIV case reporting for the United States—a defining moment in the history of the epidemic. N Engl J Med 1997;337:1162–1167.
16. Fleming PL, Ward JW, Karon JM, Hanson DL, De Cock KM. Declines in AIDS incidence and deaths in the USA: a signal change in the epidemic. AIDS 1998;12(Suppl A):S55–S61.
17. Fleming PL, MS, Wortley PM, Karon JM, DeCock KM, Janssen RS. Tracking the HIV epidemic: current issues, future challenges. Am J Public Health 2000;90:1037–1041.
18. "WARD, JOHN," *The Global Health Chronicles*, accessed January 29, 2023, https://globalhealthchronicles.org/items/show/7953.
19. CDC. Guidelines for national human immunodeficiency virus case surveillance, including monitoring for human immunodeficiency virus infection and acquired immunodeficiency syndrome. MMWR Morb Mortal Wkly Rep 1999;48(RR-13):1–27.
20. Lyss SB, Buchacz K, McClung RP, et al. Responding to outbreaks of human immunodeficiency virus among persons who inject drugs—United States, 2016–2019: perspectives on recent experience and lessons learned. J Infect Dis 2020;222(Suppl 5):S239–S249.
21. CDC. HIV surveillance report. Diagnoses of HIV infection in the United States and dependent areas 2019. https://www.cdc.gov/hiv/library/reports/hiv-surveillance/vol-32/index.html. Published May 2021. Accessed September 22, 2021.
22. Fauci AS, Redfield RR, Sigounas G, Weahkee MD, Giroir BP. Ending the HIV epidemic: a plan for the United States. JAMA 2019;321:844–845. doi:10.1001/jama.2019.1343.
23. Giroir BP. The time is now to end the HIV epidemic. Am J Public Health 2020;110(1):22–24. doi:10.2105/AJPH.2019.305380.

24. Hall, HI, Brooks JT, Mermin J. Can the United States achieve 90–90–90? Curr Opin HIV AIDS. 2019;14:464–470.
25. "MERMIN, JONATHAN," *The Global Health Chronicles*, accessed January 29, 2023, https://www.globalhealthchronicles.org/items/show/8126.
26. Author communication with Jonathan Mermin, 2021.
27. The National Center for HIV, Viral Hepatitis, STD, and TB Prevention. https://www.cdc.gov/nchhstp/.
28. Song R, Hall HI, Green TA, Szwarcwald C, Pantazis N. Using CD4 data to estimate HIV incidence, prevalence, and percent of undiagnosed infections in the United States. J Acquir Immune Defic Syndr 2017;74:3–9.
29. CDC. Vital signs: deaths among persons with diagnosed HIV infection, United States, 2010–2018. MMWR Morb Mortal Wkly Rep 2020;69:1717–1724. doi: http://dx.doi.org/10.15585/mmwr.mm6946a1external icon.
30. National Center for Health Statistics. Provisional drug overdose death counts. https://www.cdc.gov/nchs/nvss/vsrr/drug-overdose-data.htm.
31. Oster AM, Wertheim JO, Hernandez AL, Ocfemia MC, Saduvala N, Hall HI. Using molecular HIV surveillance data to Understand transmission between subpopulations in the United States. J Acquir Immune Defic Syndr 2015;70(4):444–451. doi: 10.1097/QAI.0000000000000809.
32. CDC. Social determinants of health among adults with diagnosed HIV infection, 2018. HIV Surveillance Supplemental Report 2020;25(No. 3). https://www.cdc.gov/hiv/library/reports/hiv-surveillance/vol-25-no-3/index.html. Published November 2020. Accessed September 22, 2021.

21

WHO and the Evolving AIDS Pandemic

Kevin M. De Cock

Few organizations are as misunderstood as WHO. Many expect it to be the ultimate guarantor of global health—controlling outbreaks, enforcing standards, collecting data—but that is not the organization the world created or pays for. My time as head of HIV/AIDS at WHO headquarters in Geneva from 2006 to 2009 gave insights difficult to glean from the outside. I grew to think that CDC and WHO were mirror images of each other, back-to-front opposites, where CDC was a technical organization whose work had political implications while WHO was a political organization whose work had technical implications.

WHO was established in 1948 as the specialized organization for health within the UN system,[1,2] with the objective of "the attainment by all peoples of the highest possible level of health."[3] Its core functions are leadership in global health; defining knowledge and gaps; setting norms and standards; defining health policy; providing technical support; and monitoring health trends. WHO advises rather than implements. It has neither the capacity nor the mandate to direct programs or investigate outbreaks; there is no "global EIS" program.

WHO is governed by the World Health Assembly, which comprises representatives of the organization's 194 member states. The Assembly approves WHO's policies, activities, and budget, and selects its director-general. WHO has six regional offices throughout the world, each of which have their own elected director and oversee individual country offices in their region. This three-layered structure, with regions largely autonomous from Geneva headquarters, resembles a confederation more than a single organization.[4,5] Many political and public health leaders today would agree that if we could start again, this is not the structure we would choose but also that if WHO did not exist, we would have to invent it.

WHO budgets are based on aspiration, not real money, and the organization is in constant fundraising mode. For perspective, CDC has

Kevin M. De Cock, *WHO and the Evolving AIDS Pandemic* In: *Dispatches from the AIDS Pandemic*. Kevin M. De Cock, Harold W. Jaffe, and James W. Curran and Edited by: Robin Moseley, Oxford University Press.
© Oxford University Press 2023. DOI: 10.1093/oso/9780197626528.003.0021

a congressionally guaranteed annual budget that is two to three times the uncertain one of WHO. Monies received by WHO come in two categories, "assessed" and "voluntary." Assessed contributions are like membership fees, fixed amounts that member states must pay and can be used as seen fit by WHO, but these resources account for less than one fifth of the organization's total funding. Voluntary contributions, from countries and other entities, often come with strict stipulations about how the money is to be spent. Fiscal uncertainty results in many staff being hired on short-term contracts, often to be renewed under the same adverse conditions of limited benefits and lack of long-term security.

Despite the complexities and bureaucracy, WHO has many talented and hardworking staff, committed only to trying to improve health across the world. And, too easily forgotten, especially when criticism reigns down in crisis, is who is ultimately in charge. The WHO we have is the WHO funded and directed, through the World Health Assembly, by its member states; at the end of the day, it is member states who control the money and define the WHO secretariat's leeway.

Mann to Merson

When Mike Merson succeeded Jonathan Mann as head of WHO's GPA in 1990 (Chapter 14), he inherited the headwinds already facing his predecessor. AIDS activities needed expansion at the country level, donors intended to work bilaterally with countries rather than through GPA (thus depriving GPA of some of its funding), and donors were demanding a program review. Merson worked to integrate GPA better into WHO's regular structure and to focus on epidemiology, research, and tangible programmatic interventions.[1,2] Merson provided sound management and strategic thinking and emphasized administrative order. Nonetheless, the turbulence around AIDS was too great for WHO to keep going it alone.

Continuous worsening of the pandemic, lingering resentments about internal WHO transitions, and skepticism about the impact of AIDS programs drove demands for change. UN and donor politics played their role, and criticism was levied that WHO's medical approach neglected broader social and development factors underlying AIDS. All these forces were to lead to a unique change in global health architecture: the creation of a separate UN organization to specifically address the AIDS pandemic.

Creating UNAIDS

ITM's Peter Piot (Chapter 13) had begun advising GPA when Mann was its director. Piot chaired GPA's Steering Committee on Epidemiology and Surveillance, which gave guidance, inter alia, on global estimates of HIV infection.[6] He later commented that early estimates for western Europe were too high, while those for sub-Saharan Africa and eastern Europe were too low. Piot, with a background in STIs, joined GPA full time in 1992, overseeing research and integrating the STI program into GPA's portfolio.

Relations between "AIDS people" and STI professionals were strained since the earliest days, analogous to later tensions between the HIV and TB communities. The resources and attention given to AIDS, while STIs languished in obscurity, fueled resentment. The STI community, including at WHO, saw HIV as another sexually transmitted agent and believed that only they had the required expertise. The classic STI approach was top-down, medicalized, and regimented. By contrast, the AIDS community felt that AIDS "was different," especially regarding community involvement and education, with its emphasis on prevention (including condom use). I remember Jim Curran saying that when he would be asked why HIV wasn't treated the same way as syphilis (referring to the emphasis on confidentiality and individual rights in the AIDS response), he would reply, "You mean just ignore it?"

Although Piot was respected by both the AIDS and STI groups, even he was never able to fully bridge this divide. STI control was important because STIs were shown to enhance HIV transmission.[7] A "syndromic approach" to STI treatment was introduced, defining major symptom categories, and advising antimicrobial treatment without laboratory diagnosis.[8] Unwittingly, this has contributed to lack of technical investment in the STI field over the longer term and to the development of antimicrobial resistance. Despite the evident links between the disciplines, the STI community never achieved the global influence that might have been expected in setting the AIDS agenda.

Tensions also existed across the UN. Other UN agencies, particularly the UN Development Programme (UNDP) and the United Nations Children's Fund (UNICEF), had begun their own independent AIDS work. UNDP believed that because AIDS was much more than a health issue, leadership rightly lay with them. Relations between UNICEF and GPA were tense around how to address the risk of HIV transmission from breastfeeding, which was an important component of child survival activities (Chapter 19).

Internal UN discussions and donor negotiations focused on how best to ensure interagency coordination. In July 1994, ECOSOC* passed a resolution to establish an interagency-cosponsored program with a strong secretariat, meaning WHO would not be in charge. Reasons, in addition to interagency rivalry, included lack of confidence in WHO, especially in its African regional office, and dissatisfaction with Director-General Nakajima. So UNAIDS was born, its formal title the "Joint United Nations Programme on HIV/AIDS." For the first and only time (to date), a new UN organization was established to deal with a single disease.†

The initial cosponsoring agencies were UNDP, UNICEF, the World Bank, the United Nations Educational, Scientific and Cultural Organisation (UNESCO), the United Nations Fund for Population Activities (UNFPA, now called the United Nations Population Fund), and WHO. Other agencies joining later, for a total of eleven, were the World Food Programme (WFP), the United Nations Office on Drugs and Crime (UNODC), the United Nations High Commissioner for Refugees (UNHCR), the International Labour Organization (ILO), and the United Nations Entity for Gender Equality and Empowerment of Women (UN Women).

Individual countries and interested individuals lobbied and campaigned for the directorship.[2,6] Ultimately, with support from donor countries and the cosponsoring agencies, UN Secretary-General Boutros-Ghali appointed Piot as the first executive director of UNAIDS. Governance of the new structure was through its Programme Coordinating Board, which consisted of donor countries, the cosponsoring agencies, and some NGOs. Neither the Programme Coordinating Board nor the newly appointed executive director of UNAIDS had direct oversight of the various agencies' activities and could only guide and coordinate. Administrative functions for UNAIDS, such as financial and personnel management, remained with WHO, which also housed the new entity on its Geneva campus. The intent to rationalize the AIDS response was implemented, but incompletely. UNAIDS, which became operational on January 1, 1996, had moral authority but not overall fiscal or organizational control.

* The United Nations Economic and Social Council (ECOSOC) is the UN's governing body. WHO is a specialized agency of the UN, so it falls under the ultimate (if remote) authority of ECOSOC.
† The UN Mission for Ebola Emergency Response (UNMEER) was a time-limited UN initiative to combat Ebola in Guinea, Liberia, and Sierra Leone. It was set up in September 2014 and closed in July 2015.

The End of WHO's Global Programme on HIV/AIDS

With the creation of UNAIDS, Merson returned to the United States and WHO left the AIDS scene. Donor funding for AIDS was diverted to UNAIDS, other UN agencies felt empowered, and "mainstreaming" and "the multisectoral response" became the *mots du jour*. Dismantling of GPA began and its staff dispersed, many to UNAIDS.[1,2] For much of the later 1990s only three professional staff at WHO headquarters were working full-time on HIV/AIDS, and WHO never regained overall leadership of the global AIDS agenda.

The early 1990s had been years of despair regarding AIDS and the response. WHO declared TB, including HIV-associated and multidrug-resistant disease, a global emergency.[9,10] The World Bank devoted its 1993 annual report to health, and highlighted AIDS, TB, and malaria as major obstacles to development in Africa.[11] Concern increased about heterosexual spread of HIV in Asia and the Caribbean. The results of the Concorde trial showing that zidovudine monotherapy gave no survival benefit (Chapter 19) furthered the sense of hopelessness.[12] But then, in 1996, abruptly, optimism replaced the terrible bleakness of preceding years.

Consistent with the presentations on the lifesaving impact of ART, the theme of the 1996 international AIDS conference in Vancouver was "One World, One Hope." [13] This immediately raised the question of how the benefits of this scientific advance were to be shared where needed most, that is, in sub-Saharan Africa. WHO did not initially engage in the question of treatment access, but for Piot and his nascent organization, it rapidly became the priority issue.

UNAIDS seized another opportunity by filling the void WHO had left regarding HIV/AIDS surveillance and epidemiologic estimates. Because no official body was now doing this work, like-minded public health researchers had formed a group called MAP, "Monitoring the AIDS Pandemic." This self-appointed, unofficial group, of which I was a member, would meet around major conferences, review available data, and then rapidly write a short report. This was for some time the only summary data concerning the world's then most important epidemic disease.

The MAP group met a few days before the international AIDS conference in Geneva in mid-1998. At the group's meeting, Bernhard Schwartlander of UNAIDS announced that his team had already generated a report on the global epidemic and would be publishing it under the name of UNAIDS, making the work of MAP irrelevant. The UNAIDS report received great media interest,[6] and Piot later recounted how he and Schwartlander shared a bottle of champagne to celebrate the international attention. Henceforth, UNAIDS prioritized its role as keeper of the data and generator of global reports, a role that it has maintained. I was at that time director of CDC's Division of HIV/AIDS Prevention—Surveillance and Epidemiology in Atlanta and was able to second Peter Ghys from Projet RETRO-CI (Chapter 15) in Cote d'Ivoire to UNAIDS as an epidemiologist. Ghys stayed with UNAIDS until his retirement in 2022, leading the influential and increasingly sophisticated epidemiology and mathematical modeling work extensively used for program design and funding.

The 3 by 5 Initiative and WHO's Return to AIDS

The issue that eventually brought WHO back to the AIDS table was treatment. Following the 1996 Vancouver conference, access to ART only increased as a topic of discussion. French President Jacques Chirac spoke at the AIDS in Africa conference in Abidjan in late 1997, proclaiming that the world could not tolerate *une épidémie à deux vitesses* (a two-speed epidemic), characterized by medicines in the global North but patients in the South. At the international AIDS conference in Durban in 2000 (Chapter 22), Edwin Cameron, a South African High Court judge and openly gay man living with HIV, spoke with devastating eloquence. "Amidst the poverty of Africa," he told the thousands of delegates, "I stand before you because I am able to purchase health and vigour. I am here because I can afford to pay for life itself,"[14] thereby recognizing the millions who could not.

Some statements by development officials seemed callous or out of tune with the changing environment. USAID Administrator Andrew Natsios said Africans would not adhere to therapy because of their inability to read a clock or keep to time.[15] In the early 2000s, I heard a senior health official from the United Kingdom saying she was "pro-poor" and therefore wanted money spent more usefully than on AIDS treatment.

A meeting I attended at WHO in 2002 focused on two questions: whether the world should take on provision of ART in low- and middle-income settings, which really meant in Africa, and if so, how to do it. Caution was understandable because of the potential for doing harm, specifically generating widespread drug resistance. Listening to the discussions, I concluded that there were three options: do nothing, start pilot initiatives, or go for global treatment. The latter was the only viable choice. ART would later be viewed as a disruptive intervention, as game changing as cell phones and leapfrogging earlier stages of development.[16] If people with AIDS could simply access and adhere to the drugs, they should survive. The Netherlands' Joep Lange (Chapter 15) famously argued that if it was possible to always find cold *Coca-Cola** or beer in the most remote African villages, then it should be possible to deliver medicines to the same locations.[17]

The target of having three million people on ART by 2005 ("3x5") was first discussed in a 2001 article published in the journal *Science* by Schwartlander and colleagues.[18] It was cited in WHO's first ART guidelines released in 2002; further raised by WHO Director-General Gro Harlem Brundtland, former Prime Minister of Norway, at the international AIDS conference in Barcelona in 2002; and committed to by Lee Jong-Wook (Figure 21.1) in his inaugural speech as WHO's director-general in 2003.

Widely respected and welcomed after Nakajima's unpopular tenure, Brundtland surprised the world by serving only one term as WHO's director-general. Lee, or "JW" as he was known, was a WHO long-termer from South Korea who was selected in 2003 following a brutal campaign against

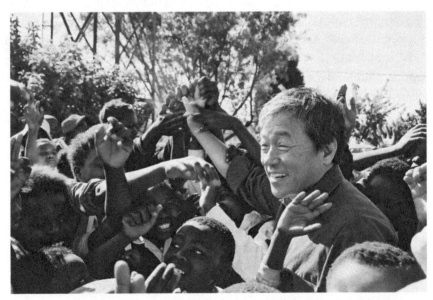

Figure 21.1. WHO Director General JW Lee in KwaMhlanga, South Africa, 2003. (WHO / Christine McNab)

UNAIDS Director Piot.[6,19,20] Although he was described in the media as "a little-known tuberculosis expert,"[21] Lee was a wily operator whose true ambition, it was rumored, was to be Secretary-General of the United Nations.

Useful ART pilot initiatives had been implemented since the late 1990s in various low-income countries, including in Cote d'Ivoire where CDC's investment in Projet RETRO-CI again proved its value. These efforts were supported by UNAIDS as well as by the "corporate responsibility" arm of Big Pharma.[22] Tense negotiations were held between diverse parties around intellectual property rights, drug prices, generic formulations, and parallel importing (the redistribution of products onto a global market to benefit from differential prices across the world). For its part, WHO included individual antiretroviral drugs in its influential list of essential medicines, instituted a quality assurance program for prequalification of generic antiretroviral medicines, enhanced capacity in procurement and supply-chain management, and kept an inventory of antiretroviral drug prices.

Lee's announcement of 3x5 was audacious, especially because consultation with other partners had been limited. The Government of Canada gave substantial funding, and a program was rapidly set up—large by WHO experience, small by the later standards of PEPFAR or the Global Fund. Perhaps the most important WHO contribution was development of the so-named "public health approach" to ART scale-up, led by the United Kingdom's Charles (Charlie) Gilks, that guided implementation of therapy without depending on laboratory capacity beyond HIV testing.[23,24,25] The initiative was first directed by Brazil's Paolo Texeira and then by Jim Yong Kim from Partners in Health, who later was nominated by President Obama to lead the World Bank.

The challenge of increasing access was steep: only 8 percent of people in need of ART globally were receiving it at that time. The initiative put WHO back on the AIDS map but was awkward for an organization whose prime functions are advisory, not operational. The greatest surprise about 3x5 was not that it went so badly but that it went as well as it did.[26,27,28] In the words of *The Economist*, what was achieved was not 3x5 but "1.3 by 5."[27] By the end of 2005, 1.3 million people were receiving ART, the target of three million being met in 2007. The experience was more important than the target, and WHO's technical guidance and advocacy for ART access had long-lasting influence.

An evaluation report for 3x5[28] was released in the spring of 2006, shortly after my arrival at WHO. The report included major recommendations concerning the need to strengthen health systems, especially human resources whose constraints were a barrier to increasing ART coverage globally.[29] The subsequent argument within WHO concerning the relative merits of disease-specific (vertical) versus overall capacity-building (horizontal) approaches—a longstanding debate in public health[30]—only became more fractious. Despite the difficulties, 3x5 gave legitimacy to global HIV treatment, which became regarded as a global public good, an individual right, and central to the long-term AIDS response.

WHO 2006–2009

My position as head of WHO's Department of HIV/AIDS in 2006 was the same position that Mann had started in 1986 (Chapter 14), though it now garnered much less authority. I was WHO's twelfth HIV director in the sixteen years since Mann resigned, indicative of the troubled environment. The World Health Assembly in May of 2006 was different from any other. Over the weekend preceding the Assembly, Director-General Lee collapsed at a meeting at the Chinese Embassy, never to regain consciousness.[31] On Monday, the Assembly started late. The Chairman announced that Lee, Director-General for just three years, had died from an intracranial hemorrhage. The usually orderly Assembly descended into chaos, facing the dual challenge of how to run the meeting and how to select a new director-general. I had spoken with Lee on only two occasions and had looked forward to following up on his outwardly genuine offer of meeting on a regular basis.

Shock and respect prevailed for an hour before naked politics took over. Anders Nordström, the Norwegian Assistant Director-General overseeing health systems work, was appointed acting director-general.[32] In a special election later in 2006, Margaret Chan from Hong Kong was elected to the definitive position, the first senior UN appointment awarded to China.[33] My last memories of that week in May were attending JW Lee's funeral in Geneva's Catholic cathedral. Jim Kim, who had served Lee faithfully, for his election campaign as well as for 3x5, was in tears.

When Chan began, she proposed a six-point agenda, focusing on development, health security, health systems, information, partnerships, and performance. A widely quoted, early remark of hers was "What gets measured gets done," an endorsement of the importance of surveillance.[34] She distanced herself from a disease-specific emphasis and recommitted the organization's support for primary health care. I sensed that organizational commitment to HIV post-3x5 was lukewarm and that my tenure might be lonely.

The WHO vision for AIDS post-3x5 was "universal access." A statement by leaders of the G8 countries who met in Gleneagles, Scotland, in July 2005 committed to "working with WHO, UNAIDS, and other international bodies to develop and implement a package of HIV prevention, treatment, and care, with the aim of as close as possible to universal access to treatment for all those who need it by 2010."[35] This goal was duly endorsed by the UN General Assembly.

Universal access required definition. Qualitatively, it meant that everyone needing HIV prevention and treatment services could get them. Somewhat arbitrarily, we decided with Ties Boerma, WHO's lead for statistics and informatics, that 80 percent coverage for treatment essentially meant unrestricted access. I asked Alan Greenberg (Chapter 15), now at George Washington University, to serve as an external advisor, and we structured departmental reorganization to meet the universal access goal around five themes: expanding HIV testing and counseling, maximizing prevention, accelerating treatment scale-up, strengthening health systems, and investing in strategic information.

Despite WHO's constraints, it also had unique strengths. Early in my tenure, Greenberg and I saw a powerful example of WHO's influence. The STI group at WHO had organized a meeting on the interaction between HIV and other STIs. Greenberg and I looked down from a balcony over a crowd of more than one hundred people gathered for coffee below. The group included some of the most eminent figures in HIV and STIs from across the world. "This is WHO's convening authority," Greenberg remarked.[36] When WHO invites, people come. Stefan Wiktor, another former Projet RETRO-CI director, similarly told me, "At CDC, we think we are. . . the real experts in all public health, but in many countries, it ain't real until they hear it from WHO."[37]

UNAIDS and WHO Collaboration

In theory, UNAIDS played a coordinating role and WHO a technical one, but these boundaries were often unclear. UNAIDS had over 750 staff, ten times greater than the number in WHO's HIV/AIDS Department. Frequent arguments from outside that both organizations faced were that weakness of health systems was the fundamental obstacle, and therefore disease-specific approaches were misplaced; that too much money was devoted to HIV/AIDS compared to other global health priorities; and that the global HIV estimates were exaggerated. Despite the challenges, WHO and UNAIDS engaged constructively on several technical issues with global impact including HIV epidemiology, male circumcision, and HIV testing policies, as outlined below.

Epidemiology and Measurement

Yves Souteyrand directed WHO's HIV/AIDS surveillance work and was responsible for an annual report on the health sector's progress toward universal access.[38] Data on the number of people on ART captured the lion's share of attention. This was apparent at a major infectious diseases conference in Washington in late 2008, where I shared a platform with Tony Fauci. By the time I spoke, at least four people, including Fauci, had shown the bar charts from WHO's report on treatment scale-up. I felt reassured we were serving a useful and unique function.

HIV/AIDS data can engender great controversy. Estimates of the number of people infected were initially based on extrapolations from sentinel surveillance in pregnant women, because the HIV prevalence in this sexually active group was considered representative of the general population. In Africa's generalized epidemics, however, women tend to have a higher HIV prevalence than men, for biological as well as social reasons. When large-scale surveys were conducted, HIV prevalence was generally found to be lower than indicated by sentinel surveillance.[39] Over the years, with improved methods and more data, global HIV estimates have been repeatedly revised.

At the end of 2007, the prior UNAIDS estimate of 40 million persons living with HIV worldwide was reduced to about 33 million, and the estimate of new infections almost halved.[40] We helped UNAIDS manage skepticism and refute accusations that data were "cooked" for advocacy and fundraising. A vociferous critic was the late Jim Chin (Chapter 13) who vigorously promoted his book claiming UNAIDS inflated HIV case numbers.[41] His criticism was especially hard because he had served as lead epidemiologist under Mann in the early days of GPA.

This collaborative experience with UNAIDS did not protect WHO from later controversy at a UN high-level meeting on HIV/AIDS in

New York in June 2008. It was clear to me that the world was divided into two epidemiologic situations concerning HIV. Southern and eastern Africa suffered self-sustaining, generalized epidemics, with heterosexual HIV transmission the dominant mode of spread. Outside of sub-Saharan Africa, HIV was largely restricted to key populations such as MSM, people who inject drugs, and sex workers and their clients. Large-scale heterosexual transmission of HIV had not occurred outside of Africa, including in the vast populations of Asia.

Prior to the 2008 high-level meeting, I was interviewed on the status of AIDS by various media. The United Kingdom's *Independent* misquoted and took my comments out of context, with a headline that read, "Threat of World AIDS Pandemic Among Heterosexuals is Over, Report Admits," with a subtitle continuing, "A 25-year health campaign was misplaced outside the continent of Africa."[42] Spin-offs from this headline reverberated around the world. UNAIDS colleagues considered me a pariah and called for my dismissal. WHO issued a press statement, I received incredulous emails, and criticism continued. Paul Delay from UNAIDS and I urgently wrote an academic piece for the *Lancet* putting this epidemiologic discussion into perspective,[43] but that hardly settled the furor, which only subsided with time. An important lesson was that it is not enough to be right—communication of the truth also must be managed.

Male Circumcision

Shortly after results of the East African randomized controlled trials of male circumcision were released (Chapter 19), WHO and UNAIDS cosponsored a global meeting to discuss implications. The focal point on this issue at UNAIDS was Cate Hankins, who until then had invested more in this topic than anyone in WHO's HIV/AIDS Department. A large constituency, including some within WHO, was hostile toward male circumcision, considering it an infringement of personal dignity and integrity. Strong feelings existed, clouded by cultural and religious perceptions. I had received a flyer the year before advertising an international conference on the human rights implications of male circumcision; I was surprised, not by the topic, but on seeing it was the sixth meeting on this subject. I recalled that Peter Piot, back in 1988, had caused controversy with an off-hand remark at the international AIDS conference dismissive of circumcision. This clearly was an emotive issue to be treated with caution.

Kim Dickson, a British public health physician, took up the mantle for WHO, strongly supported by the statistician Tim Farley and collaborating with UNAIDS' Hankins. Following the global meeting on circumcision, we recommended that it be adopted as an HIV prevention strategy in generalized, heterosexual epidemics.[44] We recommended focus on fourteen priority countries in eastern and southern Africa, where rates of HIV infection were high and male circumcision low. Noncircumcising communities and their leaders had to be persuaded. Although initial negative pronouncements by leaders like Zimbabwe's Robert Mugabe and Uganda's Yoweri Museveni were unhelpful, impressive scale-up has occurred.

This once-only intervention with sustained protective efficacy of about 60 percent is analogous to a partially effective vaccine against hetero- sexual acquisition of HIV by men. There is also indirect protective effect in women, given that surveys have repeatedly shown that female partners of circumcised men (whose HIV prevalence is lower than that of uncircum- cised men) themselves have a lower prevalence.[45] Mathematical modeling following the trials suggested that over a ten-year period in a high preva- lence setting, one HIV infection might be averted for every five to fifteen circumcisions performed.[46]

Programmatically, there should be consideration of increasing neonatal circumcision in high-burden countries, to increase coverage and acceptance of circumcision as a cultural norm. Questions arise on both sides about rights and consent—whether parents should have authority to decide on bodily al- teration of their children, or whether providing inherent protection against HIV should be considered not only a right but also a responsibility. Male circumcision is now an integral component of HIV prevention programs in Africa.

Provider-Initiated Testing and Counseling

Universal access to ART was impossible without greatly increased HIV testing but testing for clinical diagnosis was still communicated in the lan- guage of human rights, as if AIDS treatment did not exist. Well-intentioned protections against mandatory testing acted as a deterrent to testing of sick people, as was shockingly conveyed to me in London in late 1996 by an HIV- positive man with life-threatening PCP who came under my clinical care. He had been followed for over twelve months by clinicians in prominent hospitals and had undergone exhaustive investigation, but his advancing HIV disease failed to be diagnosed, not least because HIV testing was viewed as "different" and certainly not to be done as a clinical routine.[47] The inherent contradictions within UN language around HIV testing were well analyzed later in various papers by the sociologist Ron Bayer from Columbia University (Chapter 17) and colleagues.[48,49]

There had been an evolving but cautious change of attitude at WHO that acknowledged "the right to know" one's diagnosis.[50] At UNAIDS, the Reference Group on HIV and Human Rights held that pre-test counseling and informed consent for HIV testing were non-negotiable. Arguing that these requirements within medical care impeded diagnosis and treatment, thus costing lives, was considered offensive.[51] A colleague from my earlier work in Kenya, Elizabeth Marum, observed the paradox that we rightly rejected mandatory testing but enforced mandatory counseling. My comment that by failing to diagnose HIV in people presenting for care we were not protecting human rights but allowing people to die of AIDS was considered provocative. A fracturing of unity in the human rights community occurred as some leading voices called for new thinking. South African judge Edwin Cameron argued for normalizing HIV testing within medical care.[52]

In the United States the terms "opt-in" and "opt-out" had been widely used for testing in healthcare settings. "Opt-in" meant individuals had to specifically agree to be tested for HIV; "opt-out" that they had to decline, or testing would be performed as routine. At WHO, we introduced the term "provider-initiated testing and counseling" (PITC), reversing the order of the words testing and counseling, a minor victory, to emphasize that people needed a test result for personal and medical decision-making and that healthcare providers should implement the process.[53]

Ian Grubb, a gay lawyer living with HIV, was our department's senior policy advisor. He was initially skeptical but over months of collaborative writing we produced guidance stratified according to epidemiologic context, our major concern being to make clinical testing more routine in Africa's generalized epidemic. We emphasized that healthcare workers in these areas should routinely *recommend* (not *offer*) HIV testing to all persons attending healthcare settings and that patients could decline but did not have to specifically agree. In this way, clinical HIV testing was viewed similarly to other essential investigations. Individual counseling was not necessary, but information had to be provided.

We released draft testing guidance for public comment in late 2006 under the banner of both WHO and UNAIDS, with quiet support from Peter Piot and UNAIDS' in-house human rights legal advisor, Susan Timberlake. Members of the UNAIDS Reference Group were vocal in opposition, but the final document was published in 2007.[53] Other criticism followed. Bayer was somewhat scathing in assessment of the compromises reached,[49] but my colleagues and I felt that calling for strengthened protections for vulnerable populations like drug injectors in eastern Europe was needed. The main point was that the guidance allowed for greatly enhanced testing in clinical settings where HIV burden was highest and where HIV treatment was now increasingly available.

Two other developments persuaded me our course was right. In September 2006, CDC issued revised guidance on HIV testing in the United States after considerable consultation, some of which I had been involved with.[54] The CDC advice was broadly consistent with what our WHO document was recommending for generalized epidemics. Second, some countries, such as Kenya, Botswana, and Lesotho, had impatiently moved ahead on their own, so that WHO and UNAIDS risked irrelevance if we had not acted. Universal access would have remained a meaningless slogan if HIV testing in clinical settings had not been rationalized.

Test and Treat

Brian Willams and Christopher (Chris) Dye were experts in mathematical modeling at UNAIDS and WHO, respectively. Along with Charlie Gilks and Reuben Granich, the latter seconded from CDC, we debated ideas about the pandemic and potential responses that resulted in a publication that drew widespread attention. I had challenged Williams to develop a model to explain the extraordinary severity of southern Africa's HIV epidemic. Although individual risk factors are understood, the magnitude of the HIV disaster in southern Africa remains perplexing. Williams returned to say that he had instead modelled what it would take to extinguish epidemics.

The Williams model showed that if we could test everyone in an epidemic like in South Africa once yearly and then immediately initiate ART for those infected, transmission would be massively reduced and HIV-related disease and death would decline. Eventually, HIV-infected people would die from other causes without their infections being replaced. HIV prevalence would fall, and HIV/AIDS would be eliminated in less than fifty years. There were, of course, many practical caveats to this theoretical exercise that the *New York Times* highlighted as a welcome "thought experiment."[55] Our paper, released in the *Lancet* in late 2008,[56] attracted attention globally, but in Geneva things did not go well.

Our communications officer had shared the findings with a major press agency for World AIDS Day, without official clearance. UNAIDS, including its Reference Group, disapproved of the intensely biomedical approach the model considered and was irritated by the attention attracted. Director-General Chan and her advisors suspected we were simply out for media attention. At a meeting in Chan's office, senior officials seemed uncertain whether to be critical or supportive. With time, sensitivities passed and the concept of HIV treatment as prevention, continually raised over the years, gathered strength. Based on evolving science, international donors expanded their support for widespread and early diagnosis and treatment. Major research investment went into African trials of "test and treat" (Chapter 19). The several times I saw Chan in later years she always greeted me warmly saying, "You were right," while I always thought inwardly, "well, it was Brian Williams."

From Universal Access to the Sustainable Development Goals

Piot stepped down from his twelve-year tenure as UNAIDS Director at the end of 2008. At a small reception hosted by the cosponsoring agencies, I highlighted three of his contributions in particular: the annual epidemiologic reports that became universally quoted and the basis for decision-making; his judgment of when to throw the weight of UNAIDS behind ART scale-up, particularly for battles about drug prices and use of generics; and his success in bringing HIV/AIDS to the attention of the highest political levels globally.

I participated as WHO's representative on the initial search committee for Piot's replacement. The committee was chaired by Ambassador Marie-Louise Overvad from Denmark, who was surprised by the politics and diversity of constituencies claiming a stake in the selection process. UN Secretary-General Ban Ki-Moon ultimately appointed Michel Sidibe, Piot's longstanding deputy, a Malian and French citizen who had previously worked for UNICEF.[‡][57]

As science increasingly showed the prevention as well as treatment benefit from ART, a mood of perhaps excessive optimism began to take hold. Prominent figures such as Fauci wrote in nuanced fashion, but nonetheless suggested available tools were adequate to contain the pandemic.[58] Secretary of State Hillary Clinton declared that an "AIDS-free generation" was in sight.[59] Ambassador Deborah Birx, head of PEPFAR, said, "With the tools we already have, there's the historic opportunity—for the first time ever—to control a pandemic without a vaccine or a cure."[60] These optimistic assessments provided advocacy for high-level and sustained commitments but risked overpromising impact. A particular concern is that generalized assessments can overlook trends in key and marginalized populations.

As an agency of the UN, WHO activities are heavily influenced by global commitments such as the Millennium Development Goals[61] and the Sustainable Development Goals (SDGs).[62] The overarching aspiration of the SDGs was to eradicate absolute poverty by 2030. Within that framework, one aim of the only health goal, SDG 3, was to "end the epidemics of AIDS, tuberculosis, malaria and neglected tropical diseases."[62] Associated annual numeric targets were fewer than 500,000 new HIV infections globally by 2020, and fewer than 200,000 by 2030—declines of 75 percent and 90 percent, respectively, compared to 2010.

To support the quest for the SDGs, UNAIDS launched its "Fast-Track" strategy in 2014 with its 90:90:90 targets (described in Chapter 19),[63] later to be followed by respective 95 percent targets. Williams, my modeling colleague, participated in background discussions leading to this proposal, which initially was about advocacy as much as evidence-based targets. Achieving 90:90:90 or more, however, cannot be assumed to result in achieving the SDG-defined HIV incidence targets.

I left WHO in 2009 after almost three and a half years as HIV director. My replacement was the Austrian Gottfried Hirnschall, appointed after months of an acting position held by my deputy, Ethiopian Teguest Guerma. Hirnschall had previously served as HIV advisor in WHO's region of the Americas. He stayed in the director position until his retirement in 2019, thus becoming the longest serving HIV director since the creation of GPA

‡ Sidibe served as UNAIDS Director from January 2009 to May 2019. He was succeeded by Winnie Byanyima from Uganda.

in 1986. Under Hirnschall's leadership, WHO rightly focused on the scientific advances around ART (Chapter 19). Several revisions of WHO's HIV guidelines occurred between 2010 and 2016, the latter in a consolidated form bringing together prevention and treatment guidance for adults, children, and pregnant women.[64,65] The guidelines extended to operational issues such as introduction of self-testing, differentiating the intensity of monitoring required for different patients, and expansion of PrEP. Meg Docherty, who oversaw this work, followed Hirnschall as director of the HIV/AIDS Department. Hirnschall and Docherty also succeeded in integrating STIs and hepatitis into the department, with Stefan Wiktor and then Marc Bulterys seconded from CDC as technical advisors for hepatitis.[66,67,68,69,70]

Conclusions

Perhaps WHO's greatest contribution to the AIDS field today, started under 3x5, is the regular revision of HIV treatment guidelines that rapidly become accepted as best practice throughout low- and middle-income countries. Some of WHO's high-level functions, such as monitoring health trends or providing technical assistance, have become shared and sometimes largely taken over by other entities in today's crowded global health space. Chan's successor, Director-General Tedros Adhanom, has been supportive of WHO's HIV/AIDS agenda, even as his tenure has been dominated by discussions of universal health coverage, Ebola, and, more recently, COVID-19.

My last conversation with Director-General Lee in the spring of 2006, three weeks before he died, well describes WHO's difficult position. I asked him what he thought the future held, what kept him awake at night. His answer was characteristically half in jest but also serious. He reflected on how other organizations come and go while WHO would persist, and how people would continue to look to it for guidance, yet all the while criticize it for not delivering. His comments captured the ambiguous regard and unrealistic expectations the world has for this essential organization.

Notes

1. Cueto M, Brown TM, Fee E. The World Health Organization. A history. Cambridge, United Kingdom: Cambridge University Press; 2019.

2. Merson M, Inrig S. The AIDS pandemic. Searching for a global response. Cham, Switzerland: Springer; 2018.

3. International Health Conference. Constitution of the World Health Organization, 1946. Bulletin of the World Health Organization 2002;80(12):983–984. https://apps.who.int/iris/handle/10665/268688

4. Chow JC. Foreign policy: how to keep the WHO relevant. National Public Radio, December 9, 2010. https://www.npr.org/2010/12/09/131929167/foreign-policy-how-to-keep-the-who-relevant.

5. Chow JC. Is the WHO becoming irrelevant? Foreign Policy, December 9, 2010. https://foreignpolicy.com/2010/12/09/is-the-who-becoming-irrelevant/.

6. Piot P. No time to lose. A life in pursuit of deadly viruses. New York: WW Norton; 2021.

7. Laga M, Nzila N, Goeman J. The interrelationship of sexually transmitted diseases and HIV infection: implications for the control of both epidemics in Africa. AIDS 1991;5(Suppl 1):S55–S63.

8. WHO. Management of patients with sexually transmitted diseases. World Health Organ Tech Rep Ser 1991;810:1–103.

9. WHO. Tuberculosis: a global emergency. World Health 1993;46:3–31. https://apps.who.int/iris/handle/10665/52639.

10. CDC. National action plan to combat multidrug-resistant tuberculosis. MMWR Morb Mortal Wkly Rep 1992;41(RR-11):1–48.

11. Berkley S, Bobadilla J-L, Hecht R, et al. World development report 1993: investing in health. Washington, DC: World Bank Group; 1993.

12. Concorde Coordinating Committee. Concorde: MRC/ANRS randomised double-blind controlled trial of immediate and deferred zidovudine in symptom-free HIV infection. Lancet 1994;343:871–881.

13. De Cock KM, Churchill D, Grant A, et al. Summary of track B: clinical science. AIDS 1996;10(Suppl 3):S107–S113.

14. Cameron E. Witness to AIDS. Cape Town, South Africa: Tafelberg Publishers; 2005:110.

15. Committee on International Relations. The United States' war on AIDS. Hearing before the Committee on International Relations, House of Representatives, 107th Congress, 1st session, June 7, 2001. http://commdocs.house.gov/committees/intlrel/hfa72978.000/hfa72978_0.HTM.

16. De Cock KM, El-Sadr WM, Ghebreyesus TA. Game changers: why did the scale-up of HIV treatment work despite weak health systems? J Acquir Immune Defic Syndr 2011;57(Suppl 2):S61-S3. doi: 10.1097/QAI.0b013e3182217f00.

17. Yasmin S. The impatient Dr. Lange. One man's fight to end the global HIV epidemic. Baltimore: Johns Hopkins University Press; 2018.

18. Schwartländer B, Stover J, Walker N, et al. Resource needs for HIV/AIDS. Science 2001;292:2434–2436.

19. South Korea's Jong Wook Lee elected new WHO Director-General. Lancet 2003;361:399.

20. Benkimoun P. How Lee Jong-wook changed WHO. Lancet 2006;367:1806–1808. doi: 10.1016/S0140-6736(06)68787-4.

21. CBS News. S. Korean to head U.N. health agency. January 28, 2003. https://www.cbsn ews.com/news/s-korean-to-head-un-health-agency/.

22. WHO, UNAIDS. Accelerating Access Initiative: widening access to care and support for people living with HIV/AIDS: progress report, June 2002. https://apps.who.int/ iris/handle/10665/42550

23. WHO. Treating 3 million by 2005. Making it happen: the WHO strategy. Geneva, Switzerland: WHO; 2003. https://www.who.int/3by5/publications/documents/en/ Treating3millionby2005.pdf.

24. Gilks C, Crowley S, Ekpini R, et al. The WHO public-health approach to antiretroviral treatment against HIV in resource-limited settings. Lancet 2006;368:505–510.

25. Schwartländer B, Grubb I, Perriëns J. The 10-year struggle to provide antiretroviral treatment to people with HIV in the developing world. Lancet 2006;368:541–546.

26. Nemes MIB, Beaudouin J, Conway S, Kivumbi GW, Skjelmerud A, Vogel U. Evaluation of WHO's contribution to "3 by 5." Geneva, Switzerland: WHO; 2006.

27. Treating AIDS: 1.3 by 5. The Economist, April 1, 2006. https://www.economist.com/ science-and-technology/2006/03/30/13-by-5.

28. WHO, UNAIDS. Progress on global access to HIV antiretroviral therapy: a report on "3 by 5" and beyond, March 2006. https://www.who.int/hiv/fullreport_en_high res.pdf.

29. Samb B, Celletti F, Holloway J, Van Damme W, De Cock KM, Dybul M. Rapid expansion of the health workforce in response to the HIV epidemic. N Engl J Med 2007;357:2510–2514.

30. Stensland PG. Review: Health and the Developing World by John Bryant. Health and the developing world. Millbank Quarterly 1971;49:98–106.

31. Boseley S. Obituary. Lee Jong-wook. Lancet 2006;367:1812.

32. Brown H. New WHO Director-General to be appointed in November. Lancet 2006;367:1805. doi:https://doi.org/10.1016/S0140-6736(06)68786 2

33. Editorial. WHO 2007–12: the era of Margaret Chan. Lancet 2006;368:1743.

34. Address by Dr. Margaret Chan. January 22, 2007. https://www.who.int/director-gene ral/speeches/detail/address-by-dr-margaret-chan.

35. G8 Geleneagles 2005. Africa. https://data.unaids.org/topics/universalaccess/postg8_ gleneagles_africa_en.pdf

36. Alan Greenberg. Conversation with Author.

37. Stefan Wiktor. Communication with Author.

38. WHO, UNAIDS, UNICEF. Towards universal access: scaling up priority HIV/AIDS interventions in the health sector. Progress report 2008http://www.who.int/hiv/pub/ towards_universal_access_report_2008.pdf

39. Kenya Demographic and Health Survey 2003. https://dhsprogram.com/pubs/pdf/ FR151/FR151.pdf

40. UNAIDS. AIDS epidemic update: December 2007. https://data.unaids.org/pub/episli des/2007/2007_epiupdate_en.pdf.

41. Chin J. The AIDS pandemic: the collision of epidemiology with political correctness. London: Taylor and Francis; 2007.

42. Lawrence J. Threat of world AIDS pandemic among heterosexuals is over, report admits. Independent. http://www.independent.co.uk/life-style/health-and-wellbe ing/health-news/threat-of-world-aids-pandemic-among-heterosexuals-is-over-rep ort-admits-842478.html [first published June 8, 2008, online post dated October 23, 2011].

43. De Cock KM, DeLay P. HIV/AIDS estimates and the quest for universal access. Lancet 2008;371:2068–2070.

44. WHO. WHO and UNAIDS announce recommendations from expert consultation on male circumcision for HIV prevention. https://www.who.int/hiv/mediacentre/ news68/en/

45. National AIDS and STI Control Programme (NASCOP), Kenya. Kenya AIDS Indicator Survey 2012: Final Report. Nairobi: NASCOP; June 2014.

46. UNAIDS/WHO/SACEMA Expert Group on Modelling the Impact and Cost of Male Circumcision for HIV Prevention. Male circumcision for HIV prevention in high HIV prevalence settings: what can mathematical modelling contribute to informed decision making? PLoS Med 2009;6:e1000109. doi:10.1371/journal.pmed.1000109.

47. De Cock KM, Johnson AM. From exceptionalism to normalisation: a reappraisal of attitudes and practice around HIV testing. BMJ 1998;316:290–293. doi: 10.1136/ bmj.316.7127.290.

48. Oppenheimer GM, Bayer R. The rise and fall of HIV exceptionalism. Virtual Mentor 2009;11:988–992. doi: 10.1001/virtualmentor.2009.11.12.mhst1-0912.

49. Bayer R, Edington C. HIV testing, human rights, and global AIDS policy: exceptionalism and its discontents. J Health Polit Policy Law 2009;34:301– 323. doi: 10.1215/03616878-2009-002.

50. WHO. The right to know. New approaches to HIV testing and counselling. Geneva, Switzerland: WHO; 2003. https://apps.who.int/iris/bitstream/handle/10665/68131/ WHO_HIV_2003.08.pdf?sequence=1&isAllowed=y

51. De Cock KM, Mbori-Ngacha D, Marum E. Shadow on the continent: public health and HIV/AIDS in Africa in the 21st century. Lancet. 2002;360:67–72. doi: 10.1016/ S0140-6736(02)09337-6.

52. Cameron E. Normalizing testing—normalizing AIDS. Theoria 2007;112:99–108.

53. WHO, UNAIDS. Guidance on provider-initiated HIV testing and counselling in health facilities. Geneva: WHO; 2007. https://apps.who.int/iris/handle/10665/43688.

54. Branson BM, Handsfield HH, Lampe MA. Revised recommendations for HIV testing of adults, adolescents, and pregnant women in health-care settings. MMWR Morb Mortal Wkly Rep 2006;55(RR14):1–17.

55. Editorial. A breathtaking aspiration for AIDS. New York Times, December 1, 2008. https://www.nytimes.com/2008/12/01/opinion/01mon3.html.

56. Granich RM, Gilks CF, Dye C, De Cock KM, Williams BG. Universal voluntary HIV testing with immediate antiretroviral therapy as a strategy for elimination of HIV transmission: a mathematical model. Lancet 20093;373:48–57. doi: 10.1016/ S0140-6736(08)61697-9.

57. UNAIDS. Mr Michel Sidibé appointed UNAIDS Executive Director. https://www.unaids.org/en/resources/presscentre/pressreleaseandstatementarchive/2008/december/20081201prsidibeappointment.
58. Fauci A. An opportunity to end the AIDS pandemic. Washington Post, July 26, 2012. https://www.washingtonpost.com/opinions/anthony-fauci-an-opportunity-to-end-the-aids-pandemic/2012/07/26/gJQAurGKCX_story.html28.
59. The Office of the U.S. Global AIDS Coordinator. PEPFAR blueprint: creating an AIDS-free generation. Washington, DC; 2012.
60. Das P. Deborah L Birx: on a mission to end the HIV/AIDS epidemic. Lancet 2016;388:2583.
61. United Nations Development Programme. Millennium Development Goals. https://www.undp.org/content/undp/en/home/sdgoverview/mdg_goals.html.
62. United Nations. Department of Economic and Social Affairs. The 17 Goals. https://sdgs.un.org/goals.
63. UNAIDS. Understanding Fast-Track. Accelerating action to end the AIDS epidemic by 2030. https://www.unaids.org/sites/default/files/media_asset/201506_JC2743_Understanding_FastTrack_en.pdf.
64. WHO. Consolidated guidelines on the use of antiretroviral drugs for treating and preventing HIV infection. Recommendations for a public health approach. Geneva: WHO; 2013.
65. WHO. Consolidated guidelines on the use of antiretroviral drugs for treating and preventing HIV infection: recommendations for a public health approach, Second edition. Geneva: WHO; 2016. https://apps.who.int/iris/handle/10665/208825
66. WHO. Guidelines for the care and treatment of persons diagnosed with chronic hepatitis C virus infection. Geneva: WHO; 2017.
67. WHO. Guidelines for the prevention, care and treatment of persons with chronic hepatitis B infection. Policy brief. Geneva: WHO; 2015. https://www.who.int/publications/i/item/policy-brief-prevention-care-treatment-persons-chronic-hep-b-WHO-HIV-2015-5
68. WHO. Global health sector strategy on viral hepatitis 2016–2021. Towards ending viral hepatitis. Geneva: WHO; 2016. https://apps.who.int/iris/handle/10665/246177
69. WHO. Progress report on HIV, viral hepatitis and sexually transmitted infections 2019: accountability for the global health sector strategies, 2016–2021. Geneva: WHO, 2019. https://apps.who.int/iris/handle/10665/324797
70. WHO. Global hepatitis report, 2017. Geneva: WHO; 2017. https://www.who.int/publications/i/item/global-hepatitis-report-2017

22

CDC and the US President's Emergency Plan for AIDS Relief (PEPFAR)

Bess Miller and Kevin M. De Cock

As with the 1996 international AIDS conference in Vancouver where the world learned of the dramatic benefit of ART,[1,2] the 2000 conference in Durban, South Africa also proved an important milestone in the global AIDS response. With about 5 million people living with HIV, South Africa had a greater AIDS burden than any other country in the world.[3,4] For many of the thousands of international delegates, the conference was their first exposure to Africa and the African AIDS crisis. President Thabo Mbeki, South Africa's leader, had become persuaded by denialist views—both on HIV as the cause of AIDS and on the effectiveness of ART.[5] With an appearance at the conference by the legendary former president, Nelson Mandela, and demonstrations by diverse groups of AIDS activists, the occasion was charged with tension and high emotion. Increasing access to ART became an ever more visible political issue.[6,7]

The United States had been the principal donor for international AIDS activities since the 1980s, mainly through USAID.[8] Funds were mostly allocated to American nongovernmental and faith-based organizations, and to a lesser extent multilateral agencies such as WHO. CDC had technical experts detailed to various agencies, but its independent international work on AIDS was restricted to the research sites in Zaire, Cote d'Ivoire, and Thailand described in Section II.

By the late 1990s the severity of AIDS in Africa was widely recognized. President Bill Clinton's administration had increased commitment and funding to combat AIDS, including through establishment of the Office of National AIDS Policy at the White House. In July 1999, Clinton announced a new global initiative called LIFE (Leadership and Investment in Fighting an Epidemic)—a $100 million commitment to increase international efforts against the pandemic.[9] USAID was the designated coordinator, but the

Bess Miller and Kevin M. De Cock, *CDC and the US President's Emergency Plan for AIDS Relief (PEPFAR)* In: *Dispatches from the AIDS Pandemic*. Kevin M. De Cock, Harold W. Jaffe, and James W. Curran and Edited by: Robin Moseley, Oxford University Press. © Oxford University Press 2023. DOI: 10.1093/oso/9780197626528.003.0022

initiative also involved HHS, principally through CDC, and the Department of Defense.

The American effort aimed to reduce global HIV incidence by 25 percent within three to five years, provide care to 30 percent of persons with HIV, provide support for AIDS orphans, and enhance public health capacity. About half of the funds were devoted to prevention. The focus of the initiative was on fourteen countries in sub-Saharan Africa and India. Although announced near the end of his administration, LIFE was a quantum step in the history of AIDS funding, providing a basis for later, even more ambitious programs.

The Global Fund to Fight AIDS, Tuberculosis, and Malaria

The global impact of AIDS had aroused increased political interest and activist attention over the 1990s. Political pressure by UNAIDS and activists, supported by Richard Holbrooke, US Ambassador to the UN, brought AIDS to the attention of the Security Council. In early 2001, UN Secretary-General Kofi Annan called for establishment of a "war chest" to fight Africa's principal disease scourges. So it was that in January 2002 The Global Fund was launched in Geneva.[10,11] The influential British scientist Richard Feachem, former Dean of the London School of Hygiene and Tropical Medicine and later head of population and health at the World Bank, was its founding director.

The Global Fund is a financing mechanism, not an implementer of programs. It receives donations from sixty or more countries, with the United States providing about a third of all the Fund's resources—more than any other country. Since its founding, the Fund has distributed more than $45 billion in support of programs; it provides about 73 percent of all external TB funding in low- and middle-income countries, 56 percent of development assistance for malaria, and about 21 percent of external support for global AIDS programs.

PEPFAR Beginnings

In a 2018 article published in the *New England Journal of Medicine*,[12] Tony Fauci summarized fifteen years of PEPFAR impact. As others have done,

he credited [US] President George W. Bush with having the moral convic-
tion that something had to be done and recognizing that "the US could and
should design and implement a transformational and accountable program
to address the HIV/AIDS pandemic in low-income countries,"[12] all this
when estimates of persons living with HIV in such countries amounted to
approximately 30 million.

Early in his presidency Bush ordered a fact-finding mission to Africa,
and in December 2002 a group of about one hundred individuals from business, academia, government, the media, and the civil sector descended on
the continent.[13] The effort was led by HHS Secretary Tommy Thompson,
former Governor of the state of Wisconsin. Countries visited were Kenya,
Rwanda, Uganda, and Zambia. Just from the American side, apart from
the Secretary (the equivalent to any other country's Minister of Health),
the group included the directors and senior officials of CDC, NIH, and
USAID, as well as the recently appointed Global AIDS Coordinator
Randall Tobias, formerly the chief executive officer of the pharmaceutical
company Eli Lilly. With funding at stake, international dignitaries joined
in, including WHO Director JW Lee, UNAIDS Executive Director Peter
Piot, and senior officials from various nongovernmental organizations
and pharmaceutical companies.

The purpose of the trip was to examine ongoing AIDS work and to assess
what more could be done. Some critics expressed skepticism or dismissed
the trip as a photo opportunity. But, in fact, the delegation endured a grueling
schedule and uncomfortable traveling conditions. Most importantly, the
visitors were convinced by what they saw and were ready to communicate
it: the AIDS situation was awful, scale-up of interventions was necessary, and
Africa could manage HIV treatment programs.

Bush announced his AIDS initiative during the State of the Union address on January 28, 2003.[14] The world had been anxiously awaiting what
the President would say about the widely anticipated invasion of Iraq, so his
announcement of an AIDS initiative took people by surprise. "Seldom has
history offered a greater opportunity to do so much for so many," Bush said.
"We have confronted, and will continue to confront, HIV/AIDS in our own
country. And to meet a severe and urgent crisis abroad, tonight I propose the
Emergency Plan for AIDS Relief."[14] Even more surprising, and not widely
noticed, was the president's comment that the price of ART had dropped
from $12,000 to under $300 per year. One of the authors (KDC) recalled

sitting bolt upright when he heard this, thinking to himself, "he [Bush] is talking about allowing generics."

In May 2003 Congress passed the "United States Leadership against HIV/AIDS, Tuberculosis, and Malaria Act," requiring the President to formulate a five-year program to address the AIDS pandemic, the initiative known as PEPFAR. Less recognized are the important contributions made through the Act for global efforts against TB and malaria, on a bilateral basis as well as through the Global Fund. PEPFAR was bold in several ways. First, it committed to treating persons with HIV, unlike other development assistance programs that had only supported HIV prevention. Second, it would allow the use of generic medications, an important policy shift in a context of bitter international discussions about drug pricing and intellectual property. Finally, it was audacious in the money pledged—billions instead of millions of dollars—to countries that mostly had weak financial management systems.

PEPFAR was established as an interagency US government effort, housed in the newly created Office of the Global AIDS Coordinator in the Department of State,[8,15] with involvement of the White House. Agencies represented included USAID, HHS,* the Department of Defense, the Department of Commerce, the Department of Labor, and the Peace Corps. CDC and USAID took the lead in program implementation. A "principals" group of senior political appointees from the agencies involved met in person weekly to establish and coordinate overall PEPFAR policy.

PEPFAR changed the world of AIDS and global health, and many deserve credit for its success. Bush also was responsible for launching the President's Malaria Initiative—the largest funder of malaria programs globally. Fauci and his then associate Mark Dybul were highly influential in PEPFAR, as was Joe O'Neil of HRSA. Senior diplomats spoke out on the AIDS threat, including Secretary Colin Powell and ambassadors on the ground such as Jonny Carson, former Ambassador to Uganda and later Kenya. And the pressure from activists, some of them well connected politically, was palpable. To this day, PEPFAR has retained bilateral support in Congress.

---

* HHS agencies included CDC, NIH, the Health Resources and Services Administration (HRSA), FDA, and the Substance Abuse and Mental Health Services Administration (SAMHSA).

Early PEPFAR Implementation

Country-based implementation teams were established in fifteen countries across Africa, Asia, and Latin America,[†] each reporting to the US ambassador who was overall in charge of the PEPFAR program in country. However, it was well recognized by people working in AIDS internationally that ambassadors had many other responsibilities and that many diplomats were not especially knowledgeable about AIDS. That would have to change, especially in countries with smaller embassies, because PEPFAR soon dwarfed other funding streams. As CDC Country Director in Kenya, one of the authors (KDC) recommended to Ambassador Michael Bellamy, Carson's successor in Nairobi, that he appoint a coordinator for PEPFAR to advise him and ensure coordination between the US agencies involved. Bellamy appointed Buck Buckingham, an openly gay man with longstanding HIV who had been working with USAID, to this position. Buckingham and his deputy Viviane Chao established a model that became widely emulated across the PEPFAR focus countries.

PEPFAR's early targets were to treat 2 million people with ART, prevent 7 million new HIV infections, and provide care to 10 million people, including orphans and vulnerable children.[8] Pilot studies introducing the interventions were to be followed by scale-up at district, provincial, and national levels. The emphasis was on program implementation, not research; in fact, despite reference to "learning by doing," formal research was not supported, in fact, the very term was avoided.

For technical leadership and human resources, the aim was to rely on and strengthen country ministries of health and local-level capacity. In some cases, CDC staff were seconded to the health ministry to provide additional human resources. Implementation involved day-to-day collaboration with a plethora of partners and providers. These included staff of US agencies, ministries of health, global and country HIV and TB partners, community- and faith-based groups, universities, and the private sector.

PEPFAR represented a radically different approach to US development assistance for health. Instead of channeling funds through USAID, the program was run out of the State Department, not usually a program implementer.[8] The Global AIDS Coordinator had the rank of ambassador

---

[†] Initial focus countries were Botswana, Cote d'Ivoire, Ethiopia, Guyana, Haiti, Kenya, Mozambique, Namibia, Nigeria, Rwanda, South Africa, Tanzania, Uganda, Vietnam, and Zambia

and controlled all the funding and, therefore, essentially all US government global AIDS activities. For CDC, receipt of programmatic funds to independently provide services at country level also was novel; previously, CDC was restricted to providing technical assistance. Still another departure was the comprehensiveness of interventions for a single disease. CDC had previously participated in focused prevention programs, such as for smallpox and polio eradication (Chapter 12), but this broad approach to HIV/AIDS that included surveillance, laboratory diagnosis, prevention, treatment, and care was new.

A high-level concern was that this unique AIDS funding would be diverted to other purposes. In addition to precluding research, Global AIDS Coordinator Tobias laid down the limitations in memorable fashion. One of the authors (KDC) remembers seeing him gesticulating with his long arms spread out and saying, "This represents development." Bringing his arms closer together, he continued, "This represents health overall." And finally, his arms and hands closer still, "And this represents AIDS." Funds were to be used exclusively for HIV/AIDS, a statement of position by PEPFAR in the longstanding debate about the effectiveness of disease-specific vertical programs as opposed to horizontal approaches aimed at broad strengthening of health systems.

During the first five years, CDC staff played a lead role in developing and implementing the PEPFAR strategy for the initial fifteen focus countries. These efforts were at first directed out of the Global AIDS Program and later Division of Global HIV/AIDS, entities housed in CDC's domestic center dealing with AIDS. Only in 2010 was CDC's most visible international work, including for HIV, malaria, immunization, and health security, grouped together in the newly created Center for Global Health.[16]

CDC country program directors were appointed, and in-country offices established in all PEPFAR focus countries (eventually in over fifty countries) (Figure 22.1). Working with national leadership, CDC experts provided policy and on-the-ground guidance, drawing on broad domestic and international experience, especially in relation to surveillance, laboratory, and program evaluation. Efforts concentrated on prevention services, including HIV counseling and testing,[17,18,19,20,21,22,23,24,25,26,27] OI prophylaxis,[28] and prevention of mother-to-child transmission,[29] in addition to the primary focus of establishing ART programs.[30,31,32,33,34,35] Also included were TB service provision,[18,25,26,28,33,35] laboratory strengthening,[36,37] surveillance and monitoring, and evaluation.

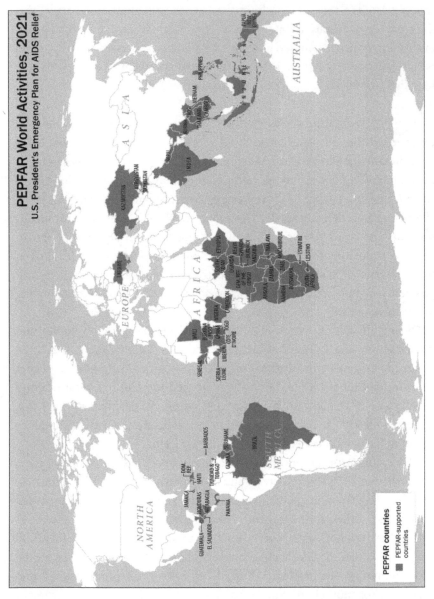

Figure 22.1. PEPFAR-supported countries, 2021. (Office of the US Global AIDS Coordinator)

Budgets were tightly earmarked: 55 percent of funds were devoted to medical care, of which 75 percent was to be spent on pharmaceuticals, including ART, and 25 percent to general care. Prevention received 20 percent of the overall budget, and at least a third of prevention funds were earmarked to support abstinence-until-marriage programs despite lack of evidence of their efficacy. Faith-based organizations were favored in terms of funding. Initially all drugs had to be FDA-approved, precluding purchase of some generic medicines prequalified by WHO. For a while, this resulted in participating healthcare sites having to track separately commodities purchased though PEPFAR or the Global Fund. Interventions for high-risk groups, that is, "key populations" such as sex workers and people who inject drugs, were hampered by restrictions on provision of harm reduction interventions such as needle and syringe services for drug users and on collaboration with groups interpreted as supporting prostitution. These early years were hard, but much was achieved.[38]

The 2003 Leadership Act that authorized PEPFAR required an evaluation of progress three years after passage of the legislation. This was undertaken by the Institute of Medicine[‡] (IOM), which provided an extensive report with detailed recommendations including acceptance of WHO prequalification of drugs and abolition of budgetary earmarks in favor of locally assessed need.[39,40] The report also called for improved local coordination, supporting the UNAIDS concept of "the three ones": one national coordinating committee, one national plan, and one monitoring and evaluation system. More general calls were for national capacity building and an emphasis on learning from experience. Importantly, the report highlighted the need for PEPFAR to transition from an emergency plan to a sustained and sustainable response and for the United States to continue to provide leadership and funding.[39,41]

Early Observations from CDC PEPFAR Staff

CDC staff members working in PEPFAR countries described the dire AIDS situation in the early 2000s, the enormity of work to be done, the associated stresses, and the challenges of coordination. Barbara Marston[42] led scale-up of HIV treatment in Kenya. As she recalled, "Funerals were the common activity. . . Most people went to a funeral every single weekend. The thriving

---

[‡] Now, the National Academy of Medicine.

business when I got to Kisumu was coffin making"[42] (Figure 22.2). This was a widespread observation: in Malawi, a research group tracked coffin sales to monitor AIDS mortality trends.

Technical support to countries was provided through extensive travel by CDC staff from Atlanta who were often shocked by what they found. One of the authors (BM) recalled visiting what were called AIDS clinics in the early days of PEPFAR's ART pilot programs:

> There were hundreds of people, with only a few chairs. People were standing or lying on the floor in clinic rooms, in the hallways, outside the facility—many severely ill, wasting, dying. . . waiting for treatment. Returning to work in Atlanta, it was impossible to forget these images. But it was motivating.

Jon Kaplan (Chapters 3 and 19), then Chief of the HIV Care and Treatment Branch at CDC headquarters in Atlanta, commented on the situation in the PEPFAR countries:

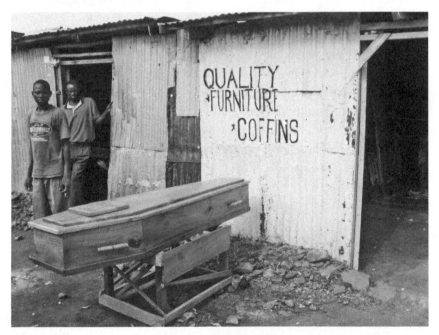

Figure 22.2. Coffin maker, Kisumu, Kenya (circa 2002). (Courtesy of Barbara Marston)

I remember (during in-country strategy sessions). . . thinking about all the things we could do and somebody just stopping the conversation with "Let's start with a good meal, that's what these people need the most, there's a lot of malnutrition". . . So food and nutrition. . . End-stage care. A lot of people dying, so-called palliative care, pain management . . . Treatment of sexually transmitted infections. These were all on the table to get to the ten million (the PEPFAR goal of providing care to 10 million persons).[43]

Generous AIDS funding contrasted with unfunded requirements such as food and clean water. Slum dwellers in Nairobi considered lack of food a barrier to adherence to treatment. One woman said succinctly, "If you give us ARVs,[§] please give us food, just food."[34]

But progress was made, despite the gap between treatment theoretically available and getting it to where it was needed. Initially, few people knew their HIV status and even fewer disclosed it. The introduction of point-of-care, rapid HIV tests in the early 2000s was an important advance.[27] These could be done without running water or electricity and performed by lay staff, not just laboratory technologists. Patients could witness their own testing and results. Eventually clinic-based testing with same-day results became possible in almost all funded countries.

Traditional voluntary counseling and testing required extensive training of counselors and lengthy sessions focusing on patients' risk factors. Privacy required separate counseling spaces, often unavailable. According to Jono Mermin (Chapter 20), then CDC country director in Uganda,

The vast majority of people with HIV in Africa. . . did not know they had HIV infection. There was a human rights movement that emphasized that you have a human right not to know your HIV status. We had to change that. . . people were inadvertently infecting partners because they didn't know they had HIV themselves.[44]

It took several years to arrive at diverse approaches, including home-based testing and routine HIV testing of ill patients (provider-initiated testing and counseling, "PITC," Chapter 21).

Marston described the impact of stigma on testing:

§ Antiretrovirals

> [F]or individuals that felt too stigmatized. . . transport became a bigger
> deal. They wouldn't . . . feel comfortable going to an HIV clinic in the village
> where they lived. . . (then) transport issues would get in the way of adher-
> ence when patients would try to. . . go to a different district hospital to get
> their treatment.[42]

Another obstacle was the inability of women to undergo a test without agreement of their husbands.

Despite initial difficulties, antenatal and TB clinics proved suitable
for HIV testing and later for ART. In some countries, such as Botswana,
up to 80 percent of TB patients were HIV-infected, so these essentially
served as AIDS clinics. One of the authors (BM) had conducted a pilot
study of HIV testing (using the rapid test kits) in TB clinics in a large
African urban area. The nurses there were trained briefly and were eager
to help address the AIDS crisis. Along with colleagues from WHO, the
ministry of health, and the TB program, she (BM) observed an early episode of such TB nurse-initiated HIV counseling and testing. The patient
was a small twelve-year-old girl, the daughter of a TB patient under care.
AIDS was explained in the local language, using adult terminology to
the child. Her blood was drawn, the results, negative, quickly apparent.
So, it was possible to use TB clinics for HIV services. But to scale this
up nationally and then throughout PEPFAR programs would require
massive training of TB nurses on counseling, including counseling of
children, drawing blood, sharps containment, and infection control. At
CDC headquarters, months and years were spent developing, piloting,
and then implementing such training programs throughout PEPFAR
countries.[18]

Beyond cost, PEPFAR programs encountered numerous practical hur-
dles to scaling up ART. These included lack of space for seeing patients, inadequate buildings and roads, supply chain management, human resources
challenges, patient transport and retention, quality of care, and record
keeping—the list seemed endless. But the biggest challenge was the sheer
enormity of the problem. As Kaplan recounted,

> Initially, we had to get things going quickly because the idea was, we have
> all this money, we want to get started right away. . . so at the beginning the
> places that either were or could become clinics were generally in the big
> cities affiliated with hospitals. . . As time went on. . . we had to get out to

more peripheral areas of the country, to districts and even communities, and find ways to develop clinics.[43]

Marston and a Kenyan colleague, Doris Macheria, initiated an ART program (Figure 22.3) in Kibera, a large slum in Nairobi.[31,32] In describing these efforts, Marston recalled,

> People were skeptical. Some patients had heard about antiretroviral therapy and were anxious to receive it. Some people were afraid of it... [After treatment] We got those viral load results back... and 85 percent of the patients were suppressed... It dispelled, basically, people's concerns about adherence to therapy and whether it could be done.[42]

An important figure in implementation of PEPFAR-funded ART programs was Tedd Ellerbrock, who later served in Kaplan's previous position overseeing HIV treatment and care. Ellerbrock, an obstetrician by training, joined the EIS program in 1986 when already in his forties and then became an epidemiologist in the agency's AIDS division. Beginning in 2003, Ellerbrock led the "Track One" program, a centrally funded initiative

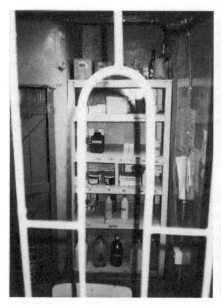
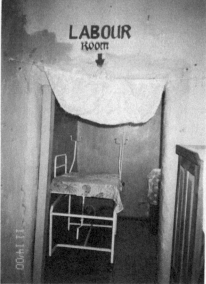

Figure 22.3. Pharmacy and labor room in a health center in Kibera, Nairobi, 2001. (Kevin De Cock, personal collection)

supervised by CDC and HRSA. Four implementing partners** received $2.2 billion over the ensuing eight years and treated 1.4 million people across fourteen countries. To identify what was working and what was not, Ellerbrock and his team traveled tirelessly around the globe, consulting with ministry of health officials, PEPFAR country implementers, ART clinical care providers, and patients.

To a limited degree PEPFAR also supported prophylaxis and treatment of OIs, which had been the mainstays of AIDS management in high-income countries in the pre-ART era (Chapter 19). Studies of the spectrum of disease in low-income settings and the efficacy of cotrimoxazole prophylaxis came late (Chapters 15 and 19), and scale-up was hampered by logistics and inconsistencies in its use. As Mermin recalled,

> [W]e developed this basic care package, and it became standard. When you got diagnosed with HIV. . . you would be provided with a package that had condoms. . . cotrimoxazole over a long time. . . a water vessel and chlorine. . . (and) ultimately. . . isoniazid prophylaxis to prevent TB.[44]

Cotrimoxazole had the added benefit of preventing malaria. But, as Mermin observed, "the total extended life expectancy from taking cotrimoxazole was still a matter of months. . . So, it helped people, but there were limits."[44] People needed ART.

PEPFAR supported diverse prevention programs, but abstinence featured prominently in early discussions. Eugene McCray (Chapter 10) was Director of CDC's Global AIDS Program in Atlanta during the 2000s. As he recalled, "There was a strong push by the conservative element to really push abstinence. . . There were some countries that did not accept this idea of having abstinence be a major pillar of their program."[45] Uganda introduced the "ABC" strategy: abstain; if you cannot, be faithful; if you cannot, use a condom. This became the focus for prevention in the initial PEPFAR five-year strategy (Figure 22.4). Although more pragmatic than an abstinence-only message, it was simplistic in relation to the realities of sexual transmission of HIV and to HIV programs more broadly.[46] Abstinence-only earmarks were lifted with PEPFAR reauthorization in 2008, but abstinence and fidelity remained reporting requirements and an area of controversy.

** The four Track One implementing partners were AIDS Relief (a Catholic Relief Services Consortium), the Elizabeth Glaser Pediatric AIDS Foundation, ICAP at Columbia University, and the Harvard School of Public Health

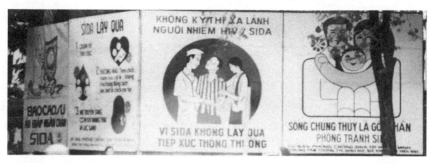

Figure 22.4. Ho Chi Minh City, Vietnam, circa 2003. Billboard with AIDS prevention messages allowing for use of condoms and advocating being faithful to family. (Bess Miller, personal collection)

A priority area for CDC, as well as its dominant strategy for preventing infection in children, was prevention of mother-to-child transmission of HIV. Nathan Shaffer (Chapter 16), who joined CDC's Global AIDS Program after returning from work in Thailand, described early challenges in Africa:

> We're talking about pregnant women being infected at rates of anywhere from four or five percent to as high as twenty-five or thirty percent... Many women came late to antenatal care... We spent a lot of time in hospitals... providing side-by-side technical assistance to understand how could the systems work... that we had people in the CDC (in country) office, that was a great strength.[47]

Facility-based interventions were the most practical, and eventually were implemented down to the level of small health centers that provided maternal and child health care. As Shaffer remarked, "The backbone of the health system really was the nurses... to introduce a rapid HIV test was not that big an issue... But... there was a tremendous drain on nurses and a constant turnover."[47]

In addition to lack of adequately trained healthcare workers, laboratory systems had long been neglected in resource-poor countries. Many diseases were managed empirically, and early attempts at scaling up ART depended on clinical rather than laboratory staging and monitoring. HIV testing was paramount for ART, with the next priority increasing access to CD4+ cell counts to guide treatment initiation. Health system strengthening, including for laboratories, was a focus of PEPFAR's second, five-year authorization starting in 2009.

The most influential figure in CDC's HIV-related laboratory work was John Nkengasong, who became chief of the Laboratory Branch of CDC's Global AIDS Program in 2005 after distinguished work at Projet Retro-CI (Chapter 15). His expertise, knowledge of Africa, and pragmatism earned him the respect of HIV laboratorians around the world. In January 2008, scientists involved with PEPFAR met in Mozambique and issued an influential declaration calling for strengthening of laboratory services as an integral part of overall health systems.

Nkengasong and colleagues elaborated on what integrated national laboratory plans should include: a framework for training and career development for laboratorians, infrastructure development, supply-chain management, laboratory information systems, and a governance structure that would address regulatory issues and reporting requirements. A key component was the development of standards for quality management systems and accreditation. Under PEPFAR, laboratory services later extended to quality assurance of HIV testing, early infant diagnosis using molecular methods, use of blood spot technology, viral load monitoring, and centralized as well as point-of-care CD4+ cell count testing.

Nkengasong, then Director of the Africa Centres for Disease Control and Prevention under the aegis of the African Union in Addis Ababa, Ethiopia, commented on these developments:

> [W]hen I just started the lab program in PEPFAR (2005), there were just over ten people. . . in the lab. Fast forward, when I left (2016) . . . , we had . . . seventy-six people in the lab. . . In the field. . . there were only about two lab people (in 2005). . . Robert Downing in Uganda and. . . Jane Mwangi in Kenya. But as I left. . . there were forty something lab advisors in the field.[48]

For CDC, PEPFAR required enormous expansion of field staff and administrative capacity. RJ Simonds (Chapter 16), then Deputy Director of the Global AIDS Program in Atlanta, commented on CDC's lack of operational agility for international work: "being in Atlanta, [we] tend to not be quite as facile [compared to the other agencies, all based in Washington, DC]."[49] Simonds's remarks encapsulated two realities: that CDC was primarily a domestic agency and that USAID felt it should oversee all of PEPFAR. CDC henceforth had to focus on management and better integration into overseas embassy structures. Apart from the international research collaborations described elsewhere, CDC's long-term global involvement had previously consisted of secondment of staff to other organizations.

Rapid expansion of various activities in Kenya, which was to become CDC's largest international platform, led to a senior State Department official complaining of "CDC splinter groups" and to one of the authors (KDC) emphasizing the concept of "One CDC." This meant that headquarters-based groups, especially those working on diseases other than HIV, had to collaborate better and respect the role of a CDC country director reporting to the US ambassador. Initially not all headquarters staff embraced this new concept with enthusiasm, but it has become a guiding theme for CDC's global work.

Although two senior CDC officials, Jeff Harris and Helene Gayle, led USAID AIDS activities in Washington in the late 1980s and early 1990s while on detail from CDC, interagency tensions were frequent in the PEPFAR world. Personality differences often colored the collaboration, but underlying structural issues were important. PEPFAR never clarified whether agencies should lead the specific "lanes" in which they had a comparative advantage, or whether everyone should do everything. USAID had greater expertise in health systems work such as procurement and commodity supply chains. By contrast, CDC staff felt they had privileged relationships with ministries of health and greater capacity in clinical services, surveillance and evaluation, and laboratory services. Friction invariably arose around funding allocations to the various agencies, and because treatment received the most resources, no one was ready to relinquish this area of work.

PEPFAR Programs Continue

PEPFAR has naturally been heavily influenced by the various White House Global AIDS Coordinators. Randall Tobias was a strong manager with vast business experience. Tobias was promoted in 2006 to oversee all US foreign assistance but resigned abruptly that year. His successors were, respectively, Mark Dybul (2006–2009), Eric Goosby (2009–2013), and Deborah Birx (2013–2021). Dybul was well connected to the Bush administration but was brusquely terminated by Secretary of State Hilary Clinton. His international influence increased, however, when he later served as director of the Global Fund from 2013 to 2017.

Goosby had served in the Clinton administration and brought with him the clinician's interest in the individual patient, easily overlooked in large public health programs. Birx succeeded Goosby, after distinguished leadership of CDC's PEPFAR program (Chapter 21). As Global AIDS Coordinator, Birx greatly centralized control of the program and increased data reporting requirements. She was selected by [US] Vice-President Pence in early 2020 as Coordinator of the White House Coronavirus Task Force and retired from US government service in early 2021.

In 2008, PEPFAR was renewed, and Congress expanded the Initiative's funds to $48 billion through 2013. In 2014, the program announced PEPFAR 3.0[50] focusing on "Sustainable Control of the AIDS Epidemic by the Year 2020." By 2014, CDC PEPFAR staff included 400 persons at headquarters and over 1,500 in the field, most of the field staff being host-country nationals employed through the local US embassy. As of September 30, 2019, the US government had invested close to $100 billion combating AIDS through PEPFAR and the Global Fund in over fifty countries.[51,52,53,54,55,56,57,58]

Over time, PEPFAR established close relations with UNAIDS and WHO's HIV/AIDS Department, its influence undoubtedly enhanced by the funding provided to these UN agencies. Representation of CDC staff at UNAIDS and WHO and on groups developing HIV guidelines served technical as well as political purposes. The approach to the global epidemic became increasingly aligned, including to the UNAIDS "Fast-Track" strategy and its 90:90:90 targets (Chapter 19).[59] Revised WHO guidelines followed research showing the benefits of immediate ART,[60,61] profoundly influencing practice and funding requirements. With stable funding, an increased proportion of PEPFAR resources was needed to support treatment, with potentially negative consequences on the rest of the AIDS portfolio.

Widely respected and credited with life-saving impact, PEPFAR retains broad support but remains susceptible to political constraints cited earlier.[62] Thanks to PEPFAR funding, the role and visibility of faith-based organizations in health service provision has been enhanced.[63,64,65] Despite their restrictions in relation to condom promotion and other measures contrary to their beliefs, such organizations often provide AIDS and other services in hard-to-reach areas, including rural settings, fragile states, and areas of conflict. And, they commit for the long term.

Despite its reach, PEPFAR may not have exploited its learning potential to the fullest. In 2004, Global fund Executive Director Richard Feachem argued for support of research into new products as well as field operations for HIV/

AIDS, TB, and malaria.[66] He observed that none of the principal funders— PEPFAR, the Global Fund, and the World Bank—prioritized operations research. Although "public health evaluations" and other cautious terms were coined to allow the quest for generalizable knowledge, PEPFAR could have done more to support implementation science to influence global health policies and practice.

Despite these limitations, CDC collaborations provided important information, including on use of cotrimoxazole and its effect on reducing the incidence of malaria; on essential care packages, including bednets for prevention of malaria and safe water interventions[67,68,69]; and on the impact of ART in reducing HIV transmission from mothers to their infants through breast feeding.[70] CDC technical expertise remained visible in five yearly population-based surveys of HIV developed in collaboration with Wafaa El-Sadr and others from ICAP at Columbia University (later referred to as Population-Based Health Impact Assessments, "PHIAs").[71,72] These surveys, as well as other CDC evaluations, have contributed to generating global HIV estimates and assessing program impact on HIV incidence and mortality.[73,74,75]

At end-2021, according to UNAIDS estimates, 38.4 million people worldwide were living with HIV, with 1.5 million people newly infected and 650,000 dying from HIV disease over that year.[76] Approximately 75 percent of all persons with HIV were accessing ART, and, overall, 68 percent were virally suppressed. PEPFAR remains committed to supporting the UN's Sustainable Development Goals (Chapter 21) and the stated aim to end the epidemic of AIDS by 2030.[77] As indicated earlier, there is divergent opinion about what "ending AIDS" means, whether it is feasible, or how to define slogans such as "epidemic control" or an "AIDS-free generation."[78,79] The world is not on track to meet the ambitious numeric targets of the SDGs, which have been criticized for inadequate focus on key populations where HIV may find refuge even as generalized epidemics decline.

PEPFAR estimates that to date its programs have provided ART to 19 million people, including nearly 700,000 children; HIV testing services to 63.4 million people; mother-to-child prevention services, allowing 2.8 million infants to be born HIV free; voluntary medical male circumcision to 28 million men and boys; and training to 300,000 healthcare workers.[51] The billions of dollars expended, and millions of lives saved have been revolutionary in global health overall, rescuing the African continent from social and demographic disruption.

What does the future hold? Development assistance for AIDS is unlikely to increase and may be challenged in the face of other emerging health priorities, especially those relating to health security as illustrated by COVID-19.[80] The year 2030 will inevitably bring assessment of performance toward the SDGs and definition of the next set of global aspirations. The global pandemic of AIDS is not close to being over, and conclusions from the 2007 IOM report,[39] namely, that the need for US leadership and funding in the effort to control the HIV/AIDS pandemic continues, remain valid. There is plenty more work for CDC to do on global AIDS.

Notes

1. De Cock KM, Churchill D, Grant A, et al. Summary of track B: clinical science. AIDS 1996;10(Suppl 3):S107–S113.
2. Williams IG, De Cock KM. The XI International Conference on AIDS, Vancouver, July 7–12, 1996: A review of clinical science Track B. Genitourin Med 1996;72:365–369.
3. WHO. World health report 1999. Making a Difference. Geneva, Switzerland: WHO; 1999. https://apps.who.int/iris/handle/10665/42167
4. UNAIDS, WHO. AIDS Epidemic Update 2003. Geneva, Switzerland: UNAIDS; 2003. https://data.unaids.org/publications/irc-pub06/jc943-epiupdate2003_en.pdf
5. International AIDS Society. History of the IAS. Episode 4—2000: AIDS denialism and treatment equity at the Durban conference. https://www.iasociety.org/Who-we-are/About-the-IAS/25th-anniversary-of-the-IAS/Episode-4.
6. Campaign for access to medicines. A matter of life and death: the role of patents in access to essential medicines. Médecins Sans Frontières, November 2001. https://www.msf.org/sites/msf.org/files/doha_11-2001.pdf.
7. Hogg R, Cahn P, Katabira ET, et al. Time to act: global apathy towards HIV/AIDS is a crime against humanity. Lancet 2002;360:1710–1711.
8. Henry J. Kaiser Family Foundation. The U.S. Government engagement in global health: a primer. February 2019. http://files.kff.org/attachment/Report-The-US-Government-Engagement-in-Global-Health-A-Primer.
9. Shaffer N, McConnell M, Bolu O, et al. Prevention of mother-to-child HIV transmission internationally. Emerg Infect Dis 2004;10:2027–2028.
10. Piot P. No time to lose. A life in pursuit of deadly viruses. New York: WW Norton; 2012.
11. The Global Fund. Global Fund overview. https://www.theglobalfund.org/en/overview/.
12. Fauci AS, Eisinger RW. PEPFAR—15 years and counting the lives saved. N Engl J Med 2018;378:314–316. doi: 10.1056/NEJMp1714773.
13. Rivers B. Tommy Thompson's Africa trip. AIDSPAN Dec 20, 2003. https://www.aidspan.org/en/c/article/178.

14. The Washington Post. Text of President Bush's 2003 State of the Union Address. Jan 28, 2003. https://www.washingtonpost.com/wp-srv/onpolitics/transcripts/bushtext_012803.html

15. Office of the U.S. Global AIDS Coordinator. The President's emergency plan for AIDS relief: U.S. five-year global HIV/AIDS strategy. Washington, DC: OGAC; 2004.

16. Frieden TR, De Cock KM. The CDC's Center for Global Health. Lancet 2012;379(9820):986–988. doi: 10.1016/S0140-6736(12)60370-5.

17. Campbell C, Marum E, Alwano-Edyegu M, et al. The role of HIV counseling and testing in the developing world. AIDS Educ Prev 1997;9(3 Suppl):92–104.

18. Bock NN, Nadol P, Rogers M, et al. Provider-initiated HIV testing and counseling in TB clinical settings: tools for program implementation. Int J Tuberc Lung Dis 2008;12(3 Suppl 1):S69–S72.

19. Creek T, Ntumy R, Seipone K, et al. Successful introduction of routine, opt-out HIV testing in antenatal care in Botswana. J Acquir Immune Defic Syndr 2007;45:102–107.

20. De Cock KM, Mbori-Ngacha D, Marum E. Shadow on the continent: public health and HIV/AIDS in Africa in the 21st century. Lancet 2002;360:67–72.

21. Grabbe K, Menzies N, Taegtmeyer M, et al. Increasing access to HIV counseling and testing through mobile services in Kenya: strategies, utilization and cost-effectiveness. J Acquir Immune Defic Syndr 2010:54:317–323.

22. Kalichman SC, Simbayi LC. HIV testing attitudes, AIDS stigma, and voluntary HIV counselling and testing in a black township in Cape Town, South Africa. Sex Transm Infect 2003;79:442–447.

23. Marum E, Taegtmeyer M, Chebet K. Scale-up of voluntary HIV counseling and testing in Kenya. JAMA 2006;296:859–862.

24. Menzies N, Abang, B, Wanyenze R, et al. The costs and effectiveness of four HIV counseling and testing strategies in Uganda. AIDS 2009;23:395–401.

25. Odhiambo J, Kizito W, Njoroge A, et al. Provider-initiated HIV testing and counselling for TB patients and suspects in Nairobi, Kenya. Int J Tuberc Lung Dis 2008;12(3 Suppl 1):S63–S68.

26. Van Rie A, Sabue M, Jarrett N, et al. Counseling and testing TB patients for HIV: evaluation of three implementation models in Kinshasa, Congo. Int J Tuberc Lung Dis 2008;12(3 Suppl 1):S73–S78.

27. Plate DK, Rapid HIV Test Evaluation Working Group. Evaluation and implementation of rapid HIV tests: the experience in 11 African countries. AIDS Res Hum Retroviruses 2007;23:1491–1498.

28. CDC. USPHS/IDSA guidelines for the prevention of opportunistic infections in persons infected with human immunodeficiency virus: a summary. MMWR Morbid Mortal Wkly Rep 1995;44(No. RR-8):1–34.

29. DeCock KM, Fowler MG, Mercier E, et al. Prevention of mother-to child transmission of HIV-1 in resource poor countries: translating research into policy and practice. JAMA 2000;283:1175–1182.

30. Gilks C, Crowley S, Ekpini R, et al. The WHO public-health approach to antiretroviral treatment against HIV in resource-limited settings. Lancet 2006;368:505–510.

31. Marston BJ, Macharia DK, N'ganga L, et al. A program to provide antiretroviral therapy to residents of an urban slum in Nairobi, Kenya. J Int Assoc Physicians AIDS Care 2007;6:106–112.

32. Kim AA, Wanjiku L, Macharia DK, et al. Adverse events in HIV-infected persons receiving antiretroviral drug regimens in a large urban slum in Nairobi, Kenya, 2003–2005. J Int Assoc Physicians AIDS Care 2007;6:206–209.

33. Koenig SP, Leandre F, Farmer, PE. Scaling up HIV treatment programmes in resource-limited settings: the rural Haiti experience. AIDS 2004;18:521–525.

34. Marston B, De Cock KM. Multivitamins, nutrition, and highly active antiretroviral therapy for HIV and AIDS in Africa. N Engl J Med 2004;351:78–80.

35. Reid A, Scano F, Getahun H, et al. Towards universal access to HIV prevention, treatment, care, and support: the role of tuberculosis/HIV collaboration. Lancet 2006;6:483–495.

36. Petti CA, Polage CR, Quinn TC. Laboratory medicine in Africa: a barrier to effective health care. Clin Infect Dis 2006;42:377–382.

37. Nkengasong JN, Nsubuga P, Nwanyanwu O, et al. Laboratory systems and services are critical in global health: time to end the neglect? Am J Clin Pathol 2010;134:368–373.

38. Vella S, Schwartlander B, Sow S, et al. The history of antiretroviral therapy and of its implementation in resource-limited areas of the world. AIDS 2012;26:1231–1241.

39. Institute of Medicine. PEPFAR implementation: progress and promise. Washington, DC: The National Academies Press; 2007. https://doi.org/10.17226/11905.

40. Waning B, Diedrichsen E, Moon S. A lifeline to treatment: the role of Indian generic manufacturers in supplying antiretroviral medicines to developing countries. J Int AIDS Soc 2010;13:35. doi: 10.1186/1758-2652-13-35.

41. Zewdie D, De Cock K, Piot P. Sustaining treatment costs: who will pay? AIDS 2007;21 (Suppl 4):S1–S4.

42. "MARSTON, BARBARA," Global Health Chronicles, accessed January 29, 2023. https://globalhealthchronicles.org/items/show/8127.

43. "KAPLAN, JONATHAN," Global Health Chronicles, accessed December 28, 2022, https://globalhealthchronicles.org/items/show/8137.

44. "MERMIN, JONATHAN," Global Health Chronicles, accessed January 29, 2023, https://www.globalhealthchronicles.org/items/show/8126.

45. "MCCRAY, EUGENE," Global Health Chronicles, accessed January 29, 2023, https://www.globalhealthchronicles.org/items/show/6470.

46. Collins CS, Coates T, Curran JW. Moving beyond the alphabet soup of HIV prevention. AIDS 2008;22:55–58.

47. "SHAFFER, NATHAN," Global Health Chronicles, accessed January 29, 2023, https://www.globalhealthchronicles.org/items/show/8131.

48. "NKENGASONG, JOHN," Global Health Chronicles, accessed December 25, 2022, https://www.globalhealthchronicles.org/items/show/8138.

49. "SIMONDS, RJ," Global Health Chronicles, accessed January 29, 2023, https://www.globalhealthchronicles.org/items/show/8139.

50. Office of the US Global AIDS Coordinator. PEPFAR 3.0. Controlling the epidemic: Delivering on the promise of an AIDS-free generation. December 2014.

https://www.state.gov/wp-content/uploads/2019/08/PEPFAR-3.0-%E2%80%93-Controlling-the-Epidemic-Delivering-on-the-Promise-of-an-AIDS-free-Generation.pdf.

51. The United States President's Emergency Plan for AIDS Relief. 2022 Annual Report to Congress. https://www.state.gov/wp-content/uploads/2022/05/PEPFAR2022.pdf.

52. Dybul M. Lessons learned from PEPFAR. J Acquir Immune Defic Syndr 2009;52(Suppl 1):S12–S13.

53. El-Sadr W, Holmes CB, Mugyenyi, et al. Scale-up of HIV treatment through PEPFAR: a historic public health achievement. J Acquir Immune Defic Syndr 2012;60(Suppl 3):S96–S104.

54. Merson MH, Curran JW, Griffith CH, Ragunanthan B. The President's Emergency Plan for AIDS Relief: from successes of the emergency response to challenges of sustainable action. Health Aff (Millwood) 2012;31:1380–1388. doi: 10.1377/hlthaff.2012.0206.

55. Simonds RJ, Carrino CA, Moloney-Kitts M. Lessons from the President's Emergency Plan for AIDS Relief: from quick ramp-up to the role of strategic partnership. Health Aff (Millwood) 2012;31:1397–1405. doi: 10.1377/hlthaff.2012.0193.

56. Goosby E. The President's Emergency Plan for AIDS Relief: marshalling all tools at our disposal toward an AIDS-free generation. Health Aff (Millwood) 2012;31:1593–1598. doi: 10.1377/hlthaff.2012.0241.

57. Chi BH, Adler MR, Bolu O, et al. Progress, challenges, and new opportunities for the prevention of mother-to-child transmission of HIV under the US President's Emergency Plan for AIDS Relief. J Acquir Immune Defic Syndr 2012;60(Suppl 3):S78–S87. doi: 10.1097/QAI.0b013e31825f3284.

58. Goosby E, Dybul M, Fauci AS, et al. The United States President's Emergency Plan for AIDS Relief: a story of partnerships and smart investments to turn the tide of the global AIDS pandemic. J Acquir Immune Defic Syndr 2012;60(Suppl 3):S51–S56. doi: 10.1097/QAI.0b013e31825ca721. Erratum in: J Acquir Immune Defic Syndr 2012;61:e24. Fauci, Anthony A [corrected to Fauci, Anthony S].

59. UNAIDS. Understanding fast-track. Accelerating action to end the AIDS epidemic by 2030. https://www.unaids.org/sites/default/files/media_asset/201506_JC2743_Understanding_FastTrack_en.pdf.

60. INSIGHT START Study Group, Lundgren JD, Babiker AG, et al. Initiation of antiretroviral therapy in early asymptomatic HIV infection. N Engl J Med 2015;373:795–807.

61. TEMPRANO ANRS 12136 Study Group, Danel C, Moh R, et al. A trial of early antiretroviral and isoniazid preventive therapy in Africa. N Engl J Med 2015;373:808–822.

62. Ditmore MH, Allman D. An analysis of the implementation of PEPFAR's antiprostitution pledge and its implications for successful HIV prevention among organizations working with sex workers. J Int AIDS Soc 2013;16:17354. doi:10.7448/IAS.16.1.17354.

63. Olivier J, Tsimpo C, Gemignani R, et al. Understanding the roles of faith-based health-care providers in Africa: review of the evidence with a focus on magnitude, reach, cost, and satisfaction. Lancet 2015;386:1765–1775.

64. US President's Emergency Plan for AIDS Relief. A firm foundation: the PEPFAR consultation on the role of faith-based organizations in sustaining community and

country leadership in the response to HIV/AIDS. Washington: US Department of State; 2012.

65. Karpf T, Ferguson JT, Swift R, Lazarus JV, Eds. Restoring hope: decent care in the midst of HIV/AIDS. London: Palgrave MacMillan; 2008.

66. Feachem RGA. The research imperative: fighting AIDS, TB and malaria. Trop Med Int Health 2004;9:1139–1141.

67. Mermin J, Lule J, Ekwaru JP, et al. Effect of co-trimoxazole prophylaxis on morbidity, mortality, CD4-cell count, and viral load in HIV infection in rural Uganda. Lancet. 2004;364:1428–1434.

68. Mermin J, Ekwaru JP, Liechty CA, et al. Effect of cotrimoxazole prophylaxis, antiretroviral therapy, and insecticide-treated bednets on the frequency of malaria in HIV-1-infected adults in Uganda: a prospective cohort study. Lancet 2006;367:1256–1261.

69. Mermin J, Were W, Ekwaru JP, et al. Mortality in HIV-infected Ugandan adults receiving antiretroviral treatment and survival of their HIV-uninfected children: a prospective cohort study. Lancet 2008;371:752–759.

70. Thomas TK, Masaba R, Borkowf CB, et al. Triple-antiretroviral prophylaxis to prevent mother-to-child HIV transmission through breastfeeding—the Kisumu Breastfeeding Study, Kenya: a clinical trial. PLoS Med 2011;8:e1001015. doi:10.1371/journal.pmed.1001015.

71. De Cock KM, Rutherford G, Akhwale W, Eds. Kenya AIDS Indicator Survey 2012. J Aquir Immune Defic Syndr 2014;66(Suppl 1):S1–S137.

72. Justman JE, Mugurungi O, El-Sadr WM. HIV population surveys—bringing precision to the global response. N Engl J Med 2018;378:1859–1861.

73. Borgdorff MW, Kwaro D, Obor D, et al. Reduction of HIV incidence in western Kenya during scale up of antiretroviral therapy and voluntary medical male circumcision, a population-based cohort analysis. Lancet HIV 2018;5:e241–e249.

74. Young PW, Kim AA, Wamicwe J, et al. HIV-associated mortality in the era of antiretroviral therapy scale-up—Nairobi, Kenya, 2015. PLoS One 2017;12:e0181837. https://doi.org/10.1371/journal.pone.0181837.

75. Otieno GO, Whiteside YO, Achia T, et al. Decreased HIV-associated mortality rates during the scale-up of antiretroviral therapy in western Kenya (2011–2016): a population-based cohort study. AIDS 2019;33:2423–2430.

76. UNAIDS. Global HIV & AIDS statistics—fact sheet. https://www.unaids.org/en/resources/fact-sheet.

77. United Nations. The 17 Goals. https://sdgs.un.org/goals.

78. Jones J, Sullivan PS, Curran JW. Progress in the HIV epidemic: identifying goals and measuring success. PLoS Med 2019;16:e1002729. doi: 10.1371/journal.pmed.1002729.

79. Office of the Global AIDS Coordinator. PEPFAR blueprint: creating an AIDS-free generation. Washington, DC: A/GIS/GPS; 2012. https://www.avac.org/sites/default/files/resource-files/PEPFAR%20Blueprint.pdf.

80. De Cock KM, Jaffe HW, Curran JW. Reflections on 40 years of AIDS. Emerg Infect Dis 2021;27:1553–1560. doi: 10.3201/eid2706.210284.

Epilogue

The Authors

The story of the AIDS pandemic is both remarkable and tragic. Who but a science fiction writer could have imagined that a virus originating in chimpanzees and gorillas would lead to the greatest global health threat of the last half of the twentieth century? And who but the most wide-eyed optimist would have predicted that AIDS could be transformed from a death sentence to a chronic disease that can be managed with as little as one pill a day? Yet the lives of millions of people were cut short by AIDS and millions more are living with HIV infection, their lives dependent on uninterrupted access to treatment.

In this book, we have examined AIDS through our own experiences and those of many of the other individuals involved in CDC's efforts to confront the disease—from its first description to the present. The book has also described the scientific and public health advances toward understanding and stemming the pandemic.

Former CDC Director Bill Foege describes epidemiology as the basic science of public health. Epidemiology and surveillance were essential to CDC's initial response to AIDS, providing objective data to show the increasing magnitude of the problem, clarify the modes of transmission, and propose prevention measures—even before the causative agent was identified.[1,2] These early achievements were followed by other seminal advances, including the discovery of the AIDS virus in 1983,[3] the widespread introduction of diagnostic tests for HIV in 1985,[4] the proof that azidothymidine (AZT) could prevent mother-to-child transmission in 1993,[5] and the discovery of the efficacy of ART in 1996.[6] Research later refined guidance on how best to treat HIV (start ART immediately) and how it could be used for prevention, both by reducing infectiousness and in the form of PrEP.[7]

The availability of ART, fifteen years after the first description of AIDS, was stunning and evoked patients and clinicians to speak almost miraculously of a Lazarus effect. In his book, *How to Survive a Plague*, David France described his own reaction, while attending a presentation at New York University in 1995, to hearing that ART might allow HIV-infected people to lead normal lives.

> It had been many years since I cried—but now tears rolled down my cheeks. . . was it over? Was the long nightmare passed?. . . I was thirty-five years old. I've lived my entire adult life in the age of unrelenting death. We all had. The feeling of relief overwhelmed me."[8]

What are the lessons from the AIDS pandemic and how well have we learned them? Perhaps most importantly, we are reminded that despite ongoing scientific and medical advances we remain at risk of diseases from new and reemerging infections. Examples are numerous and include Ebola, hantavirus, West Nile virus, H1N1 influenza ("swine flu"), Zika virus, the catastrophic COVID-19 pandemic, and, most recently, monkeypox, now named mpox. Like HIV, many of these infections emerged because of human interactions with the animal hosts of these agents.[9] With each epidemic come after-action reports calling for increased response capabilities and international collaboration.[10,11,12] Although improvements continue to be made, we still find ourselves surprisingly unprepared for the next pandemic.

AIDS also taught us, often profoundly, the importance of community involvement and activism. In the United States, the response to the AIDS pandemic was energized and facilitated by persons with HIV and members of at-risk communities at a scale and an effectiveness not seen with other diseases previously or since. Gay men were dying, and governments and much of the establishment seemingly ignored their plight. The angry community responded politically, technically, and socially. Self-help and support groups sprang up to care for the ill and the dying. Organizations such as the AIDS Coalition to Unleash Power (ACT UP) and the Gay Men's Health Crisis demanded involvement and increased response from government, industry, and the civil sector. They used publicity-generating tactics with CDC, NIH, industry, and other establishments, including a demonstration against the New York Archdiocese that left St. Patrick's Cathedral littered with condoms. In an ACT UP supported protest at CDC, an individual chained himself to the office door of one of the authors (JWC). The personal interactions with activists were sometimes painful for those of us working in AIDS, but we recognized that the intent and overall impact of the activism was crucial and eminently understandable. On more than one occasion, we would note the absence of a prominent activist at an AIDS meeting, only to learn later that the individual had died of AIDS.

Increasing recognition of the international extent of the epidemic led to activism globally. Alliances between American and European MSM occurred early. Linkages with Africa's heterosexual epidemic were not immediate, but activism nonetheless globalized around issues of discrimination and especially access to treatment. Perhaps the first and best-known activist group in Africa was The AIDS Support Organization (TASO) in Uganda. The Treatment Action Campaign (TAC) also exerted important influence in South Africa on treatment policies and access. Community pressure and activism remain necessary for successful and equitable HIV prevention and treatment.

AIDS also clearly showed us that high-level political leadership is critical to respond to major epidemics. In the United States, the lack of leadership from the Reagan administration during the early 1980s delayed critically needed funding to investigate the AIDS epidemic and support prevention programs. The restrictions in the availability of ART and denialism of HIV by South African President Thabo Mbeki and his government had catastrophic consequences. Harvard researchers estimated that their restrictions caused more than 330,000 avoidable deaths, 35,000 HIV-infected infants, and at least 3.8 million person-years of life lost over the period 2000–2005.[13] In contrast, the establishment of The Global Fund resulted from extensive negotiation and pressure at the United Nations. And the leadership of President George W. Bush led to the creation of PEPFAR and the nation's commitment to this life-saving initiative. These two developments changed the face of global AIDS and global health and yielded results. ART now reaches over three fourths of HIV-infected persons worldwide.[14]

At a time when COVID-19, rather than AIDS, is seen as the greatest infectious disease threat to global health, mpox has unexpectedly spread in epidemic fashion. Related to smallpox but fortunately less severe, the disease has long been endemic in Central and western Africa. In late spring 2022, however, infections were diagnosed in countries not previously affected, reaching approximately 20,000 mpox cases reported from nearly eighty countries by late July and prompting WHO to declare the outbreak a Public Health Emergency of International Concern.[15] An unusual feature of this outbreak—and one harking back to the early days of AIDS and reigniting concerns over stigma—has been its high (>95%) concentration among MSM; in the United States approximately 40 percent of MSM with mpox also have HIV.[16] Although mpox has not been considered an STI, its spread among MSM—particularly across sexual networks—suggests that it can be transmitted during intimate contact with infected partners.

Although the response to mpox is still in its early phases, comparing the public health responses to HIV, COVID-19, and mpox may be instructive for future health emergencies. For any epidemic, understanding the biology, transmission, and natural history of the etiologic agent remains essential. Yet, as we continue to be reminded, control of epidemics is highly dependent on public health preparedness, science-based action, political leadership, community involvement, and clear messaging.

Surgeon General Koop's 1988 report *Understanding AIDS*[17] still stands as a model for effective communication of the public health risks of a new disease, providing authoritative guidance to enable the public to make informed health decisions. In contrast, during the COVID-19 pandemic lack of clear messaging along with widespread disinformation on social media—platforms that did not exist during the early years of AIDS—impacted the public's reaction to the SARS-COV-2 threat. For mpox, the history of AIDS reminds us about the importance of communicating targeted and specific information about transmission risks while avoiding potentially stigmatizing language.

Given the central role of governments in epidemic response, public trust in governmental organizations and officials is critical. In recent years, however, and particularly during the COVID-19 pandemic, this trust has eroded—fueled in part by misinformation but also by missteps and mistakes early on, such as CDC's release of a flawed COVID-19 test and its shifting advice on masking and social distancing. Evolving scientific information and changing public health guidance, however, are inherent in responses to new infections. But some remarks, including those made by President Trump about unproven treatments for COVID-19, were misleading and even dangerous.[18] The spread of misinformation also led to criticism of government officials and even threats against their lives.

The public is justified in expecting governments to provide the most up-to-date technologies in responding to epidemics. The development of effective COVID vaccines, underwritten by the government, was a remarkable achievement. However, public views about the vaccine were highly politicized. For mpox, despite the existence of an effective vaccine, initial delays in distribution resulted in vaccine rationing for those most likely to benefit. And, although CDC's early testing of mpox was criticized for being too slow, this was quickly remedied by transferring the technology to large commercial laboratories.

At CDC, the early years of AIDS occurred in an atmosphere of political neglect and social disdain toward affected populations. Nonetheless, the agency was able to complete its public health work with less constraints compared with today. The COVID-19 outbreak highlighted serious gaps in the nation's public health infrastructure, including the inadequacy of current surveillance and reporting systems. To better anticipate the magnitude and trajectories of infectious disease threats, CDC has established a new Center for Forecasting and Outbreak Analytics.[19]

For HIV/AIDS, the global fight continues—with important successes yet persistent gaps. Two thirds of new HIV infections worldwide are in populations, such as MSM and sex workers, that remain stigmatized, discriminated against, or otherwise marginalized.[14] Homosexuality remains illegal in sixty-nine countries, almost half of them in Africa, and in a few it is legally punishable by death.[20] Sex work occurs everywhere but remains outlawed in most countries. And, despite abundant evidence showing the benefits of harm-reduction activities, ([21,22]) such as syringe exchange, for persons who inject drugs, these services are often unavailable because of local or national politics or scarcity of resources.

In the fifth decade of AIDS, the world is substantially different than it was in 1981. Younger people, including those at risk for HIV, are mostly unaware of the history of AIDS, the suffering endured, or the fears engendered. With the welcome scientific and medical advances, many consider the AIDS epidemic to be over and a dangerous complacency has descended. Those who claim the epidemic of HIV has ended or that HIV is under control are prematurely declaring victory.[23] In low-income countries presentation with advanced HIV disease remains frequent, high HIV incidence persists in various groups, and the virus remains an important cause of death.[24]

Efforts to combat AIDS and discrimination must be continuous. Our former CDC colleague, Ronald (Ron) Valdiserri wrote a moving book in memory of the twin brother he lost to AIDS. In it he equates the fight against discrimination to weeding a garden—the job is incessant and only successful if it is maintained.[25] Without an effective vaccine and curative therapy, claims that elimination of AIDS as a public health threat is in sight are more likely to eliminate program resources than to end HIV.

The next chapters of the AIDS story remain to be written. The most gratifying and successful aspects to date have been the continued demonstration of countless people in collaboration—working toward the same goal of controlling HIV. The authors have been privileged to have played a role in the first forty years of the response to the pandemic. It is for the next generation of physicians, scientists, activists, and others to write these new chapters.

Notes

1. CDC. Acquired immune deficiency syndrome (AIDS): precautions for clinical and laboratory staffs. MMWR Morbid Mortal Wkly Rep 1982; 31:577–580.
2. CDC. Prevention of acquired immune deficiency syndrome (AIDS): report of inter-agency recommendations. MMWR Morbid Mortal Wkly Rep 1983;32:101–103.
3. Barre-Sinoussi F, Chermann JC, Rey F, et al. Isolation of a T-lymphotropic retrovirus from a patient at risk for acquired immune deficiency syndrome (AIDS). Science 1983;220:868–871.
4. CDC. Update: Public Health Service workshop on human T-lymphotropic virus type III antibody testing—United States. MMWR Morb Mortal Wkly Rep 1985;34:477–478.
5. Connor EM, Sperling RS, Gelber R, et al. Reduction of maternal-infant transmission of human immunodeficiency virus type 1 with zidovudine treatment. N Engl J Med 1994;331:1173–1180.
6. De Cock KM, Churchill D, Grant A, et al. Summary of Track B: clinical science. AIDS 1996;10(Suppl 3):S107–S113.
7. NIH. Clinical guidelines. https://clinicalinfo.hiv.gov/en/guidelines
8. France D. How to survive a plague. New York: Alfred Knopf; 2016.
9. Allen T, Murray KA, Zambrana-Torrelio C, et al. Global hotspots and correlates of emerging zoonotic diseases. Nat Commun 2017;8:1124. https://doi.org/10.1038/s41 467-017-00923-8.
10. National Academy of Medicine. The neglected dimension of global security: a framework to counter infectious disease crises. Washington, DC: The National Academies Press; 2016. https://nap.nationalacademies.org/catalog/21891/the-neglected-dimens ion-of-global-security-a-framework-to-counter.
11. WHO Ebola Response Team. After Ebola in West Africa—unpredictable risks, preventable epidemics. N Engl J Med 2016;375:587–596.
12. The Independent Panel for Pandemic Preparedness & Response. COVID-19: Make it the Last Pandemic. https://theindependentpanel.org/wp-content/uploads/2021/05/COVID-19-Make-it-the-Last-Pandemic_final.pdf.
13. Chigwedere P, Seage G, Gruskin S, Lee T-H, Essex M. Estimating the lost benefits of antiretroviral drug use in South Africa. J Acquir Immune Defic Syndr 2008;49:410–415. doi: 0.1097/QAI.0b013e31818a6cd5
14. UNAIDS. Global HIV & AIDS statistics—fact sheet. https://www.unaids.org/en/resources/fact-sheet.

15. WHO. WHO Director-General declares the ongoing monkeypox outbreak a Public Health Emergency of International Concern. News release, July 23, 2002. https://www.who.int/europe/news/item/23-07-2022-who-director-general-declares-the-ongoing-monkeypox-outbreak-a-public-health-event-of-international-concern

16. Philpott D, Hughes CM, Alroy KA, et al. Epidemiologic and Clinical Characteristics of Monkeypox Cases—United States, May 17–July 22, 2022. MMWR Morb Mortal Wkly Rep. ePub: 5 August 2022. doi: http://dx.doi.org/10.15585/mmwr.mm7132e3.

17. "Understanding AIDS," *The Global Health Chronicles*, accessed November 12, 2022, https://www.globalhealthchronicles.org/items/show/8156.

18. Rogers K, Hauser C, Yuhas A, Haberman M. Trump's suggestion that disinfectants could be used to treat coronavirus prompts aggressive pushback. New York Times, April 24, 2020.

19. CDC. CDC Stands Up New Disease Forecasting Center. Press release, August 18, 2021. https://www.cdc.gov/media/releases/2021/p0818-disease-forecasting-center.html.

20. BBC. Homosexuality: the countries where it is illegal to be gay. May 12, 2021. https://www.bbc.com/news/world-43822234.

21. Barre-Sinoussi F, Abdool Karim SS, Albert J, et al. Expert consensus statement on the science of HIV in the context of criminal law. J Int AIDS Soc 2018;21:e25161. https://onlinelibrary.wiley.com/doi/epdf/10.1002/jia2.25161.

22. Lambert EY, Normand JL, Volkow ND. Prevention and treatment of HIV/AIDS among drug-using populations: a global perspective. J Acquir Immune Defic Syndr 2010;55 (Suppl1):S1–S4.

23. De Cock KM, Jaffe HW, Curran JW. Reflections on 40 years of AIDS. Emerg Infect Dis 2021;27:1553–1559.

24. Fauci AS, Redfield RR, Sigounas G, Weakhee MD, Giroir M. Ending the HIV epidemic: a plan for the United States. JAMA 2019;321:844–845.

25. Valdiserri R. Gardening in clay: reflections on AIDS. New York: Cornell University Press; 1994.

Acknowledgments

We thank the following friends and colleagues for providing helpful discussions or reviews regarding topics covered in the book: Marc Bulterys, Jon Cohen, Bob Colebunders, Bill Darrow, Bruce Evatt, Judy Gantt, Alan Greenberg, Beatrice Hahn, Harry Haverkos, Mary Hilpertshauser, Joyce Johnson, Lydia Kline, Tim Mastro, Gene Matthews, Jono Mermin, Meade Morgan, Tom Quinn, Taraz Samandari, Mike St. Louis, Tom Starcher, Polly Thomas, and Stefan Wiktor. We also thank Nancy Sterk for exceptional administrative contributions.

ACKNOWLEDGMENTS

Index